Richard P Schmidt

Recent Advances in
**EPILEPSY**

TIMOTHY A. PEDLEY MD
*Professor and Vice-chairman, Department of Neurology, College of Physicians & Surgeons of Columbia University; Director, Clinical Neurophysiology Laboratories, Columbia-Presbyterian Medical Center, New York*

BRIAN S. MELDRUM MA MB BChir PhD
*Professor of Experimental Neurology, Department of Neurology, Institute of Psychiatry, London*

# Recent Advances in
# EPILEPSY

EDITED BY
TIMOTHY A. PEDLEY
BRIAN S. MELDRUM

NUMBER FOUR

CHURCHILL LIVINGSTONE
EDINBURGH LONDON MELBOURNE AND NEW YORK 1988

CHURCHILL LIVINGSTONE
Medical Division of Longman Group UK Limited

Distributed in the United States of America by Churchill Livingstone Inc., 1560 Broadway, New York, N.Y. 10036, and by associated companies, branches and representatives throughout the world.



First published 1988

ISBN 0 443 03915 1
ISSN 0264–7400

**British Library Cataloguing in Publication Data**
Recent advances in epilepsy.—No. 4
1. Epilepsy—Periodicals
616.8'53'005 RC372.A1

**The Library of Congress has cataloged this serial publication as follows:**
Recent advances in epilepsy.—No. 1—Edinburgh : New York : Churchill Livingstone, 1983–
v. ill. 24 cm
Editors: Timothy A. Pedley, Brian S. Meldrum
1. Epilepsy—Periodicals. I. Pedley, Timothy A. II. Meldrum, Brian S.
[DNLM: W1 RE105ULAH]
RC372.A1R43 616.8'53—dc19 84-641834
AACR 2 MARC-S

Printed in Great Britain at The Bath Press, Avon

# Preface

This fourth volume continues the practice established in the first three of presenting critical reviews of major topics related to epilepsy. Most contributions rely heavily on new information that has become available only recently. As in previous volumes, both basic and clinical subjects are included.

The first three chapters offer summaries of anatomical, physiological and biochemical factors that affect brain excitability, and relate to the evolution and consequences of seizure discharges. EEG remains the most widely applied laboratory test in patients with epilepsy and a cornerstone of clinical diagnosis. Previous volumes included chapters on specialized types of EEG recording; this one offers an assessment of routine EEG and its role in seizure classification, prognosis and choice of treatment. Management of women with epilepsy during pregnancy presents clinicians with special problems including potential teratogenic effects of antiepileptic drugs. These issues are discussed in two related chapters. Parasitosis is a major cause of epilepsy in third world countries, and a thorough account of this is overdue, especially for European, North American and Japanese readers. Increased knowledge of mechanisms of epileptogenesis on the one hand, and of cellular mechanisms of action of existing agents on the other, are changing the way anticonvulsant drugs are developed. Thus, a chapter summarizing new compounds, most still investigational and not yet ready for general clinical use, is timely. Advances are also being made in the surgical treatment of epilepsy, and there is renewed interest in corpus callosotomy for carefully selected patients who are intractable to medical management and are not candidates for standard resective procedures. We include a comprehensive description of the interrelation of depression and epilepsy, a common and often unrecognized accompaniment to seizures. Finally, we offer some considerations on the interface between epilepsy and the law.

We are grateful to our distinguished contributors who provided authoritative reviews in a timely fashion, and complied willingly with editorial requests for revisions. We hope that our readership will continue to find this series useful in the management of their patients with epilepsy.

New York and London, 1988

T.A.P.
B.S.M.

# Contributors

PAULO ROGÉRIO M. BITTENCOURT MD PhD
Head, Clinical Neurology Unit, Hospital Nossa Senhora das Graças, Curitiba, Paraná, Brazil

ASTRID G. CHAPMAN PhD
Honorary Senior Lecturer, Department of Neurology, Institute of Psychiatry, London

P. B. C. FENWICK MB BChir(Cantab) DPM FRCPsych
Consultant Psychiatrist, Maudsley Hospital and St Thomas' Hospital, London; Senior Lecturer, Institute of Psychiatry, London

JACQUELINE A. FRENCH MD
Clinical Fellow in Epilepsy, Mount Sinai School of Medicine and Bronx Veterans Administration Medical Center, New York

CLEVERSON M. GRACIA MD
Clinical Neurology Unit, Hospital Nossa Senhora das Graças, Curitiba, Paraná, Brazil

ILO E. LEPPIK MD
Professor of Neurology and Director of Research, Comprehensive Epilepsy Program of Minnesota, University of Minnesota, Minneapolis, Minnesota

PABLO LORENZANA MD
Assistant Professor, Department of Neurology, Universidad Nacional de Colombia, Bogotá, Colombia

NANDOR LUDVIG
Research Associate, Department of Pediatrics, Albert Einstein College of Medicine, Bronx, New York

BRIAN S. MELDRUM MA MB BChir PhD
Professor of Experimental Neurology, Department of Neurology, Institute of Psychiatry, London

SOLOMON L. MOSHÉ MD
Associate Professor of Neurology and Pediatrics, and Director of Clinical Neurophysiology, Albert Einstein College of Medicine, Bronx, New York

ROGER J. PORTER MD
Chief, Medical Neurology Branch, National Institutes of Health, Bethesda, Maryland

MARY M. ROBERTSON MB ChB MD DPM MRCPsych
Senior Lecturer, Academic Department of Psychiatry, University College and Middlesex School of Medicine, Middlesex Hospital, London

A. JAMES ROWAN MD
Professor of Neurology, Mount Sinai School of Medicine, New York; Chief, Department of Neurology, Veterans Administration Medical Center, Bronx, New York

RICHARD PENROSE SCHMIDT MD
Distinguished Physician, Veterans Administration Medical Center, Gainesville; Professor Emeritus of Neurology, University of Florida College of Medicine, Gainesville, Florida

SUSAN S. SPENCER MD
Associate Professor of Neurology, Yale University School of Medicine, New Haven, Connecticut; Consultant, Epilepsy Unit, Veterans Administration Medical Center, West Haven, Connecticut

BUNA J. WILDER MD
Chief, Neurology Service, Veterans Administration Medical Center, Gainesville; Professor of Neurology and Neuroscience, University of Florida College of Medicine, Gainesville, Florida

MARK S. YERBY MD MPH
Attending Neurologist and Clinical Associate Professor of Neurology, Comprehensive Epilepsy Program of Minnesota, University of Minnesota, Minneapolis, Minnesota

# Contents


1. Initiation and neuroanatomical spread of seizure activity *B. S. Meldrum* 1

2. Kindling *S. L. Moshé* *N. Ludvig* 21

3. Amino acid abnormalities in plasma, CSF and brain in epilepsy
*A. G. Chapman* 45

4. The role of the electroencephalogram in the diagnosis and management of epilepsy *A. J. Rowan* *J. A. French* 63

5. Teratogenicity of antiepileptic drugs *M. S. Yerby* 93

6. Management of seizures during pregnancy *I. E. Leppik* 109

7. Epilepsy and parasitosis of the central nervous system
*P. R. M. Bittencourt* *C. M. Gracia* *P. Lorenzana* 123

8. New antiepileptic drugs: prospects for improved treatment of seizures
*R. J. Porter* 161

9. Corpus callosotomy in the treatment of intractable seizures *S. S. Spencer* 181

10. Depression in patients with epilepsy reconsidered *M. M. Robertson* 205

11. Epilepsy and the law *P. Fenwick* 241

12. Epilepsy and the law: a commentary from the United States perspective
*R. P. Schmidt* *B. J. Wilder* 253

Index 259

# 1. Initiation and neuroanatomical spread of seizure activity

*B. S. Meldrum*

## INTRODUCTION

The first major contributions to understanding the anatomical basis of epilepsy in terms of the intracerebral sites of origin and patterns of spread of abnormal activity were made by Hughlings Jackson approximately 100 years ago (see Jackson 1931). His conclusions about the intracortical spread of activity associated with focal motor seizures were based on clinical observation and post-mortem identification of focal lesions (Jackson 1873) allied to the experimental observations of David Ferrier (1886) in the monkey, dog and rabbit. His conclusions about the temporal lobe origin of seizure activity in cases of 'dreamy state' or 'uncinate fits' (with gustatory automatisms) were also based on clinico-pathological correlations (Jackson & Beevor 1889, Jackson & Colman 1898). Over the subsequent 90 years new understanding came principally from the development of neurosurgical techniques for the treatment of epilepsy in man, notably by Penfield, and the introduction of electro-encephalographic procedures, with major contributions from Jasper and Gastaut. Experimental studies in animals involving surgical procedures with focal pharmacological manipulation were performed by Hayashi (1952, 1953). He demonstrated in dogs and monkeys the subcortical pathways responsible for the spread of abnormal activity to the final common path in the brain stem or spinal cord.

In the past 10 years research in this area has been transformed by two new developments. One is the introduction of imaging techniques which allow the study of regional changes in blood flow, cerebral metabolism or electrical or magnetic activity either in patients or in experimental models of epilepsy. The second is the growth in understanding of the synaptic systems in the brain, in terms of the mechanisms of inhibition and excitation and of the patterns of interconnection of such systems, and the aberrant events responsible for certain types of epileptic discharge. These recent developments make it important to re-assess older accounts of the anatomical basis of epilepsy. Consideration has to be given to each of the major clinical forms of epilepsy as they involve different sequences of anatomical activation. We shall look in some detail at focal motor seizures, limbic seizures, primary generalised seizures of the absence type, tonic clonic seizures, and reticular seizures in the newborn. We shall also discuss seizures with sensory induction because the afferent pathway and the physiological parameters of the stimulus can be accurately defined both in man and in experimental animals.

It is first necessary to define the abnormal activity we are considering and how it may spread.

## ICTAL AND INTERICTAL DISCHARGES

The concept of interictal and ictal discharges derived from electrographic-clinical correlations which contrasted brief electrical events occurring focally (spikes, sharp waves, spikes and waves) without clinical correlations, with sustained paroxysmal discharges occurring in association with clinically manifest seizures. Extracellular and intracellular recordings in vivo and in vitro have shown that the interictal event is usually associated with a paroxysmal depolarising shift of the membrane potential and a brief rapid burst of action potentials in primary neurons of cortex or hippocampus (Ayala et al 1970). The initial excitatory event is followed by inhibitory phenomena (seen as an after-hyperpolarisation that is partly due to electrogenic pumps and partly to both fast and slow GABA-mediated inhibition). These interictal events can be produced by spontaneously bursting neurons (Miles & Wong 1983), readily found — in uninjured tissue — among hippocampal CA3 pyramidal neurons or among cortical pyramidal neurons at the junction between lamina IV and lamina V (Connors 1984). Recruitment occurs within such a primary neuronal aggregate but it tends to remain localised, partly because of inhibitory mechanisms which limit the interictal event spatially and temporally. Interictal events can spread within the same class of neurons or they can spread via axons and synapses to other classes of neurons e.g. from CA3 to CA1 pyramidal neurons or from deep pyramidal neurons to superficial neurons within the same cortical column or to distant pyramidal neurons by commissural or cortico-cortical pathways. In neocortical slices paroxysmal events propagate horizontally in a saltatory fashion i.e. synchronous bursts are triggered sequentially in adjacent neuronal aggregates (Gutnick 1987). The mechanisms synchronising interictal events are not understood but may include electrical connections (gap junctions) between neurons, ephaptic spread, extraneuronal ionic changes, and synaptic connections (Dichter & Ayala 1987). Recurrent excitation to inhibitory interneurons within and around the epileptic aggregate may limit the spread of synchronous bursting activity but it may also facilitate further synchronisation of phases of excitability. Projection areas of a primary focus may show inhibitory activity during interictal or ictal discharges. This is seen contralaterally to a cortical focus induced by penicillin (Crowell 1970). Asymmetrical cortical foci induced by oestrogen in the cat are mutually inhibitory through callosal pathways (Mutani & Durelli 1980).

The synchronous interictal firing of a neuronal aggregate may be brought about by properties of the afferent input — which may itself show no epileptic features. In reflex epilepsy this property relates to the way highly specific (usually visual or auditory) inputs are transmitted or filtered. In generalised seizures of the absence type intrinsic properties of the thalamus may favour synchronous interictal events in the cortex (see below).

Synaptic spread of interictal events to other neuronal aggregates occurs to a variable extent, increasing as the events become more intense and rhythmically recurrent.

The transition to an ictal event has been much studied in model systems. Characteristically the initial excitatory depolarisation becomes more severe and more sustained and instead of being followed by an inhibitory potential is followed by repetitive excitatory events, often resembling interictal events but without their inhibitory components (Ayala et al 1970). Some research workers refer to such activity as 'tonic' when recorded in a slice. However the transmission between aggregates may not be true. If we consider a sequence of aggregates leading from the one in which epileptogenesis occurs ('aggregate A') to the final common path ('aggregate Z'), assumed for motor seizures to be brain stem or spinal motoneuronal aggregates, at each stage the epileptic events may be transformed either towards normal patterns of activity or towards more severe ictal patterns.

Interictal events (by definition) fade out or are subject to inhibition before being transmitted to the final common path. Of course abnormal movements could occur as a result of epileptic activity in aggregates A, B, etc without specifically epileptic activity occurring in aggregate Z. Indeed it is a property of motoneurons that they can show patterns of fast firing readily but epileptic discharges are not easily induced. We therefore may look for an earlier aggregate (aggregate X) whose sequential patterns of epileptic activity determine the motor patterns observed. There may of course be only one such aggregate or a number of aggregates whose sequential interactions determine the pattern of motor events. Direct evidence for all the above hypothetical phenomena is available. We shall discuss evidence from hippocampal slices here. The concept of 'aggregate X' is reconsidered in relation to the role of the midbrain motor areas in tonic clonic and neonatal 'reticular' seizures below.

In hippocampal slices the occurrence of interictal events in the CA3 region can be favoured by small adjustments to the ionic environment such as a very small increase in potassium concentration. These interictal events have the characteristic features described above i.e. brief burst + inhibitory afterpotentials. Such interictal events in CA3 can trigger ictal events in CA1 (i.e. showing a sustained depolarisation, and closely repetitive bursts without inhibition). These ictal events are nevertheless driven by and dependent on the interictal events in CA3. This provides evidence that transmission from one aggregate to another can produce not only diminution but also enhancement of the severity of the epileptic phenomena. A series of events initially driven from a primary aggregate can evolve to become independent at any subsequent aggregate.

Spread of epileptic activity involves interrelated time and frequency dependent phenomena that permit recruitment of further neuronal aggregates. These are the progressive potentiation or opening up of latent excitatory pathways and the loss of inhibitory feedback. The relationship of these phenomena has been elegantly demonstrated in hippocampal slices by Miles & Wong (1987). Blockade of inhibition by picrotoxin permits transmission of burst discharges via connections not previously functional. In the presence of initially normal inhibitory function repetition of brief tetanii delivered via afferent (mossy) fibres to CA3 neurons leads to a progressive suppression of recurrent inhibition that reveals latent excitatory connections which transmit burst firing.

## PHARMACOLOGY OF INITIATION AND SPREAD OF SEIZURE ACTIVITY

This is too complex a topic to be reviewed here but it is necessary to summarise some key points. The initiation of interictal or ictal events and their spread can be favoured or induced by pharmacological agents acting in three major ways:

1. On membrane properties to decrease stability of resting membrane potential (e.g. decreasing potassium conductance, increasing calcium conductance).

2. Decreasing inhibitory processes especially GABA-mediated inhibition and,
3. Enhancing excitation, especially at the various glutamate receptors (subtypes classified as N-methyl-D-aspartate, kainate and quisqualate preferring).

Conversely seizure initiation and spread is inhibited by drugs producing membrane stabilisation or enhancing inhibition or decreasing excitation. Synaptic transmission from one aggregate to another appears to depend principally on fast excitation induced by acidic amino acids such as glutamate and aspartate. The NMDA receptor system is of particular interest in that its activation in normal cells of cortex, striatum or hippocampus induces intermittent paroxysmal depolarisation and burst discharges very similar to the activity recorded intracellularly in interictal discharges. Specific antagonists acting at this receptor (such as 2-amino-7-phosphono-heptanoate, APH, and 2-amino-5-phosphono-valerate APV) are effective anticonvulsants in a wide range of seizure models (Meldrum 1984, 1985). Transmission from one aggregate to another appears to depend in the first instance on non-NMDA receptors (kainate or quisqualate preferring) and secondarily on NMDA receptors. In hippocampal slices an NMDA antagonist such as APV shortens the duration of paroxysmal events rather than preventing their spread (Dingledine et al 1986). Intrinsic GABA-mediated inhibition appears to prevent the recruitment of a new neuronal aggregate into interictal or ictal activity. Repetition of the epileptic input seems progressively to overcome this. The focal injection of a GABA A agonist such as muscimol can delay or prevent the recruitment of an aggregate into epileptic activity. GABA and muscimol or excitatory amino acid antagonists produce antiepileptic effects when focally injected into many different neuronal aggregates, including some relay nuclei that are unlikely to have a primary involvement in epileptogenesis but serve as pathways for transmission or recruitment. A few sites show opposite effects with clear anticonvulsant effects of excitatory agents (e.g. NMDA or bicuculline injected in the neostriatum), presumably due to activation of important inhibitory pathways (Turski et al 1987a).

## FOCAL MOTOR SEIZURES

Spread of seizure activity takes two forms, one is to other cortical regions via intracortical and transcallosal pathways, the other is to the final common path in brain stem nuclei or spinal cord via subcortical centres. The intracortical spread (Jackson's 'cortical march') could involve non-synaptic mechanisms of synchronisation. Transcallosal spread appears to be the major route for interhemispsheric spread. The evidence for this is the effect of callosal section on seizure spread, first reported in animals by Erickson (1940) and in man by Van Wagenen & Herren (1940). In patients with both partial and generalised seizures there is a marked reduction in the frequency of generalised seizures following callosotomy, although in some patients the number of partial seizures also decreases (Reeves & O'Leary, 1985).

A pattern of subcortical spread of focal motor seizure activity involving the thalamus and basal ganglia was definitively demonstrated by Hayashi (1952, 1953) in his classic experiments in dogs and monkeys. He observed clonic motor activity following the focal injection of excitant agents (such as nicotine, strychnine, pentylenetetrazol, picrotoxin or glutamate) into the cortex or into subcortical nuclei. Sectioning the pyramids at the level of the olive did not prevent focal or generalised clonic activity induced by intracortical injection of convulsants. However, clonic convulsions were blocked by bilateral lesions of either the globus pallidus or the rostral midbrain (substantia nigra). Furthermore clonic convulsions could be induced by the focal injection of nicotine into the globus pallidus or the substantia nigra pars reticulata. Hayashi interpreted these and other data in terms of a descending pathway relaying initially in either the thalamus (nucleus ventralis lateralis, from whence it spread to the opposite thalamus and to the globus pallidus, bilaterally) or the globus pallidus ipsilaterally, and from the globus pallidus to the substantia nigra pars reticulata, and from there to the contralateral brain stem and spinal cord (see Fig. 1.1). That this summary

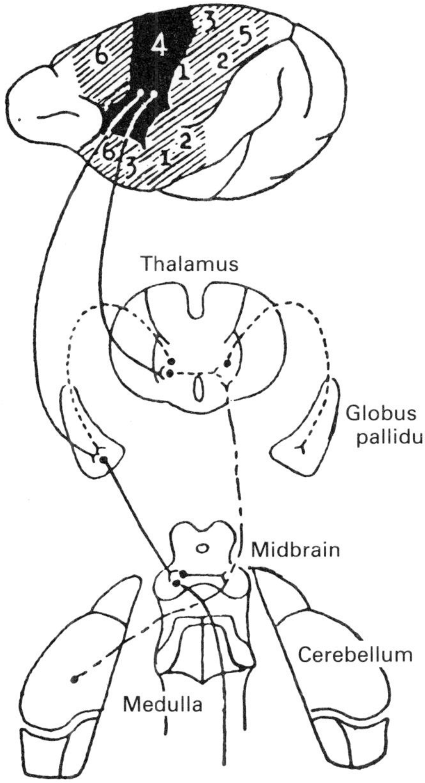


**Fig. 1.1** Levels which elicit clonic convulsions and the presumed descending pathway for cortically-induced clonus, as defined by Hayashi on the basis of experiments in dogs and monkeys. (Redrawn from Hayashi 1953, reproduced from Meldrum 1988.)

of the subcortical pathway of seizure spread is broadly correct was supported, initially, by neurosurgical treatments (lenticotomy and section of the fields of Forel) designed to interrupt the output from the globus pallidus (Gillingham et al 1980) and, subsequently, by regional metabolic studies in animal models.

Autoradiographic procedures utilising frozen sections of the brain following injection of compounds labelled with $^{3}H$ or $^{14}C$ allow the measurement of regional blood flow or metabolic rate for glucose. These values are elevated by local seizure discharges so that the regional pattern of seizure activity can be visualised. In a series of such studies in the monkey Caveness and his colleagues induced focal motor activity by the intracortical injection of penicillin and used $^{14}C$ antipyrine or $^{14}C$ deoxyglucose to measure blood flow and metabolic rate. The metabolic activation involved, ipsilaterally, the putamen, globus pallidus, substantia nigra and the ventrolateral and ventromedial thalamic nuclei, and, contralaterally, the cerebellar hemispheres and dentate nucleus (Ueno et al 1975, Caveness et al 1980). With seizure activity confined to the face-hand area of the neocortex activation occurs somatotopically in the putamen, globus pallidus and substantia nigra (Hosokawa et al 1983).

**Myoclonus of striatal origin**

In the rat, focal contralateral myoclonus follows the injection into the striatum of GABA antagonists (either acting directly such as picrotoxin and bicuculline, or indirectly by blocking GABA synthesis such as allylglycine (Tarsy et al 1978)). This effect is facilitated by cortical lesions, and is prevented by lesions of the globus pallidus. Pallidal lesions do not prevent myoclonus induced by intracortical injection of picrotoxin (Patel & Slater 1987). A circuit involving striatal outputs to globus pallidus, entopeduncular nucleus and substantia nigra with a relay to the ventral thalamus and then to motor cortex appears to be involved in striatally evoked myoclonus. Whether a purely striatal myoclonus exists in man is unknown.

## LIMBIC SEIZURES

Jackson's 'dreamy states' were renamed 'psychomotor epilepsy' by Gibbs et al (1937). The term limbic epilepsy was introduced by Fulton (1953). The pattern of spread of limbic seizure activity in man has been studied by recording from depth electrodes during evaluation for neurosurgical treatment or in the course of partial temporal lobectomy. Such studies have recently been reviewed by Wieser (1983, 1986). They show that in mesio-basal limbic seizures initiation most commonly occurs, with a high frequency discharge, simultaneously in hippocampus and amygdala. Purely hippocampal initiation is next most common with amygdala initiation least common. Hippocampal seizure discharges commonly propagate into the retrosplenial and parietal cingulate cortex. An arrest reaction i.e. a lapse of awareness with staring is commonly the accompaniment of the hippocampal discharge but may be seen with other discharge localisations. Oral-alimentary automatisms are prominent in seizures with amygdala-hippocampal origin. Complex partial seizures with movements of the trunk or limbs (postural or automatisms) have an extratemporal origin.

Experimental studies have concerned a wide range of in vitro and in vivo models, including hippocampal slices (see above), kindling with sub-threshold electrical stimulation, focal electrical stimulation, focal injections of convulsant agents, and systemic injections of convulsants acting preferentially on the limbic system (e.g. kainate or pilocarpine).

**Kindling**

'Kindling' was the name given by Goddard et al (1969) to the process whereby daily or intermittent electrical stimulation of susceptible brain areas (amygdala, hippocampus, entorhinal or pyriform cortex) at a strength which initially triggers only an after-discharge eventually initiates a seizure discharge that involves the limbic system bilaterally. In rodents this is associated with a characteristic motor sequence beginning with gustatory automatisms, progressing to clonus of the face and forelimbs and finally to rearing and falling. Activation of the substantia nigra during kindled seizures has been shown both by regional metabolic studies employing $^{14}C$-deoxyglucose (Engel et al 1978) and by electrical recording of nigral unit activity (Bonhaus et al 1986). The focal injection of GABAergic agents ($\gamma$-vinylGABA, which inhibits GABA-transaminase, or muscimol, a GABA A agonist) bilaterally into the substantia nigra partially or completely suppresses amygdala kindled seizures (LeGal La Salle et al 1983, McNamara et al 1984). Bilateral destruction of the substantia nigra (by focal injection of a neurotoxin) also suppresses the limbic seizures (McNamara et al 1984). Bilateral electrical stimulation of the substantia nigra pars reticulata (at a strength less than that inducing tonic seizures) prior to stimulation of the amygdala delays and diminishes kindled responses (Morimoto & Goddard 1987). If the electrical stimulation of the SN reticulata is primarily activating intrinsic inhibitory terminals, then all these results can be interpreted as showing that decreasing the output from the SN reticulata prevents the build up of limbic seizure activity. More detailed evidence on this point has been obtained using a chemically-induced model of limbic seizures.

**Limbic seizures induced in rats by pilocarpine**

High doses of the muscarinic agonist pilocarpine given systemically to rats induce sustained seizures whose motor pattern is similar to that of kindled limbic seizures induced by amygdala stimulation (described above). The motor and electrical seizure activity is commonly sustained for 3–5 hours and leads to neuronal loss in the hippocampus, amygdala, thalamus, neocortex and substantia nigra (Turski et al 1983).

This seizure syndrome is not an optimal model for pharmacological studies of complex partial seizures, as diphenylhydantoin and carbamazepine are relatively ineffective at suppressing the seizures (and the brain damage) whereas clonazepam, phenobarbital and valproate are effective (Turski et al 1987a). These seizures are, however, very useful for establishing the pathways involved in the initiation and development of limbic seizures.

We have studied the effect of focal injections of muscimol (a GABA agonist), of N-methyl-D-aspartate (a selective agonist at one subtype of glutamate receptor), and of two selective excitatory amino acid antagonists (2-amino-7-phosphono-heptanoic acid, 2-APH, acting on the NMDA receptor, and $\gamma$-D-glutamylamino-methylsulphonate, $\gamma$-D-GAMS, acting with partial selectivity on the kainate receptor) (Patel et al 1986, 1987, Meldrum et al 1987, De Sarro et al 1987) (see Fig. 1.2).

Focal injection of muscimol or 2-APH into the substantia nigra pars reticulata completely prevents the motor limbic seizures and the secondary pathology induced by a convulsant dose of pilocarpine (Turski et al 1986). Focal EEG recordings show that isolated spikes occur in the hippocampus following the systemic injection of pilcarpine, but they fail to develop into a sustained discharge. Injection of N-methyl-D-aspartate into the SN pars reticulata can convert a subconvulsant dose of pilocarpine into a fully convulsant dose. These experiments were interpreted as showing that decreasing the output from the SN pars reticulata has an inhibitory effect on the limbic system whereas enhancing its output facilitates seizure activity in the limbic system. The outputs involved are probably GABAergic, relaying in either the superior colliculus, the ventral tegmental area or the thalamus (ventromedial nucleus) (see Garant & Gale 1987).

The other major output nucleus for the basal ganglia is the globus pallidus. In the rat the entopeduncular nucleus is homologous with the internal part of the globus

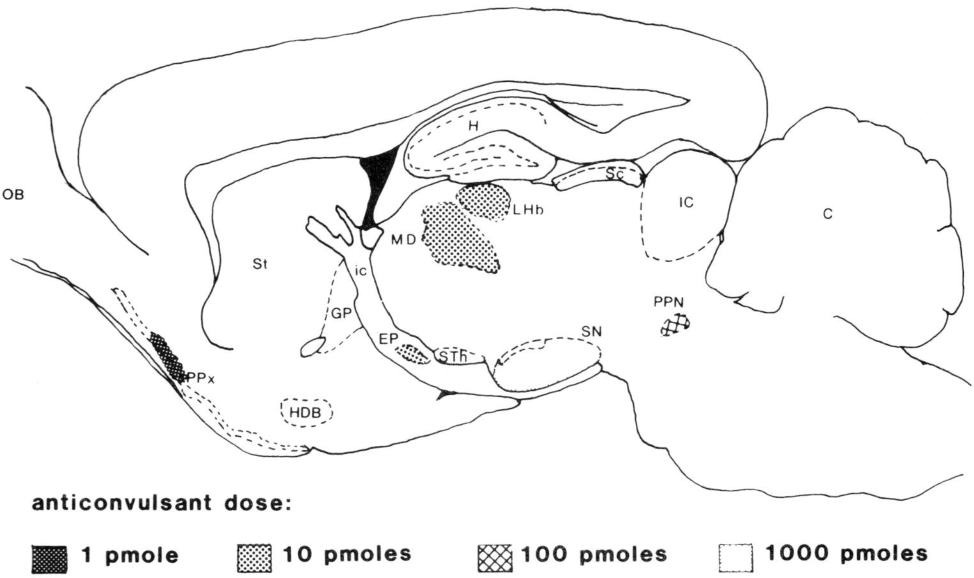


**Fig. 1.2** Sagittal diagram of the rat brain showing sites at which focal injections of 2-amino-7-phosphono-heptanoic acid have an anticonvulsant action against limbic seizures induced by systemic injection of pilocarpine. The threshold dose producing an anticonvulsant effect is indicated by the pattern of crosshatching. The prepyriform cortex (PPx) is the most sensitive region, the lateral habenula (LHb) the medio-dorsal nucleus of the thalamus (MD) and the entopeduncular nucleus (EP) are the next most sensitive. The pedunculopontine nucleus (PPN) is less sensitive and the substantia nigra, pars reticulata (SN) is the least sensitive. (From Patel et al 1987 with permission.)

pallidus in the primate or cat. Focal injection of muscimol or of 2-APH into the entopeduncular nucleus potently protects against seizures induced by pilocarpine. Indeed the effective dose of 2-APH at this site is some 100-fold lower than that required in the substantia nigra (Patel et al 1986). Interestingly γ-D-GAMS which acts preferentially on the kainate receptor is nearly as effective as 2-APH in the substantia nigra pars reticulata but very much less effective in the entopeduncular nucleus (De Sarro et al 1987). An important output of the entopeduncular nucleus is to the lateral habenula which in turn relays to the thalamus (including the mediodorsal nucleus). Protection against limbic seizures induced by pilocarpine is also seen after focal injection of 2-APH into either the lateral habenula or the mediodorsal nucleus of the thalamus (see Fig. 1.2).

However the site which is most sensitive to the protective action of 2-APH lies deep in the prepiriform cortex (see Fig. 1.3) (Millan et al 1986a). This area has been described by Piredda & Gale (1985) as a crucial epileptogenic site on the basis of its high sensitivity to the epileptogenic action of various convulsants including bicuculline (a GABA antagonist) kainic acid, or carbachol (cholinergic agonist). It is possible that pilocarpine-induced limbic seizures begin here and spread to the amygdala and hippocampus.

N-methyl-D-aspartate is convulsant when given systemically and is proconvulsant in the pilocarpine-limbic seizure model when injected into the SN pars reticulata. When injected focally into the ventral caudate/putamen, however, it is anticonvulsant (Turski et al 1987b). This protective effect can be abolished by the simultaneous

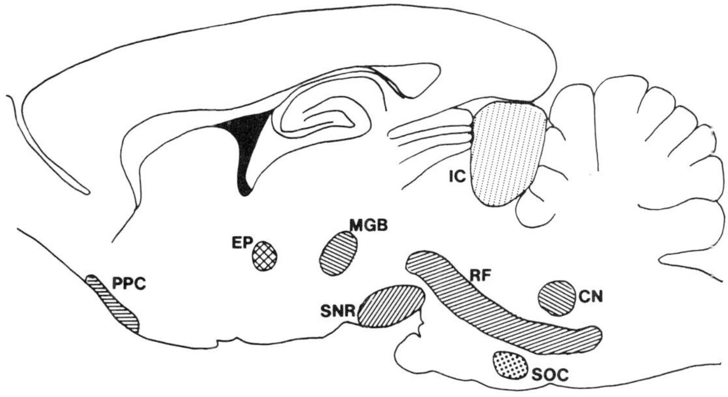


**Fig. 1.3** The sensitivity of brain areas to protective action of APH against the AGS in the GEP rat. *Key*: PPC, prepiriform cortex; EP, entopeduncular nucleus; MGM, medial geniculate body; SNR, substantia nigra pars reticulata; IC, inferior colliculus; RF, reticular formation; CN, cochlear nucleus; SOC, superior olivary complex. (From Millan 1988, with permission.)

microinjection of GABA antagonists into the SN or entopeduncular nucleus. Thus it is probable that NMDA protects against limbic seizures by activating the GABAergic inhibitory pathways that run from the striatum to the nigra and entopeduncular nucleus.

These experiments provide clear evidence that the output of the basal ganglia tonically influences excitability within the limbic system. This tonic activity apparently facilitates the development of seizure activity; reducing it suppresses seizure development. The pathways involved are clearly polysynaptic and involve relays in the habenula and thalamus, and possibly also the medial septal nucleus and the tegmentum.

## THE BASAL GANGLIA IN NEONATAL SEIZURES

The pattern of metabolic activation during focal motor seizures in newborn monkeys is similar to that occurring in pubescent monkeys, but more ipsilateral deep structures show an increased metabolism (Kato et al 1980). These include the ventrocaudal parts of the putamen and the globus pallidus, the substantia nigra and the ventroposterolateral nucleus of the thalamus. Experiments in rat pups suggest that the functional relationships are different, however, in the new born period. Kindled seizures in rat pups are not associated with enhanced glucose metabolism in the globus pallidus and substantia nigra (Ackermann et al 1982). Further bilateral injection of muscimol into the substantia nigra decreases the motor component of flurothyl seizures in adult rats but facilitates such seizures in 15 day old pups (Moshe & Albala 1984).

## SECONDARY GENERALISATION OF FOCAL SEIZURES

Focal motor seizures spread transcortically rather slowly. They are thought to generalise by three major routes:

1. Callosal spread (which is limited to the homologous cortical area)
2. Via the thalamus (ventromedial and ventrolateral nuclei and the thalamic commissure) and

3. Via the midbrain reticular formation.

It is a widely held belief that the latter route of generalisation is involved in cases with a relatively rapid transition from focal motor to generalised tonic activity. The evolution of limbic seizures into generalised clonic-tonic seizures is similarly believed to involve generalisation via the ventral thalamus or the mid-brain or upper brain stem reticular formation.

Given that these pathways are always present it is appropriate to ask why many cases show pure focal motor seizures or pure complex partial seizures without ever showing secondary generalised seizures. Inhibitory activity evoked in relay nuclei and acting locally or at a distance may be responsible for the failure to generalise. It is also possible that more widespread cerebral dysfunction is required for spread of seizure activity (to produce either partial or secondarily generalised seizures) than is implied in the concept of an epileptogenic focus (Engel 1987). There is much evidence from studies of kindling that changes in synaptic function occur at many anatomical sites. There are also studies of focal cortical seizures showing similar phenomena. For example the establishment of an alumina focus in the sensorimotor cortex of the cat is preceded by focal signs of epileptogenesis in subcortical structures (Morillo et al 1982).

## SEIZURES WITH SENSORY INDUCTION

The major form of sensory or reflex epilepsy in man is photically-induced epilepsy, which is usually expressed as a form of primary generalised epilepsy. A similar syndrome is found in the Senegalese baboon, *Papio papio*.

Sound-induced seizures occur in certain inbred strains of rodents such as DBA/2 mice and Genetically-Epilepsy Prone Rats. These are remarkable in that a complex sequence of motor manifestations occurs but there is no participation of the cortex in the seizure process.

### Photosensitive epilepsy

In man photosensitive epilepsy takes two principal forms, (Hishikawa et al 1967, Newmark & Penry 1979).

1. Some children or adults with primary generalised epilepsy show precipitation of their seizures by stroboscopic stimulation or equivalent oscillating inputs as provided by a maladjusted TV set.

2. Some patients show a classical photoconvulsive response that can be triggered by stroboscopic stimulation but also commonly by static or moving grid patterns, in which EEG recordings show that seizure activity is initiated in the occipital cortex. Studies of the effect of a range of static and moving patterns indicate that epileptogenicity can be linked to the intensity of stimulation of individual neurons in the visual cortex and the area of cortex involved (Binnie et al 1985a, Meldrum & Wilkins 1985). The population of neurons concerned with seizure initiation includes binocularly innervated neurons with complex properties.

Photically-induced seizures with occipital initiation are presumably comparable to focal motor seizures in terms of intracortical and subcortical generalisation.

Primary generalised seizures precipitated by stroboscopic stimulation were widely presumed to depend on activation of non-specific diffuse projection systems (Jasper

1949, Gastaut & Hunter 1950, Brazier 1953) but can just as readily be considered to depend on 'cortico-thalamic' mechanisms for their initiation (see below). Little direct evidence concerning site of epileptogenesis is available in man. Animal experiments concern convulsant drug administration in non-epileptic animals and electrophysiology in baboons, *Papio papio*, with genetically-determined photosensitive epilepsy. Infusion of pentylenetetrazol or bicuculline (which facilitate photically-induced seizures) in dogs produces a high frequency discharge in the lateral geniculate nucleus prior to cortical seizure activity (Binnie et al 1985b).

Over the last 20 years extensive electrophysiological and anatomical studies have been performed in the photosensitive baboon, *Papio papio* (Menini 1976, Naquet et al 1988). Depth electrode studies have firmly established that paroxysmal discharges originate within the superior frontal gyrus, an area receiving afferents from the occipital cortex (Catier et al 1973) and also somatosensory inputs relating to periorbital tissues. Laminar multiunit and current source density studies (Silva-Barrat et al 1986, 1987) show the earliest changes associated with paroxysmal discharges to be in the third lamina in the motor and premotor areas and also in the motor area at the junction of laminae five and six. Synaptic inputs from cortico-cortical (visual) and thalamic pathways are presumed to contribute to epileptogenesis, in the presence of locally impaired GABAergic inhibition (see Meldrum & Wilkins 1985, Brailowsky et al 1986) or enhanced excitatory (NMDA-mediated) responsiveness (see Meldrum 1986, Pumain et al 1985).

Ablation of the visual cortex protects against photically-induced frontorolandic paroxysmal discharges and myoclonus, emphasising the importance of the contribution of cortico-cortical afferents.

**Sound-induced seizures in rodents**

Various inbred strains of rats and mice show sound-induced seizures, which can be triggered by exposure to a loud sound of mixed frequencies and characteristically show a fixed sequence of motor elements commencing with propulsive activity ('wild running') followed by clonic and then tonic components. Many biochemical and pharmacological studies have been performed in DBA/2 mice but the principal anatomical studies concern genetically-epilepsy prone rats (GEPR) derived from the Sprague-Dawley strain. There is a similar colony (Krushinsky-Molodkina) derived from Wistars. The syndrome can be enhanced or reproduced by priming procedures which involve exposure to a loud sound or an ototoxic agent at an early age. A peripheral lesion involving cochlear receptors appears to be important in both genetically-determined and acquired forms of AGS (Penny et al 1983). There is also evidence for a deficiency in noradrenergic systems throughout the brain. In the inferior colliculus there is an enhanced number of GABAergic interneurons in the central nucleus (Roberts et al 1986) and an impaired responsiveness to locally applied GABA agonists and antagonists (Faingold et al 1986).

Electrophysiological studies show no evidence for cortical discharges during the seizures. Lesion studies suggest that structures above the midbrain are not crucial to the development of the seizures. Lesions of the inferior colliculus or of the midbrain reticular formation can abolish all or some of the motor components of the seizure (see Millan 1988). The focal injection of a GABA agonist into the inferior colliculus can block the seizure responses in a GEPR whereas a GABA antagonist, bicuculline, can make a normal rat show sound-induced seizures (Millan et al 1986b). Study of the minimal dose of the NMDA antagonist, 2-amino-7-phosphono-heptanoate, that will suppress sound-induced seizures when focally injected into different brain regions shows that the inferior colliculus is by far the most sensitive area. The superior olivary complex, the midbrain reticular formation and the substantia nigra pars reticulata also show a protective effect of NMDA receptor blockade (see Fig. 1.3). Electrolytic or mechanical lesions of the midbrain reticular formation, particularly those involving the nucleus reticularis pontis oralis abolish the tonic phase of the sound-induced seizures (and indeed of electroshock and pentylenetetrazol seizures (Browning 1985, 1987, Browning et al 1985, Kesner 1966).

Overall the data indicate that epileptic activity is initiated within the inferior colliculus in response to powerful inputs, probably because of changes in excitability induced by some degree of deafferentation. When a sufficient aggregate within the inferior colliculus is recruited there is spread of seizure activity to motor areas within the midbrain that are situated just ventral to the tegmentum, and that generate propulsive motor activity. Spread is thence to other parts of the reticular formation and the spinal cord. The substantia nigra pars reticulata has a modulating influence either by its projections to the superior colliculus or by acting on other descending pathways such as those to the pedunculopontine nucleus.

## GENERALISED EPILEPSY WITH SPIKE AND WAVE OR TONIC-CLONIC SEIZURES

The two major forms of epilepsy that constitute the primary generalised epilepsies characteristically show loss of consciousness at the beginning of the attack and a diffuse onset of seizure activity in cortical EEG records. Two influential and historically important accounts of the pathophysiology of epilepsy (Penfield & Jasper 1954, Gastaut & Fischer-Williams 1959) attributed this apparently generalised onset to initiation within the reticular core of the brain stem. Penfield formulated this 'centrencephalic theory' involving 'a region where the neural activities converge which are the indispensable substratum of consciousness' before the classical electrophysiological studies that attributed a special role in the maintenance of consciousness to the ascending reticular formation (Moruzzi & Magoun 1949, Magoun 1952). The brain stem and thalamic reticular system was assumed to be the system that provided the synchronous diffuse cortical discharges and the loss of consciousness in primary generalised epilepsies. The only direct evidence presented by Penfield & Jasper (1954) was recordings from cortex and hypothalamus in a 7 year old child with petit mal seizures (Case H.C., p. 627) which were interpreted as showing seizure onset in the hypothalamus preceding that in the cortex. The absence of decisive depth recordings showing seizure onset in the brain stem or mid brain reticular formation in primary generalised seizures must be considered a weakness in the centrencephalic theory. There has also been a widespread failure to initiate generalised seizures accompanied by appropriate cortical EEG activity using focal electrical or chemical stimulation within the brain stem. Reticular seizures can be induced in rats, rabbits and cats but they have different motor and EEG signs. Thus Kreindler et al (1958) observed in rats and cats following prolonged high-voltage stimulation of the bulbo-ponto-mesencephalic reticular formation seizures with prominent tonic elements associated with cortical arousal on the

EEG. Burnham et al (1981) observed motor patterns in rats that resembled those seen in sound-induced seizures in genetically-susceptible mice and rats (i.e. including wild-running and clonic components as well as tonic extension). Rather massive injections of penicillin in the midbrain reticular formation in cats however induce both focal spike discharges and simultaneous generalised cortical spiking (Ralston & Langer 1965). The associated clinical sign was frequent myoclonic jerking.

There is an extensive and complex literature on the involvement of various thalamic nuclei in primary generalised epilepsy. The intralaminar nuclei were proposed as part of the centrencephalic system as a result of the observation by Jasper & Droogleever Fortuyn (1977) that stimulation of the intralaminar nuclei in the kitten at 3 Hz produced a cortical discharge resembling 3 per second spike and wave. Subsequently many studies reported antiepileptic effects of thalamic lesions. Lesions of the lateral posterior thalamic nucleus in cats have a powerful protective effect against seizures induced by electrical stimulation of the cortex (Van Straaten 1975). In a rather mixed group of patients Mullan et al (1967) lesioned the lateral nuclear mass (sometimes involving the mammillothalamic tract and the fields of Forel) with moderate therapeutic success. Although stimulation of the centromedian thalamic nucleus at low frequency can induce cortically discharges mimicking 3 Hz spike and wave, high frequency stimulation induces cortical desynchronisation and blocks epileptic discharges (Velasco & Velasco 1982). This has lead to the trial of electrical stimulation of the centromedian nucleus in patients with generalised or multifocal seizures (Velasco et al 1987).

Various Italian authors (Mutani, La Grutta and colleagues) have used depth electrodes in the cat to study the effect of focal stimulation in the basal ganglia on cortical or limbic seizure activity. Prior high-frequency electrical stimulation of the head of the caudate nucleus decreases electrically-induced after discharges in the amygdala or hippocampus (La Grutta et al 1971, 1985). Electrically-induced after discharges or seizures in the amygdala are more powerfully suppressed by conditioning stimulation of the globus pallidus or substantia nigra than of the striatum (Amato et al 1982). Lesions in the globus pallidus or substantia nigra decrease the inhibitory effect on amygdala discharges of striatal stimulation, implying that the basal ganglia output pathway is responsible for this inhibitory effect (Amato et al 1982). Using the intravenous administration of penicillin to induce 'interictal' spikes in the hippocampus somewhat different results have been obtained (Sabatino et al 1986). Stimulation of the substantia nigra pars compacta suppresses the spikes whereas stimulation of the globus pallidus pars interna facilitates their evolution into seizure discharges. Destruction of the medial septal nucleus prevented both these effects (Sabatino et al 1986) suggesting that a pallido-habenula-septal pathway could be providing a means for basal ganglia output to control hippocampal excitability.

Many conclusions about the probable mechanisms underlying generalised epilepsy with spike and wave discharge have been drawn from animal experiments with models employing oestrogens, penicillin or pentylenetetrazol as the epileptogenic agent. In particular Gloor (1979) has utilised penicillin epilepsy in the cat to study the relationship between the thalamic and cortical discharges.

The 'cortico-reticular' theory of Gloor (1968, 1979) provides an explanation for the synchronous discharges in primary generalised epilepsy of the absence type. It is supported not only by experiments using systemic penicillin, but also by numerous electrophysiological studies of thalamic and cortical function. The bilaterally synchronous spike-and-wave discharges are seen as an abnormal response to afferent thalamocortical volleys (normally involved in the elicitation of spindles). Intrinsic properties of thalamic neurones and the pattern of connection within the thalamus produce certain synchronous oscillations in excitability that filter afferent activity so that it causes synchronous excitation in cortical neurons which is followed by synchronous inhibition because of recurrent activation of GABAergic interneurons. The cortical event is similar at the cellular and neuronal aggregate level to an interictal event in an epileptogenic focus but its synchronous occurrence over a large area and its rhythmic repetition produce a clinical ictal event through a mechanism not involving epileptic activation of motor pathways. The primary abnormality is the hyperexcitability of cortical neurons that causes them to generate an increased excitatory response to the afferent volley. The synchronous oscillation between excitation and inhibition within the cortex disrupts the pattern of activity that sustains normal motor and cognitive function which is therefore arrested during the spike and wave discharge. Evidence for gradations in the loss of consciousness during absence attacks supports this interpretation. This is thus the minimal form of epilepsy both in that it involves only one neuronal aggregate and in that it involves one type of discharge which does not develop the characteristics associated with most self-sustaining forms of seizure.

Evidence for a crucial role in pentylenetetrazol seizures of an ascending pathway passing via the mammillary bodies and anterior thalamus has been provided by experiments in guinea pigs and rats (Mirski & Ferrendelli 1984, Mirski et al 1986). Discrete electrolytic lesions of the mammillothalamic tract block the induction of seizures by pentylenetetrazol, suggesting that this pathway is a relay from a more caudal initiating site (such as the ventral tegmental area). Injection of $\gamma$-vinyl GABA into the anterior thalamus also blocks the seizures indicating that enhanced inhibition within this relay nucleus prevents spread to cortex.

Human data concerning focal pathology in primary generalised epilepsy of the absence type are very sparse.

## BRAIN STEM SEIZURES IN MAN

Gastaut (1969) described generalized tonic-clonic seizures not associated with forebrain EEG discharges as 'reticular epilepsy'. Syndromes that probably fall into the category of brain stem seizures include seizures in the neonatal period that are not associated with corresponding EEG signs of epilepsy. These are seen in infants with hypoxic-ischaemic encephalopathy. Their clinical characteristics include 'motor automatisms' (oral-buccal-lingual movements, ocular movements, and progression or locomotor movements) and tonic seizures (hyperextension of the upper and lower extremities or hyperextension of the legs with flexion of the arms). Reasons for considering these as manifestations of seizure activity occurring at the midbrain level include their similarity to the range of motor activities that can be induced in rodents or other animals by electrical stimulation of the motor areas of the midbrain reticular formation (e.g. propulsive movements, wild running, tonic extension, see Burnham 1987).

In has been argued that these clinical syndromes are not epileptic in nature, but brain stem reflexes or release phenomena revealed when cortical control is lost (Kellaway & Hrachovy 1983, Mizrahi & Kellaway 1987). The arguments for this view include the poor epileptogenicity of brain stem structures and the response of the clinical phenomena to sensory stimulation. Thus in the infants with hypoxic/ischaemic encephalopathy tactile stimulation will commonly trigger the abnormal movements, the response being proportional to the stimulation and remaining stimulus dependent. Abnormal movements can often be terminated by restraint of the limb or by postural adjustment of the head and neck. Although these phenomena demonstrate a role for somatosensory inputs in controlling the abnormal movements, they do not prove that they are 'reflex' and not 'epileptic' because very similar effects (of stimulus dependence and of facilitation and arrest by somatosensory stimulation) can be demonstrated in relation to facial myoclonus during stroboscopic stimulation in *Papio papio*, a phenomenon that is undoubtedly related to epileptic activity in the cortex.

## CONCLUSIONS

The clinical manifestations of an epileptic attack — abnormal motor activity or disturbances of consciousness — depend on spread of abnormal neuronal discharges from their site of initiation to involve either motor output neurons in the brain stem and spinal cord or to regions of the brain subserving consciousness (limbic or cortical areas). The routes of spread are complex involving multiple interactions and transformations (relay, recruitment and inhibition). A suppressive effect on seizure phenomena is seen following blockade of excitatory transmission in very many central nuclei. Inhibitory processes may be intrinsic to a particular region or activated via multisynaptic pathways. The basal ganglia provide an important relay system for focal and generalised seizures with motor manifestations. For a cortical discharge the sequential relays are: (1) the striatum; (2) globus pallidus or substantia nigra pars reticulata; (3) mesencephalic locomotor region (pedunculopontine nucleus); (4) further reticular relays; (5) spinal cord. The midbrain and brain stem motor areas play a crucial role in determining the motor pattern and sequential nature of seizure phenomena.

The basal ganglia also provide tonic modulatory influences on limbic seizures and certain motor components of generalised seizures. The pathways involved may include relays in the habenula, thalamus and medial septum.

## REFERENCES

Ackermann R F, Moshe S L, Albala B J, Engel J 1982 Anatomical substrates of amygdala kindling in immature rats demonstrated by 2-deoxyglucose autoradiography. Epilepsia 23: 434–435

Amato G, Crescimanno G, Sorbera F, LaGrutta V 1982 Relationship between the striatal system and amygdaloid paroxysmal activity. Experimental Neurology 77: 492–504

Ayala G F, Matsumoto H, Gumnit R J 1970 Excitability changes and inhibitory mechanisms in neocortical neurons during seizures. Journal of Neurophysiology 33: 73–85

Binnie C D, Findlay J, Wilkins A J 1985a Mechanisms of epileptogenesis in photosensitive epilepsy implied by the effects of moving patterns. Electroencephalography and Clinical Neurophysiology 61: 1–6

Binnie C D, Van Emde Boas W, Wauquier A 1985b Geniculate spikes during epileptic seizures induced in dogs by pentylenetetrazol and bicuculline. Electroencephalography and Clinical Neurophysiology 61: 40–49

Bonhaus, D W, Walters J R, McNamara J O 1986 Activation of substantia nigra neurons: role in the propagation of seizures in kindled rats. Journal of Neuroscience 6: 3024–3030

Brailowsky S, Menini C, Silva-Barrat C, Naquet R 1986 Epileptogenic γ-aminobutyric — withdrawal syndrome after chronic intracortical infusion in baboons. Neuroscience Letters 74: 75–80

Brazier, M A B 1953 A review of physiological mechanisms of the visual system in relation to activation techniques in electroencephalography. Electroencephalography and Clinical Neurophysiology 4 93–107

Browning R A 1985 Role of the brain-stem reticular formation in tonic-clonic seizures: Lesion and pharmacological studies. Federation Proceedings 44: 2425–2431

Browning R A 1987 Effect of lesions on seizures in experimental animals. In: Fromm G H, Faingold C L, Browning R A, Burnham, W M (eds) Epilepsy and the reticular formation: the role of the reticular core in convulsive seizures. Liss, New York, p 137–162
Browning R A, Nelson D K, Mogharreban N, Jobe P C, Laird H E 1985 Effect of midbrain and pontine tegmental lesions on audiogenic seizures in genetically epilepsy-prone rats. Epilepsia 26: 175–183
Burnham W M 1987 Electrical stimulation studies: generalized convulsions triggered from the brain stem. In: Fromm G H, Faingold C L, Browning R A, Burnham W M (eds) Epilepsy and the reticular formation: the role of the reticular core in convulsive seizures. Liss, New York, p 25–38
Burnham, W M, Albright P, Schneiderman J, Chiu P, Ninchoji T 1981 'Centrencephalic' mechanisms in the kindling model. In: J A Wada (ed) Kindling 2. Raven Press, New York, p 161–178
Catier J, Charmasson G, Christolomme A 1973 Study of ipsilateral cortico-cortical connections from the occipital lobe in the photosensitive baboon. Journal de Physiologie Paris 66: 93–100
Caveness W F, Kato M, Malamut, B L, Hosokawa S, Wakisaka S, O'Neill R 1980 Propagation of focal motor seizures in the pubescent monkey. Annals of Neurology 7: 213–221.
Connors B W 1984 Initiation of synchronized neuronal bursting in neocortex. Nature 310: 685–687.
Crowell R M 1970 Distant effects of a focal epileptogenic process. Brain Research 18: 137–154
De Sarro G, Patel S, Meldrum B S 1987 Anticonvulsant action of a kainate antagonist $\gamma$-D-glutamyl aminomethylsulphonic acid injected focally into the substantia nigra and entopeduncular nucleus. European Journal of Pharmacology 132: 229–236
Dichter M A, Ayala G F 1987 Cellular mechanisms of epilepsy: a status report. Science 237: 157–164
Dingledine R, Hines M A, King G L 1986 Involvement of N-methyl-D-aspartate receptors in the rat hippocampal slice. Journal of Physiology 380: 175–189.
Engel J 1987 New concepts of the epileptic focus. In: Wieser H G, Speckmann E J, Engel J (eds) The epileptic focus. Libbey, London, p 83–94
Engel J, Wolfson L, Brown L 1978 Anatomical correlates of electrical and behavioral events related to amygdaloid kindling. Annals of Neurology 3: 538–544
Erickson T C 1940 Spread of the epileptic discharge. An experimental study of the after discharge induced by electrical stimulation of cerebral cortex. Archives of Neurology and Psychiatry 43: 429–452
Faingold C L, Gelbach M A, Travis M A, Caspary D M 1986 Inferior colliculus neuronal response abnormalities in genetically epilepsy prone rats: evidence for a deficit of inhibition. Life Science 39: 869–878
Ferrier D 1886 The functions of the brain 2nd edn. Smith, Elder & Co, London, p 498
Fulton J F 1953 Discussion of Gastaut H. So-called 'psychomotor' and 'temporal' epilepsy. Epilepsia 2: 77
Garant D S, Gale K 1987 Substantia nigra-mediated anticonvulsant actions: role of nigral output pathways. Experimental Neurology 97: 143–159
Gastaut H 1969 Introduction to the study of generalized epilepsies. In: Gastaut H, Jasper H, Bancaud J, Waltregny A (eds) The physiopathogenesis of the epilepsies. Thomas, Springfield, Illinois, p xi–xvi
Gastaut H, Fischer-Williams M 1959 The physiopathology of epileptic seizures. In: J Field (ed) Handbook of Physiology, neurophysiology vol 1. American Physiological Society, Washington, p 329–363
Gastaut H, Hunter J 1950 An experimental study of the mechanism of photic activation in idiopathic epilepsy. Electroencephalography and Clinical Neurophysiology 2: 263–287
Gibbs F, Gibbs E, Lennox W 1937 Epilepsy, a paroxysmal cerebral dysrhythmia. Brain 60: 377–388
Gillingham F J, Watson W S, Chung S, Yates L 1980 Central brain lesions for the control of intractable epilepsy. In: Watson J A, Penry J K (eds) Advance in epileptology: The Xth Epilepsy International Symposium. Raven Press, New York, p 251–255
Gloor P 1968 Generalized cortico-reticular epilepsies: Some considerations on the pathophysiology of generalized bilterally synchronous spike and wave discharge. Epilepsia 9: 249–263
Gloor P 1979 Generalized epilepsy with spike-and-wave discharge: a reinterpretation of its electrographic and clinical manifestations. Epilepsia 20: 571–588
Goddard G V, McIntyre D C, Leech C K 1969 A permanent change in brain function resulting from daily electrical stimulation. Experimental Neurology 25: 295–330
Gutnick M J 1987 Circuitry of cortical and hippocampal epilepsy. Neuroscience 22: S196
Hayashi T 1952 A physiological study of epileptic seizures following cortical stimulation in animals and its application to human clinics. Japanese Journal of Pharmacology 3: 46–64
Hayashi T 1953 The efferent pathway of epileptic seizures for the face following cortical stimulation differs from that for limbs. Japanese Journal of Pharmacology 4: 306–321
Hishikawa Y, Yamamoto J, Furuya E, Yamada Y, Miyazaki K, Kaneko Z 1967 Photosensitive epilepsy: relationships between the visual evoked responses and the epileptiform discharges induced by intermittent photic stimulation. Electroencephalography and Clinical Neurophysiology 23: 320–334

Hosokawa S, Kato M, Kuroiwa Y 1983 Topographical distribution of propagation of seizure activity in the basal ganglia during focal motor seizures in the monkey. Neuroscience Letters 38: 29–33

Jackson J H 1873 On the anatomical investigation of epilepsy and epileptiform convulsions. British Medical Journal i: 573–557

Jackson J H 1931 In: Taylor J (ed) Selected writings, vol I. Hodder & Stoughton, London, p 500

Jackson J H, Beevor C E 1889 Case of tumour of the right temporo-sphenoidal lobe bearing on the localization of the sense of smell and on the interpretation of a particular variety of epilepsy. Brain 12: 346–357

Jackson J H, Colman W S 1898 Case of epilepsy with tasting movements and 'dreamy state'— very small patch of softening in the left uncinate gyrus. Brain 21: 580–590

Jasper H H 1949 Diffuse projection systems: the integrative action of the thalamic reticular system. Electroencephalography and Clinical Neurophysiology 1: 405–420

Jasper H, Droogleever Fortuyn J 1947. Experimental studies on the functional anatomy of petit mal epilepsy. Proceedings of the Association for Research of Nervous Mental Disorders 26: 272–298

Kato M, Malamut B L, Caveness W F, Hosokawa S, Wakisaka S, O'Neill R R 1980 Low cerebral glucose utilization in newborn and pubescent monkeys during focal motor seizures. Annals of Neurology 7: 204–212

Kellaway P, Hrachovy R A 1983 Status epilepticus in newborns: a perspective on neonatal seizures. In: Delgado-Escueta A V, Wasterlain C G, Treiman D N, Porter R J (eds) Advances in Neurology vol 34. Status epilepticus. Raven Press, New York, p 93–99

Kesner R P, 1966 Subcortical mechanisms of audiogenic seizures. Experimental Neurology 15: 192–205

Kreindler A, Zuckerman E, Steriade M, Chimion J 1958 Electro clinical features of convulsions induced by stimulation of brain stem. Journal of Neurophysiology 21: 430–436

La Grutta V, Amato G, Zagami M T 1971 The importance of the caudate nucleus in the control of convulsive activity in the amygdaloid complex and the temporal cortex of the cat. Electroencephalography and Clinical Neurophysiology 31: 57–69

La Grutta V, Sabatino M, Gravante G, La Grutta G 1985 Effects of caudate nucleus on paroxysmal activity in hippocampus of cat. Electroencephalography and Clinical Neurophysiology 61: 416–421

Le Gal La Salle G, Kajima M, Feldblum S 1983 Abortive amygdaloid kindled seizures following microinjection of γ-vinylGABA in the vicinity of substantia nigra in rats. Neuroscience Letters 36: 69–743

McNamara J O, Galloway M T, Rigsbee L C, Shin C 1984 Evidence implicating substantia nigra in regulation of kindled seizure threshold. Journal of Neuroscience 4: 2410–2417

Magoun H W 1952 The ascending reticular activating system. Proceedings of the Association for Research of Nervous Mental Disorders 30: 480–492

Meldrum B 1984 Amino acid neurotransmitters and new approaches to anticonvulsant drug action. Epilepsia 25: S140–S149

Meldrum B 1985 Possible therapeutic applications of antagonists of excitatory amino acid neurotransmitters. Clinical Science 68: 113–122

Meldrum B 1986 Is epilepsy a disorder of excitatory transmission? In: Trimble M R, Reynolds E H (ed) What is epilepsy?, Churchill Livingstone, Edinburgh, p 293–302

Meldrum B S 1988 The basal ganglia and the development and motor expression of partial seizures. In: M Swash, C Kinnard (ed) Hierarchies of the brain. In press

Meldrum B S, Wilkins A J 1984 Photosensitive epilepsy in man and the baboon: integration of pharmacological and psychophysical evidence. In: P A Schwartzkroin, H V Wheal (eds) Electrophysiology of epilepsy. Academic Press, London, p 51–77

Meldrum B, Millan, M, Patel S, De Sarro G 1987 Anti-epileptic effects of focal micro-injection of excitatory amino acid antagonists. Journal of Neural Transmission. In press

Menini C 1976 Role du cortex frontal dans l'epilepsie photosensible du singe Papio papio. Journal de Physiologie, Paris 72: 5–44

Miles R, Wong R K S 1983 Single neurons can initiate synchronized population discharge in the hippocampus. Nature 306: 371–373

Miles R, Wong R K S 1987 Latent synaptic pathways revealed after tetanic stimulation in the hippocampus. Nature 329: 724–726

Millan M H 1988 Audiogenic seizures in rodents. In: Meldrum B S, Ferrendelli J A, Wieser H G (eds) Anatomy of epileptogenesis. Libbey, London. In press

Millan M H, Patel S, Mello L M, Meldrum B S 1986a Focal injection of 2-amino-7-phosphonoheptanoic acid into prepiriform cortex protects against pilocarpine-induced limbic seizures in rats. Neuroscience Letters 70: 69–74

Millan M H, Meldrum, B S, Faingold C L 1986b Induction of audiogenic seizure susceptibility by focal infusion of excitant amino acid or bicuculline into the inferior colliculus of normal rats. Experimental Neurology 91: 634–639
Mirski M A, Ferrendelli J A 1984 Interruption of the mammillothalamic tract prevents seizures in guinea pigs. Science 226: 72–74
Mirski M A, McKeon A C, Ferrendelli J A 1986 Anterior thalamus and substantia nigra: two distinct structures mediating experimental generalized seizures. Brain Research 397: 377–380
Mizrahi E M, Kellaway P 1987 Characterization and classification of neonatal seizures. Neurology 37: 1837–1844
Morillo L E, Ebner T J, Bloedel J R 1982 The early involvement of subcortical structures during the development of a cortical seizure focus. Epilepsia 23: 571–585
Morimoto K, Goddard G V 1987 The substantia nigra is an important site for the containment of seizure generalization in the kindling model of epilepsy. Epilepsia 28: 1–10
Moruzzi G, Magoun H W 1949 Brain stem reticular formation and activation of the EEG. Electroencephalography and Clinical Neurophysiology 1: 455–473
Moshe S L, Albala B J 1984 Nigral muscimol infusions facilitate the development of seizures in immature rats. Developmental Brain Research 13: 305–308
Mullan S, Vailati G, Karasick J, Mailis M 1967 Thalamic lesions for the control of epilepsy. Archives of Neurology 16: 277–285
Mutani R, Durelli L 1980 Mechanisms of interaction of asymmetrical bilateral epileptogenic foci in neocortex. Epilepsia 21: 549–556
Naquet R, Menini C, Riche D, Silva-Barrat C, Valin A 1988 Cerebral structures and pathways involved in photic epilepsy. In: Meldrum B S, Ferrendelli J A, Wieser H G (eds) Anatomy of epileptogenesis. Libbey, London
Newmark M E, Penry J K 1979 Photosensitivity and epilepsy: a review. Raven Press, New York, p 220
Patel S, Millan M H, Mello L M, Meldrum B S 1988 2-amino-7-phosphonoheptanoic acid (2-APH) infusion into entopeduncular nucleus protects against limbic seizures in rats. Neuroscience Letters 64: 226–230
Patel S, Chapman A G, Millan M H, Meldrum B S 1987 Epilepsy and excitatory amino acid antagonists. In: D. Lodge (ed) Excitatory amino acid in health and disease. Wiley, London, p 353–378
Patel S, Slater P 1987 Analysis of the brain regions involved in myoclonus produced by intracerebral picrotoxin. Neuroscience 20: 687–693
Pellegrini A, Armani M, Testa G 1985 Involvement of cortical, thalamic and midbrain reticular formation neurons in spike and wave discharges. Extracellular study in feline generalized penicillin epilepsy. Experimental Neurology 89: 465–478
Penfield W, Jasper H, 1954 Epilepsy and the functional anatomy of the human brain Little Brown, Boston
Penny J E, Brown R D, Hodges K B, Kupetz S A Glenn D W, Jobe P C 1983 Cochlear morphology of the audiogenic-seizure susceptible (AGS) or genetically epilepsy prone rat (GEPR). Acta Oto-laryngologica 95: 1–12
Piredda S, Gale K 1985 A crucial epileptogenic site in the deep prepiriform cortex. Nature 317: 623–625
Pumain, R, Menini C, Heinemann, U, Louvel J, Silva-Barrat C. 1985 Chemical synaptic transmission is not necessary for epileptic seizures to persist in the baboon, Papio papio. Experimental Neurology 89: 250–258
Ralston B L, Langer H 1965 Experimental epilepsy of brain-stem origin. Electroencephalography and Clinical Neurophysiology 18: 325–333
Reeves A G, O'Leary P M 1985 Total corpus callosotomy for control of medically intractable epilepsy. In: Reeves A G (ed) Epilepsy and the corpus callosum, Plenum Press, New York, p 269–280
Roberts R C, Ribak C E, Oertel W H 1986 Increased numbers of GABAergic neurons occur in the inferior colliculus of an audiogenic model of genetic epilepsy. Brain Research 361: 324–338
Sabatino M, Savatteri V, Liberti G, Vella N, La Grutta V 1986 Effects of substantia nigra and pallidum stimulation on hippocampal interictal activity in the cat. Neuroscience Letters 64: 293–298
Silva-Barrat C, Menini C, Bryere P, Naquet R 1986 Multiunitary activity analysis of cortical and subcortical structures in paroxysmal discharges and grand mal seizures in photosensitive baboons. Electroencephalography and Clinical Neurophysiology 64: 455–468
Silva-Barrat C, Brailowsky S, Levesque G, Menini C 1987 Epileptic discharges induced by intermittent light stimulation in photosensitive baboons: a current source density study. Epilepsy Research 2: 1–8
Tarsy D, Pycock C J, Meldrum B S, Marsden C D 1978 Focal contralateral myoclonus produced by inhibition of GABA action in the caudate nucleus of rats. Brain 101: 143–162

Turski W A, Cavalheiro E A, Schwarz M, Czuczwar S J Kleinrok Z, Turski L 1983 Limbic seizures produced by pilocarpine in rats: a behavioural, electroencephalographic and neuropathological study. Behavioural Brain Research 9: 315–335

Turski L, Cavalheiro E A, Turski W A, Meldrum B S 1986 Excitatory neurotransmission within substantia nigra pars reticulata regulates threshold for seizures by pilocarpine in rats: effects of intranigral 2-amino-7-phosponoheptanoate and N-methyl-D-aspartate. Neuroscience 18: 61–77

Turski W A, Cavalheiro, E A, Coimbra C, Berzaghi, M D P, Ikonimidou-Turski C, Turski L 1987a Only certain antiepileptic drugs prevent seizures induced by pilocarpine. Brain Research Review 12: 281–305

Turski L, Meldrum B S, Cavalheiro E A, Calderazzo-Filho L S, Bortolotto Z A, Ikonomidou-Turski C, Turski C, Turski W A 1987b Paradoxical anticonvulsant activity of the excitatory amino acid N-methyl-D-aspartate in the rat caudate-putamen. Proceedings of National Academy of Sciences 84: 1689–1693

Ueno H, Yamashita Y, Caveness W F 1975 Regional cerebral blood flow pattern in focal epileptiform seizures in the monkey. Experimental Neurology 47: 81–96

Van Straaten J J 1975 Abolition of electrically induced cortical seizures by st ereotactic thalamic lesions. Neurology 25: 141–149

Van Wagenen W P, Herren R Y 1940 Surgical division of commissural pathways in the corpus callosum, relation to spread of an epileptic attack. Archives of Neurology and Psychiatry 44: 740–759

Velasco M, Velasco F 1982 State related brain stem regulation of cortical and motor excitability: effects on experimental focal motor seizures. In: Sterman M B et al (eds) Sleep and epilepsy. Academic Press, Orlando, p 53–61

Velasco F, Velasco M, Ogarrio C, Fanghanel G 1987 Electrical stimulation of the centromedian thalamic nucleus in the treatment of convulsive seizures: a preliminary report. Epilepsia 28: 421–430

Wieser H G 1983 Electroclinical features of the psychomotor seizure. G. Fischer-Butterworths, Stuttgart–London, p 242

Wieser H G 1986 Psychomotor seizures of hippocampal-amygdalar origin In: Pedley T A, Meldrum B S (eds) Recent advances in epilepsy vol 3. Churchill Livingstone, Edinburgh, p 57–79

# 2. Kindling

*S. L. Moshé N. Ludvig*

## INTRODUCTION

In the late sixties, Goddard (1967) and Goddard, et al (1969) sparked interest in epilepsy circles by introducing a new model they aptly named 'kindling' from the analogy to kindling a fire. In this paradigm, localized intracranial, repetitive low intensity, usually electrical, stimulations lead to the development of focal afterdischarges (ADs) (Fig. 2.1), behavioral automatisms, and eventually, generalized motor

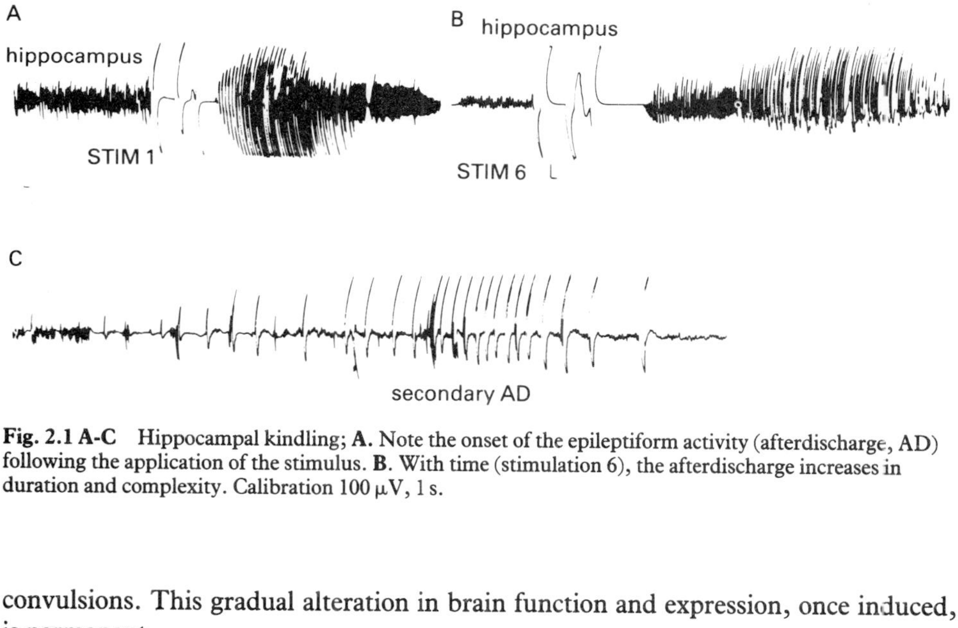


**Fig. 2.1 A-C** Hippocampal kindling; **A.** Note the onset of the epileptiform activity (afterdischarge, AD) following the application of the stimulus. **B.** With time (stimulation 6), the afterdischarge increases in duration and complexity. Calibration 100 μV, 1 s.

convulsions. This gradual alteration in brain function and expression, once induced, is permanent.

Over the next two decades, this model captured the imagination of many scientists investigating basic mechanisms of epileptogenesis. As a result, there are now over 700 publications on the kindling model. The interest derives from the theory that epilepsy in general, and 'psychomotor' epilepsy in particular, is a progressive disease in which early, subtle seizure manifestations can escape medical attention. With time, as generalized convulsions emerge, the epileptic engram becomes permanently engraved in the brain, and the seizures may become intractable to treatment. Kindling can be conceived as a possible mechanism by which epileptogenesis in humans is established.

For researchers, kindling offers several unique opportunities to study some aspects of epileptogenesis in animals and, perhaps by extrapolation, to understand the pathophysiology of certain human epileptic syndromes. In the kindling model, the investigator has precise control over the initiation of the seizures, their development and maintenance. The induced convulsive patterns are easily recognizable and reproducible, and the seizures can be quantified by severity (Table 2.1) and duration (electrographic ADs). Since there are no pathological changes in the area of stimulation other than those associated with electrode insertion (Goddard et al 1969, Goddard & Douglas 1975), the epileptic dysfunction can be dissociated from a structural lesion that may introduce confounding influences. Finally, after a certain period of time spontaneous seizures may occur (Pinel & Rovner 1978, Wada et al 1974). Thus, kindling satisfies most of the prerequisite characteristics of an 'ideal' model of epilepsy (Wada 1986).

**Table 2.1** Staging of amygdala-induced kindled seizures in adult rats. (Modified from Racine 1972a and Pinel & Rovner 1978.)

| Stage | Signs |
|---|---|
| 0 | Behavioral arrest |
| 1 | Chewing |
| 2 | Head nodding |
| 3 | Contralateral forelimb clonus |
| 4 | Bilateral forelimb clonus with rearing |
| 5 | Loss of balance |
| 6 | Wild running, jumping and rolling |
| 7 | Tonic posturing |
| 8 | Spontaneous seizures |

## THE BASICS

### *Species specificity*

Kindling can be induced experimentally in a variety of animal species (Table 2.2).

**Table 2.2** Animals that can be kindled

| Animal | Reference |
|---|---|
| Frogs | Morrell Tsuru (1976) |
| Reptiles | Rial & Gonzalez (1978) |
| Mice | Leech & McIntyre (1976) |
| Rats | Goddard et al (1969) |
| Gerbils | Cain & Corcoran (1980) |
| Rabbits | Tanaka (1972) |
| Cats | Wada et al (1974) |
| Dogs | Wauquier et al (1979) |
| Baboons | Wada & Osawa (1976) |
| Monkey | Wada et al (1978) |

In general, the lower the animal is on the phylogenetic scale, the greater its susceptibility to kindled seizures. In rats, 10–20 daily electrical stimulations, delivered to the amygdala, suffice for the development of generalized and symmetrical seizures. In contrast, symmetrically generalized seizures can not be induced in rhesus monkeys even after an average of 196 stimulations have been administered (Wada et al 1978). On the other hand, symmetrically generalized kindled convulsions can be induced after an average of 72 daily amygdala stimulations in *Papio papio* baboons, a primate species with a genetic susceptibility to photically induced seizures (Wada & Osawa, 1976). In interpreting these data, Wada et al (1978) point out that the 'abrupt onset of human epilepsy with a fully developed seizure pattern, may reflect an extraordinary pathophysiologic event in the brain, resulting from an overwhelming endogenous or exogenous insult that interacts with some genetically predisposed seizure susceptibility.'

*Agents*

Kindling can be produced in animals by various chemical means including the systemic or intracranial localized, periodic, administration of pharmacological agents such as pentylenetetrazol (Mason & Cooper 1972, Fabisiak & Schwark 1982, Diehl et al 1984), cocaine (Post 1977, Stripling & Ellingwood 1977), lidocaine (Post, et al 1975), penicillin (Collins 1978), and carbachol (Vosu & Wise 1975, Wasterlain & Jonec 1983, Cain 1983). Use of a drug stimulus is termed chemical kindling.

Repeated administration of electroconvulsive shocks (ECS) can lead to progressive intensification of the ensuing seizures (Ramer & Pinel 1967, Pinel & Van Oot 1975). Classically, however, kindling is produced by the repeated application of electrical stimuli to discrete areas of the brain.

To induce kindling the electrical stimuli must be delivered periodically. In adult animals, continuous stimulation or stimulations delivered at less than 20–30 min intervals fail to induce kindling (Goddard et al 1969, Racine et al 1973, Peterson et al 1981, Moshé et al 1983). The efficacy of the stimulus increases with interstimulus periods of 1 hour or longer (Goddard et al 1969, McIntyre et al 1987). The most common form of stimulation consists of sinusoidal or rectangular current at about 60 Hz delivered for 1–2 s; however all frequencies above 25 Hz are equally effective (Goddard et al 1969, Racine 1978). Although initially it was stated that low frequency stimulation may fail to induce kindling, recent studies have revealed that kindling can be produced with frequencies as low as 1.5–3 Hz provided that the current is delivered for a longer period of time (10–60 s) and the stimulus intensity is increased (Cain & Corcoran 1981, Corcoran & Cain 1980, Lothman et al 1985, Minabe et al 1986).

*Site specificity*

The susceptibility to electrical kindling varies with the stimulation site. Limbic and anterior neocortical sites can be readily kindled but midbrain sites (geniculate bodies, red nucleus, tegmentum, superior colliculus, substantia nigra) and the cerebellum cannot be kindled (Racine 1978). The original study of Goddard et al (1969) indicated that within the limbic system the amygdala is especially prone to kindling. Subsequent studies suggested that the prepiriform (Morimoto et al 1986, Zhao & Moshé 1987) and piriform cortex as well as the olfactory bulb (Cain 1977) are also quite sensitive, while the hippocampus and entorhinal cortex are relatively more resistant (Goddard et al 1969, Racine 1978). Within the hippocampus, the ventral part is more responsive than the dorsal (Racine et al 1977).

As a rule, triggered ADs are required for kindling to occur (Racine 1972a). While stimuli that are subthreshold for AD generation can gradually decrease the AD threshold (defined as the lowest current intensity capable of eliciting an AD), the repeated failure to induce an AD usually indicates that the site can not be kindled. Thus, determination of the AD threshold can be considered as an index of the epileptogenicity of the stimulated site although the AD threshold does not accurately predict the speed with which generalized kindled seizures will emerge (Zaide 1974, Racine et al 1977, Moshé et al 1982).

The behavioral manifestations of kindled seizures depend on the stimulated site and the animal species. In rats, the development of amygdala-kindled seizures progresses through predictable and characteristic stages, first described by Racine (1972b) (Table 2.1). Stages 0–3 represent focal (partial) seizures although by the time stage 3 seizures occur, the seizure activity has propagated to involve the ipsilateral hemisphere. Stages 4 and 5 represent frank generalized seizures of different severity. Pinel & Rovner (1978) have shown that further stimulations induce progressively more severe seizures which they classified as stages 6–8. In fact, after an average of 348 stimulations, spontaneous seizures have occurred in rats (Pinel & Rovner 1978), satisfying the important criterion necessary to establish kindling as a key animal model of epilepsy (Wada 1986, McNamara et al 1986). Spontaneous seizures have also been observed in cats (Wada et al 1974). Traditionally, however, most investigators consider the development of stage 4 or 5 generalized seizures as an end point. The number of stimulations required for the development of a generalized convulsion has been labelled as the kindling rate and is a measure of the ability of the focus to spread to distant sites involved in the behavioral expression of seizures as well as the ability of surrounding and remote brain regions to limit this propagation. Animals with short kindling rates are more seizure prone than animals with long kindling rates.

The behavioral manifestations of convulsions triggered from other limbic sites are similar to those induced by amygdala kindling (Le Galle La Salle 1982). Convulsions elicited by neocortical stimulation have different characteristics, at least initially. Burnham (1978) has described a typical tripartite seizure configuration consisting of early clonus followed by tonus culminating in late clonus. The latter component resembles that of amygdala-kindled generalized seizures and has been classified as such (Wong & Moshé 1987). The kindling rate of neocortical-induced kindled seizures is usually 2–4 times greater than that of amygdala-induced convulsions, although stimulations of the corpus callosum can produce generalized seizures within 1–5 stimulations (Goddard et al 1969 and personal observations, Figure 2.2).

### *Status epilepticus*

A modification of kindling, described first by Engel & Ackermann (1980) permits the study of another aspect of epileptogenesis, namely the capacity of CNS to resist recurrent seizures. In this paradigm, eight electrical stimulations are delivered to the focus at 2 min intervals in previously kindled animals. The severity of the seizures during the 16 min period is rated by a seizure index, obtained by adding the values of the behavioral seizure stages and dividing by the number of stimulations. A high seizure index is indicative of decreased postictal suppression and a predisposition to the development of status epilepticus. McIntyre et al (1982) have described a model of status epilepticus based on kindling in which status epilepticus was produced in

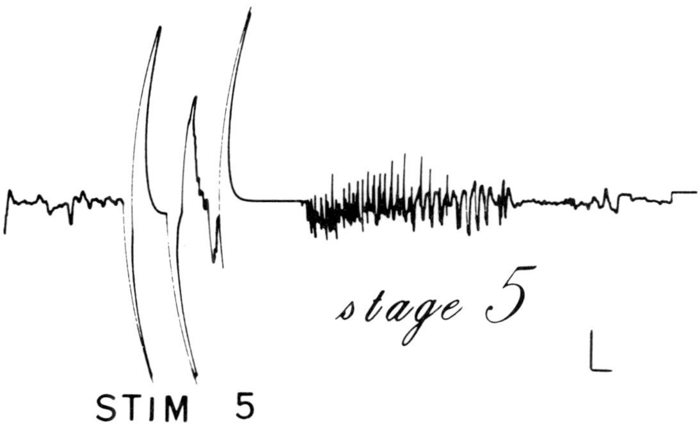


**Fig. 2.2** Kindling of corpus callosum. A short duration stage 5 seizure is elicited after 5 stimulations. Calibration 50 μV, 1 s.

previously kindled animals by delivering continuous stimulation for 1 h using the same stimulation parameters as for routine kindling. The observed status consisted mainly of stage 1 and 2 seizures and lasted for 10–24 h before spontaneously subsiding. Interestingly, this is the only type of kindling related seizure activity capable of producing structural brain damage confined to the limibic structures of the hemisphere ipsilateral to the stimulation site. However, the damage is more related to status than kindling, since Ackermann et al (1986) have shown that continuous stimulation can induce status and structural brain damage in rats that have not been previously kindled.

## KINDLING IN DEVELOPING ANIMALS

Development of kindling is age-related, and there are ontogenetic differences in every aspect of kindling. In rats, amygdala AD thresholds vary with age but can be consistently elicited by 15 days of life (Moshé 1981a, Moshé et al 1981, Gilbert & Cain 1982, Holmes & Weber 1986, Lee et al 1986). At this time, the AD threshold is high compared to older rats. In a small percentage of 15 day-old rat pups (15–25%), an AD cannot be elicited with conventional stimulation parameters, and such pups do not kindle. With maturation, AD thresholds decrease and reach a low point by 30–35 days. Thereafter, AD thresholds increase again to assume intermediate values that remain stable through adulthood (Moshé et al 1981).

Amygdala kindling can be produced in 15 day old pups using frequent stimulations, e.g. every 15 min (Moshé et 1983, Lee et al 1986). In adults, this type of stimulation either significantly retards or fails to induce kindling (Goddard et al 1969, Racine et al 1973, Peterson et al 1981, Moshé et al 1983). Furthermore, kindled seizures in rat pups exhibit different behavioral features compared to older animals, including 35-day old rats (Table 2.3). A particular aspect is the more rapid evolution in rat pups from focal to bilateral although asynchronous motor convulsions (Moshé et al 1986).

Finally, rat pups are more prone to develop recurrent kindled seizures and status epilepticus than adult rats (Moshé & Albala 1983). The ability to suppress recurrent kindled convulsions improves as the rats grow older since with maturation the same

**Table 2.3** Staging of amygdala-induced kindled seizures in rat pups (Modified from Moshé 1981b)

| Stage | Signs |
|---|---|
| 0 | Behavioral arrest |
| 1 | Facial movements |
| 2 | Rhythmic head movements or turning of body to stimulated site |
| 3 | Alternating independent forelimb clonus during the same trial, or unilateral clonus of either forelimb on consecutive stimulations; intermittent hind limb clonus |
| 4 | Bilateral clonus or rotatory movements of tonically extended forelimbs; occasional rearing |
| 5 | Loss of balance |

rats that previously exhibited frequent seizures as pups become more resistant. Once the adult level of postictal suppression has been achieved, it remains remarkably stable (Engel & Ackermann, 1979, Moshé & Albala, 1983).

In summary, these observations suggest that there is a period early in life during which the developing CNS is most susceptible to kindled seizures. Since focal AD thresholds are highest during the same period, it can be assumed that the increased seizure susceptibility is related to factors responsible for the propagation of seizures rather than to local increases in epileptogenicity. With maturation, mechanisms for limiting the spread and recurrence of convulsions become progressively more efficient.

Kindling in immature animals produces effects which persist in the mature CNS. Rats that have been kindled as pups are more susceptible to the development of kindled seizures as adults, (Moshé & Albala 1982). In adulthood, the rekindled seizures can be easily triggered either from the same site initially kindled in infancy (Moshé & Albala 1982) or from the homologous contralateral site (Moshé & Albala 1983).

## MECHANISMS

Despite many years of research, the pathophysiology of kindling is still not clear. In this section, we review some of the more commonly proposed hypotheses concerning the fundamental kindling mechanisms. For the sake of clarity, we divide kindling into four distinct although interrelated processes. Initially, we discuss the mechanisms involved in the development of the epileptic focus, followed by the substrates responsible for the propagation of seizures away from the stimulated site. Next, we describe factors that may be responsible for the arrest of seizures, and finally some of the changes that may underlie the permanence of the kindling phenomenon.

### The kindling focus

Detailed morphological studies of the stimulated site have failed to reveal any pathological changes beyond those associated with insertion of the stimulating electrode (Goddard et al 1969, Goddard & Douglas 1975). To date, there is no evidence demonstrating that the local kindling changes are either due to loss of normally present synapses or to formation of new synapses. McNamara et al (1986) have proposed that kindling may be associated with structural modification of pre-existing synapses similar to those induced when long term potentiation (LTP) is established. In LTP, repeated stimulus trains applied to a site such as the perforant path potentiate the responses evoked in a target site (dentate granule cells) by test pulses to the primary site, in this case the perforant path (Bliss & Lømo 1973). A similar mechanism may underlie the progressive growth in amplitude and frequency of ADs that occur with kindling. Yet, several studies have revealed that structures that are prone to kindling provide no LTP to target sites while the hippocampus kindles slowly despite showing the strongest LTP effects (McIntyre & Racine 1986). Furthermore, the development of kindling requires the elicitation of ADs and LTP can be induced without evoking ADs; LTP decays with time, while kindling is permanent. These observations suggest that LTP may not be responsible for the emergence of kindling (McIntyre & Racine 1986).

The neurotransmitter system(s) associated with local synaptic changes has not been defined. A role has been proposed for the cholinergic system based on the observation that repeated administration of initially subconvulsive doses of cholinergic agents leads to the development of kindled seizures (Vosu & Wise 1975, Wasterlain & Jonec 1983). Moreover, cross-sensitization between cholinergic and electrical kindling has been demonstrated (Girgis, 1980, 1981, Westerberg & Corcoran 1987). Burchfiel et al (1979) reported that an electrically induced hippocampal AD produces a state of prolonged supersensitivity to micro-iontophoretically applied acetylcholine in pyramidal cells. This supersensitivity was selective for acetylcholine since applications of glutamate or gamma-aminobutyric acid (GABA) failed to show any consistent changes in neuronal sensitivity. These results suggest that the cholinergic muscarinic (Wasterlain & Jonec 1983) system may affect local epileptogenesis, although it has been repeatedly demonstrated that systemic atropine (a muscarinic antagonist) does not alter AD thresholds despite inducing a profound delay in the development of electrical kindling (Arnold et al 1973, Albright et al 1979).

Likewise, there is contradictory evidence concerning the effects of noradrenaline on the development of a kindling focus. Spehlmann & Norcross (1984) suggested that both dopamine and noradrenaline may be involved in the early events of kindling since they found that depression of glutamate-induced firing of neurons in the amygdala induced by either catecholamine was significantly reduced after an AD was elicited. On the other hand, numerous lesion studies have revealed that norepinephrine but not dopamine depletion can enhance the emergence of generalized kindled seizures without affecting AD threshold (McIntyre et al 1979, McIntyre 1980, Corcoran & Mason 1980, Albala et al 1986).

There is some evidence to support the involvement of GABA in the creation of the local AD. Kamphuis et al (1986) found a significant decrease in the number of GABA immunoreactive-positive cell bodies in the stimulated CA1 region of the hippocampus of kindled rats compared to the contralateral site. Morimoto & Goddard (1986) suggested that a collapse of GABA-mediated recurrent inhibition may occur within the stimulated focus. This conclusion was derived from EEG analysis of the AD morphology and systemic pharmacological manipulations. However, Burchfiel et al (1979) did not demonstrate any neuronal effects following the micro-iontophoresis of either GABA or glutamate.

Cortical slices, prepared from rats kindled from the frontal cortex and stimulated in vitro by exposure to veratrine, had more endogenous glutamate and aspartate released than slices obtained from non-kindled controls (Leach et al 1985). A loss of the high affinity uptake site for aspartate has been identified in similarly prepared cortical slices (Leach et al 1987) suggesting perhaps that kindling may induce an in situ modification of existing synapses. Recently, Stelzer et al (1987) reported that kindling-like electrical stimuli administered to guinea pig hippocampal slices produced a progressive reduction of both spontaneous and stimulation-evoked GABAergic inhibitory postsynaptic potentials associated with decreased sensitivity of CA1 pyramidal neurons to iontophoretically applied GABA. In contrast, sensitivity of the pyramidal cells was increased to application of n-methyl-d-aspartate (NMDA). If the kindling-like stimuli were delivered in the presence of an NMDA receptor antagonist, the decrease in IPSPs and GABA sensitivity was prevented. These results suggest that modulation of GABAergic inhibition by activation of NMDA receptors may be directly involved in synaptic plasticity induced by kindling.

Intra-amygdala or intrahippocampal infusions of low doses of the opiates, beta-endorphin or methionin-enkephalin, produce ADs, and their repeated administration leads to the development of generalized seizures in a manner reminiscent of other forms of kindling (Cain & Corcoran 1984). The participation of opiates in the development of the kindling focus is questionable, since neither morphine nor naloxone have any effect on the AD threshold (Frenk et al 1979), and beta-endorphin levels are unchanged in the focus (Kato et al 1983).

In summary, the reported effects of several neurotransmitter systems on the development of the kindled focus have not yet enhanced our understanding of local epileptogenesis. The findings are inconsistent, or at best transient, perhaps reflecting the different methodologies used by various investigators. However, recent evidence linking up-regulation of NMDA receptors to the excitatory changes associated with kindling offers a new and potentially very fruitful avenue for further investigation.

Another hypothesis suggests that kindling may affect sensitive cells in the focus by altering their intrinsic membrane characteristics, thereby destabilizing these cells to produce synchronized epileptic bursts such as those described by Schwartzkroin & Wyler (1980) in other models. These cells may be located either in the stimulated site itself or may be associated with a nearby aggregate of neurons which may serve as the primary focus even if these neurons are not directly activated by the kindling stimulus.

In a recent review, McIntyre & Racine (1986) mention preliminary findings obtained in Racine's laboratory, indicating that several brain areas, including the piriform cortex, amygdala and entorhinal cortex, can become burst generators during kindling. However, there are no studies describing single cell responses of the neurons in the stimulated site early in kindling when ADs first appear.

More information is available concerning the properties of neurons in the vicinity of or in the stimulated focus after secondarily generalized kindled seizures have occurred. Several investigators studied the responses of hippocampal neurons following hippocampal kindling (Kairiss et al 1984, Oliver et al 1980, King et al 1985). There were few differences between kindled and control hippocampal slices in terms of most measures, including resting potential, membrane resistance and EPSP amplitude. Some cells, however, did respond with stronger bursts after the application of depolarizing currents, suggesting an increased probability of epileptiform activity.

Recent studies have implicated the amygdala-piriform cortex region as an area that may contain a 'pacemaker population' of neurons that perhaps are important in synchronizing epileptiform discharges (Kairiss et al 1984, McIntyre & Wong 1985). These cells do not appear to have distinctly different intrinsic characteristics from other neurons, but after amygdala kindling they exhibit spontaneous burst discharges and a prolongation of the burst responses to stimulation. McIntyre & Racine (1986) proposed that these cells are located in the piriform cortex rather than the amygdala but their exact location remains unknown. They speculated on the possible relationship of their findings to the site identified by Gale's group in the prepiriform cortex. The latter site is a small area, also known as endopiriform nucleus, that is susceptible to the development of generalized seizures following the administration of minute doses of chemoconvulsants (Piredda & Gale 1985, 1986a,b). However, this site is no more susceptible to kindling than the amygdala (Morimoto et al 1986, Zhao & Moshé 1987) and damage restricted to this area does not influence the development of amygdala kindling (Ludvig & Moshé 1988).

**Propagation and secondary generalization**

Kindling provides the opportunity to determine the structures that are sequentially involved in the spread of seizures. Two methodological approaches have been used, electroencephalography and 2-deoxyglucose autoradiography. The latter permits identification of structures that participate in the expression of seizures by revealing changes in their metabolic activity during seizures (Ackermann et al 1986).

Studies of amygdala-kindled seizures in rats using both approaches have yielded essentially similar results. Electrographic ADs readily propagate to other limbic sites ipsilateral to the stimulated amygdala, as well as to the contralateral homotopic regions. With repeated stimulations, the ADs increase in amplitude and frequency and the seizures become progressively more severe. Eventually, ADs spread to the basal ganglia including the neostriatum and the substantia nigra and to the neocortex (Wada et al 1975, Bonhaus et al 1986). This spread correlates with the emergence of generalized seizures (Wada et al 1975). This sequence of events was confirmed by Engel et al (1978) who studied autoradiographically the progressive patterns of metabolic activation during different phases of amygdala kindling in the rat. EEG studies in cats, monkeys and baboons indicate that the patterns of kindled seizure propagation appear to be the same in all species (Wada et al 1975, Wada & Sato 1974, Wada et al 1978).

Kindling of other sites appears to involve first the establishment of connections with the limbic system and especially the amygdala. Thus, the late phase of neocortical kindling includes behavioral manifestations that replicate those observed early in amygdala kindling. Kindling of the olfactory bulb, stria terminalis and hypothalamus also appears to operate via the amygdala (Cain 1977, Le Gal La Salle 1979, Cullen & Goddard 1975). Furthermore, lesions of the amygdala inhibit the development of kindling from either the olfactory bulb or stria terminalis (Cain 1977, Le Gal La Salle 1979). Kindling of the prepiriform cortex reveals a rapid spread of the ADs to the ipsi- and contralateral amygdala but not vice versa (Zhao & Moshé 1987). The temporal sequence of hippocampal kindling suggests that the behavioral manifestaions are similar to those observed with amygdala kindling (Aihara et al 1982). However lesions of the amygdala facilitate the rate of hippocampal kindling suggesting that in this case the amygdala may play an inhibitory role (McIntyre, et al 1982, Araki et al 1985). These results seem to implicate the structures involved in amygdala kindling in a network that may be responsible for the final expression of kindled seizures.

Lesion studies have revealed that the major transsynaptic changes associated with limbic kindling occur within the ipsilateral hemisphere and propagate downstream to brainstem structures (McIntyre 1975, Nobrega & Gaito 1978, McCaughran et al 1977, 1978). The forebrain commissures do not appear to be critical for the development of generalized convulsions, but they may play a significant role in 'transferring' the epileptiform activity to homotopic sites of the contralateral hemisphere (McCaughran et al 1978). The term 'transfer' is used to describe the observation that the establishment of kindling at a primary site results in fewer stimulations required to establish kindling in a secondary site (Goddard et al 1969). Transfer effects have been encountered among various ipsilateral sites including amygdala and neocortex (Seidel & Corcoran 1986) or hippocampus (Aihara et al 1982) and prepiriform cortex and amygdala (Zhao & Moshé 1987) as well as contralaterally (Goddard et al 1969, McIntyre & Goddard 1973, Zhao & Moshé 1987). Destruction of the primary focus does not reduce the epileptogenicity of the secondary site (Goddard et al 1969) which is now capable, upon stimulation, to support kindled seizures on its own, utilizing the kindling network already established (McIntyre & Goddard 1973). According to some investigators (Morrell & de Toledo-Morrell 1986), this observation may be the substrate for the development and persistence of mirror foci, defined as secondary sites of epileptogenesis that have been induced by, but become completely independent of, the original focus (Morrell 1969).

Several neurotransmitter systems have been implicated in mediating the propagation of kindled seizures. The similarities between cholinergic and electrical kindling (Vosu & Wise 1975, Wasterlain & Jonec 1983) suggest an involvement of the cholinergic system in the kindling process. The activity of choline acetyl transferase, the synthetic enzyme for acetylcholine, was decreased in several brain sites that may participate in the expression of kindled seizures (Noda et al 1982, Dasheiff & McNamara 1980). This decrease may only reflect a compensatory mechanism affecting the rate of synthesis of acetylcholine. On the other hand, neither acetyl cholinesterase activity nor choline uptake is altered following kindled seizures (Dasheiff et al 1981). Furthermore, the reported decreases in muscarinic receptor binding (Noda et al 1982, Byrne et al 1980) are transient and not specific for kindling (McNamara et al 1986). It is therefore quite possible that these cholinergic changes may reflect a consequence of repeated seizures and are probably not etiologically related to kindling.

The evidence for a catecholaminergic involvement is based on lesion studies that deplete forebrain norepinephrine. This depletion markedly facilitates the emergence of kindled seizures (McIntyre et al 1979, McIntyre 1980, Corcoran & Mason 1980, Ehlers et al 1980, Albala et al 1986, McIntyre et al 1987) but the effect is not limited to kindling since other types of experimentally induced seizures such as pentylenetetrazol and electroconvulsive shock seizures can also be potentiated (Mason & Corcoran 1979). Transient decreases of norepinephrine concentrations and in the number of postsynaptic beta-adrenergic receptors have been reported following kindling (Callaghan & Schwark 1979, McIntyre & Roberts 1983, McNamara 1978a). However, it is not clear whether these changes are the result of kindling or seizures per se.

The role of the GABA-ergic system has not been elucidated although a failure of GABA mediated inhibition could conceivably account for the development of kindling. Available information does not support this hypothesis since there are several reports (Tuff et al 1983, Oliver & Miller 1985) that kindling may actually increase

**Table 2.4** Benzodiazepine receptor changes with kindling

| Stimulated site | Type of change | Location of changes | Time-course of changes | Reference |
|---|---|---|---|---|
| Amygdala | Decreased binding | Hypothalamus<br>Cortex | 60 days after kindling | Burnham et al (1983) |
| Amygdala, entorhinal cortex | No change | Dentate gyrus | 28 days after kindling | Shin et al (1985) |
| Amygdala | Decreased binding (unwashed homogenates)<br>Increased binding (washed homogenates) | Hypothalamus<br>Cortex<br>Amygdala<br>Hippocampus | 14 days after kindling | Niznik et al (1984) |
| Amygdala, entorhinal cortex | Increased binding | Amygdala<br>Hippocampus | 14 days after kindling | Tuff et al (1983) |
| Olfactory bulb | No change<br>Increased binding | Hippocampus<br>Amygdala<br>Olfactory bulb | 7 days after kindling | Ben-Attia et al (1984) |
| Amygdala | Increased binding<br>No change | Hippocampus<br>Amygdala | 24 hours after kindling | McNamara et al (1980) |
| Amygdala | Increased binding<br>No change | Hippocampus<br>Amygdala | 24 hours after kindling | Tietz et al (1985) |
| Entorhinal cortex | Increased binding | Dentate gyrus | 24 hours after kindling | Fanelli & McNamara (1986) |

GABA inhibition in the hippocampus. In addition, the reported changes of benzodiazepine receptors, an integral component of the GABA-chloride ionophore complex, are transient, inconsistent and often contradictory (Table 2.4). These differences may be in part due to the various methodologies used to determine the benzodiazepine receptor changes (Niznik et al 1984).

The observation that amygdaloid kindling can produce a gradual elevation of the pain threshold (Frenk & Yitzhaky 1981) suggests that opioid peptidergic pathways are activated in areas remote from the focus. The establishment of kindling causes a marked elevation in leucine- and methionine-enkephalin (Vindrola et al 1981a,b), a-neoendorphin and dynorphin (Prezewlocki et al 1983) and methionine-enkephalin $Arg^6$-$Gly^7$-$Leu^8$ content (Iadarola et al 1986) in several brain regions outside the kindled focus indicating a possible role for opiates in the propagation of kindled seizures. However, these changes have not been reflected in receptor binding data (Ashton et al 1980). Furthermore, neither morphine nor naloxone have any effects on the rate at which kindling develops (Post et al 1979), and McNamara et al (1986) have concluded that endogenous opiates have little to do directly with kindling.

The concentration of somatostatin, a neuropeptide containing 14 aminoacids, is elevated in the focus and the contralateral homologous structure either during amygdala (Kato et al 1983) or cortical (Higuchi et al 1986) kindling. Cysteamine, an agent that depletes brain immunoreactive somatostatin, delays the development of kindled seizures (Higuchi et al 1986). The role of somatostatin, however, cannot be considered unique to the kindling process since similar changes have been observed in other models of epilepsy (Kato et al 1982).

**Arrest of seizures**

Kindled seizures, like most seizures, are short-lived rarely lasting more than 2 min. The very important question of how seizures spontaneously stop has not received the attention it deserves.

Recent evidence has implicated the substantia nigra as an important site involved in the expression of generalized seizures including kindled convulsions (Gale 1985, McNamara et al 1986, Moshé et al 1986). It has been repeatedly demonstrated by both electrical (Wada et al 1974, Bonhaus et al 1986) and autoradiographic (Engel et al 1978, Ackermann et al 1986, Albala et al 1984, Ben-Ari et al 1981, Lothman & Collins 1981, Watson et al 1983) techniques that epileptiform activity in adult animals propagates into the substantia nigra. Furthermore, there is information that in adult rats, GABA-sensitive substantia nigra pars reticulata (SNR) neurons may be responsible in part for terminating seizures. Infusions of GABA agonists into the SNR reduce the duration or severity of many types of seizures (Iadarola & Gale 1982, Gonzalez & Hettinger 1984, Moshé & Albala 1984, Okada et al 1986) including kindled convulsions (Le Gal La Salle et al 1983, McNamara et al 1984). Substantia nigra lesions (Garant & Gale 1983, McNamara et al 1984) or electrical stimulation (Morimoto & Goddard 1987) can also suppress seizures. The effect of electrical stimulation can be reversed by picrotoxin, a GABA antagonist (Morimoto & Goddard 1987).

These observations suggest that treatments which decrease the GABAergic output of the substantia nigra attenuate or terminate seizures, probably by disinhibiting post-synaptic neurons in nigral projection sites. These include the thalamus, corpus striatum, superior colliculus and pontine reticular formation (Dray 1980). There is evidence that kindled seizures can deplete nigral levels of the GABA synthesizing enzyme glutamic decarboxylase (Löscher & Schwark 1985). This may indicate that accelerated production of GABA in the substantia nigra during seizures represents an endogenous compensatory mechanism of the brain to stop ictal activity. Bonhaus et al (1986) showed that during an AD the firing pattern of SNR cells changed drastically. The cells fired in bursts of action potentials often time-locked with the AD. However, careful inspection of the data shown in their Figure 2 reveals that the overall firing rate diminished during the electrographic seizure suggesting increased GABA release (Waszczak et al 1980). The end result is decreased GABA-sensitive nigral output similar to that observed with local microinfusions of the GABA agonists, muscimol or gamma-vinyl GABA.

The presumed inhibitory role of the substantia nigra in seizures in adult animals is further supported by developmental data. Autoradiographic studies have demonstrated a lack of substantia nigra activation during kindling of 16 day old rat pups (Ackermann et al 1986). Similar findings have been reported with kainic acid seizures (Albala et al 1984). Furthermore, nigral microinfusions of muscimol in rat pups facilitate the development of seizures instead of suppressing them (Okada et al 1986). Since rat pups are more prone to status epilepticus than adult rats (Moshé & Albala 1983, Albala et al 1984), these results imply that the immature substantia nigra may not be capable of exerting its anticonvulsant effect like its mature counterpart. Nevertheless, it should be emphasized that the nigral effects are not specific for kindling but operate in other models of epilepsy as well (Gale 1985, Moshé et al 1986).

The commonly considered neurotransmitter systems do not appear to participate in mechanisms involved in the suppression of kindled seizures. For example, depletion of norepinephrine does not affect already established kindled convulsions (Westerberg et al 1984, McIntyre et al 1987). However, opiates may play a role in the maintenance of the postictal state considered by some to be an active process that prevents seizure recurrences (Caspers & Speckmann 1972, Engel et al 1981). In the kindling model, naloxone significantly shortens postictal depression, while morphine has the opposite effect (Frenk et al 1979). Furthermore, the strong postictal depression that follows massed kindling stimuli of the enkephalin-rich globus pallidus can be reversed by naloxone (Kelsey & Belluzzi 1982).

**Maintenance of permanence**

The search for mechanisms underlying the long-term changes in brain function that occur with kindling has not been successful. Following the emergence of generalized kindled seizures, relatively long-lasting changes have been reported in several putative neurotransmitter systems. These include, among others, decreased activity of tyrosine-hydroxylase (the synthetic enzyme for catecholamines) in the focus (Farjo & Blackwood 1978), decreased somatostatin receptors in the hippocampus (Higuchi et al 1986) and calcium-mediated changes in synaptic transmission. Alterations in calcium-dependent enzymes have been identified (Wasterlain et al 1986, Miller et al. 1986). Levels of a specific calcium-binding protein are reduced early in the kindling process, even before the onset of electrographic seizures. This change is relatively long-lasting (Miller et al 1986). Once again, though, it is uncertain whether any of the above changes is a simply a consequence of seizures or related more specifically to the kindling engram.

Amygdala kindling can selectively decrease the density of phencyclidine (PCP)/sigma receptors in hippocampus (Sircar et al 1987). This effect appears to be due directly to the kindling process itself rather than to a consequence of generalized seizures, since flurothyl-induced seizures did not produce significant changes in PCP/sigma receptor density compared to controls. In conjunction with modification of hippocampal NMDA receptors (Stelzer et al 1987), this decrease in the PCP/sigma receptor population may explain the long-lasting transsynaptic alterations that occur with kindling. Indeed, NMDA receptors on dentate gyrus granule cells participate in synaptic transmission once kindling has been established (Mody & Heinemann 1987).

## CLINICAL IMPLICATIONS

Since the original description of the kindling phenomenon, there are several questions that have been raised and only partially answered (Table 2.5).

**Table 2.5** The million dollar questions

1. Does kindling occur in humans?
2. Is kindling the means via which an epileptic lesion is formed in humans?
3. Does secondary epileptogenesis happen in humans?
4. Do kindling and human epilepsies (especially partially complex seizures) share some common features?
5. What is kindling good for?

There are two reports of kindling in humans following repeated direct electrical stimulations of the brain using intracerebral electrodes (Monroe 1970, Sramka et al 1977). Certainly, these two rare occurrences are not sufficient to permit a positive answer to the question whether human kindling occurs. Another form of kindling in humans could consist of a progressive worsening of seizure severity. There is no doubt that some partial seizures are difficult to control. However, while such seizures may occur frequently, they are not necessarily more severe. Many remain auras (Engel & Cahan 1986). In fact, with age the incidence of secondarily generalized seizures diminishes (Gastaut et al 1975) and those that do occur are not longer lasting than before. Tonic seizures are not observed (Engel & Cahan 1986), whereas tonus is a frequent feature of repeated generalized convulsions of 'overkindled' animals (Pinel & Rovner 1978). Finally, there are well described electroclinical syndromes characterized by a period in time during which many epileptic seizures occur before subsiding completely. If kindling were operative, it might be expected that the seizures would continue.

It has been proposed that kindling-like processes may take place in the development of epilepsy. Kindling could explain the latent period that exists between the occurrence of a causative insult such as head trauma and the actual onset of epilepsy (Goddard 1983). During the latent period, new neuronal connections may be formed leading to increased local excitability, repetitive firing with progressive increments in the severity of electrographic discharges, and eventually to the emergence of clinical seizures (McNamara et al 1986). Similarly, a kindling-like mechanism may be postulated to explain the occurrence of intractable partial seizures in children who have experienced many febrile seizures in infancy. However, others have questioned whether the number of febrile convulsions is causally related to the subsequent development of epilepsy (Nelson & Ellenberg 1978). Furthermore, in neither clinical situations does the typical progression from focal to generalized seizures observed in kindled laboratory animals occur. Generalized seizures often precede the onset of partial seizures, and this is not the case with classical kindling.

It can be argued that the transition from generalized to focal seizures may still be a form of kindling in the sense that the partial seizures are more frequent. Furthermore, it is quite possible that the expression of generalized convulsions may be suppressed by powerful inhibitory processes that become more apparent with maturation (Moshé & Albala, 1983). The development of such inhibitory mechanisms may underlie the differences in kindling observed along the phylogenetic scale (Table 2.2). Thus rhesus monkeys seldom have generalized kindled seizures despite numerous stimulations (Wada et al 1978).

Another clinical condition that may use a kindling like mechanism (transfer) for its development is the phenomenon of secondary epileptogenesis. In this case, the continuous electrical bombardment initiated at a primary site seems to alter the excitability of a target site. As a sequel, the secondary site may now independently generate epileptiform activity and perhaps, eventually clinical seizures. Morrell (1985) reported four patients with putative secondary foci developing opposite a primary focus due to a well-localized tumor. He speculated that in these very few cases the propensity for the development of such secondary foci is directly related to the duration of the epileptic illness and inversely related to the patient's age (Morrell & de Toledo-Morrell 1986). However, this correlation with age is not evident in developmental kindling studies in animals (Moshé & Albala 1982, 1983). Furthermore, others have argued that it is unclear whether these secondary foci in humans are truly capable of initiating a seizure after the primary focus has been removed (Torres & Jacome 1982, Goldensohn 1984). In this respect, human secondary epileptogenesis, if it occurs, may differ from that observed in lower mammals.

What, then is the relationship of kindling to human partial seizures? Table 2.6

**Table 2.6** Evidence that kindling may not be relevant to clinical epilepsy

1. Mammals high in the phylogenetic scale can not be easily kindled.
2. Kindling implies permanence. Human seizures can spontaneously resolve.
3. The severity of partial seizures does not increase with the duration of the illness.
4. Kindling can be most easily elicited from the amygdala. Partial seizures emanate from the hippocampus.
5. Lack of neuropathological changes in kindled focus.
6. Kindled seizures undergo a regular sequence of events culminating in secondary generalization. Symptoms of partial seizures do not follow a stereotypic sequence and generalization does not frequently occur.
7. Seizure propagation patterns are consistent only in kindling.
8. Phenytoin does not alter the development of kindling while it is quite effective against partial seizures.

contains features that provide some evidence that kindling may not be relevant to the human condition. Kindling becomes progressively more difficult to elicit the higher the animal is along the phylogenetic scale (Wada et al 1978). This implies that it may not occur in humans. Seizures in humans occur abruptly often without the characteristic march observed with kindling. Focal epileptic phenomena in humans are more variable and typically lack the stereotypic events of kindling (Engel & Cahan 1986). Consequently, the patterns of metabolic activation reported with PET scan studies of human focal seizures are not consistent (Engel & Cahan 1986) in contrast to the predictable changes seen with kindled seizures in animals (Engel et al 1978). Finally, partial complex seizures most frequently arise from the hippocampus (Babb et al 1984), and neuropathological changes are common (Brown 1973). The hippocampus is more difficult to kindle than other limibic sites (McIntyre & Racine 1986), and there is no evidence of any neuropathological changes at kindled sites (Goddard et al 1969).

Table 2.7 summarizes several features that may support the validity of kindling

**Table 2.7** Evidence implicating kindling in partial seizures

1. Two case reports of kindling occurring in humans.
2. Similarities in the behavior expression of seizures.
3. Age-related differences in seizure susceptibility.
4. Existence of a latency period before the full expression of a generalized convulsion.
5. Enhancement of evoked potentials and excitability of distant sites.
6. Secondary epileptogenesis.
7. Existence of spontaneous interictal spikes.
8. Similarities in the response to antiepileptic drugs.

as a model of human partial epilepsies. Some of the behavioral characteristics of kindling bear significant similarities to certain clinical manifestations of human complex partial seizures. These include the transient behavioral arrest, chewing movements and the motor aspect of the secondarily generalized kindled seizure which lacks a tonic component (Engel & Cahan 1986). In addition, kindling in developing animals

**Table 2.8** Effects of antiepileptic drugs on the development of kindling and on generalized kindled seizures

| Drug | Kindling | Kindled seizure | Species | Reference |
|---|---|---|---|---|
| *A. Amygdala induced* | | | | |
| Phenobarbital | | Suppression | Rat | Callaghan & Schwark (1980) |
| | | Suppression | Rat | Albertson et al (1980) |
| | | Suppression | Rat | Albright & Burnham (1980) |
| | Retardation | Suppression | Rat | Wise & Chinerman (1974) |
| | Retardation | | Cat | Turner et al (1977) |
| | Retardation | | Cat | Wada et al (1976a) |
| | | Suppression | Dog | Wauquier et al (1979) |
| | | Suppression | Baboon | Wada et al (1976) |
| Phenytoin | | Suppression | Rat | Albright & Burnham (1980) |
| | Facilitation | Slight suppression | Rat | Racine et al (1975) |
| | | Suppression[a] | Rat | Babington & Wedeking (1973) |
| | | Exacerbation | Rat | Callaghan & Schwark (1980) |
| | | No effect | Rat | Albertson et al (1980) |
| | | No effect | Rat | Ehle (1980) |
| | No effect | No effect | Rat | Wise & Chinerman (1974) |
| | No effect | | Cat | Turner et al (1977) |
| | No effect | | Cat | Wada et al (1976b) |
| | No effect | | Dog | Wauquier et al (1979) |
| | | Suppression | Cat, Baboon | Wada et al (1976a) |
| Carbamazepine | No effect | Suppression | Rat | Post et al (1984) |
| | No effect | Suppression | Rat | Albertson et al (1984) |
| | | Suppression | Rat | Albright & Burnham (1980) |
| | Retardation | | Cat | Wada et al (1976b) |
| | | Suppression | Baboon | Wada et al (1976a) |
| Valproic acid | | Suppression | Rat | Albertson et al (1981) |
| | | Suppression | Rat | Albright & Burnham (1980) |
| | | Suppression | Rat | Tulloch et al (1982) |
| | Retardation | Suppression | Cat | Leviel & Naquet (1977) |
| Diazepam | | Suppression | Rat | Albertson et al (1980) |
| | | Suppression | Rat | Callaghan & Schwark (1980) |
| | | Suppression | Rat | Albright & Burnham (1980) |
| | Retardation | Suppression | Rat | Racine et al (1975) |
| | Retardation | Suppression | Rat | Wise & Chinerman (1974) |
| | | Suppression | Dog | Wauquier et al (1979) |
| Ethosuximide | | No effect | Rat | Albertson et al (1980) |
| | | No effect | Rat | Albright & Burnham (1980) |
| | No effect | | Cat | Turner et al (1977) |
| Trimethadione | | No effect | Rat | Albertson et al (1980) |
| | | Suppression | Rat | Callaghan & Schwark (1980) |
| Phenacemide | | No effect | Rat | Albertson et al (1980) |
| | | Suppression[a] | Rat | Babington & Wedeking (1973) |
| Acetazolamide | | No effect | Rat | Albertson et al (1980) |
| | No effect | | Cat | Turner et al (1977) |
| Dexamethasone | No effect | | Cat | Turner et al (1977) |
| Cinromide | | Suppression | Rat | Chiu et al (1982) |
| Progabide | | Suppression[a] | Rat | Joy et al (1984) |
| *B. Cortically induced* | | | | |
| Phenobarbital | | Suppression | Rat | Albright & Burnham (1980) |
| | Retardation | | Cat | Turner et al (1977) |
| Phenytoin | Retardation | Suppression | Rat | Racine et al (1975) |
| | | Suppression[a] | Rat | Babington & Wedeking (1973) |
| | Retardation | | Cat | Turner et al (1977) |
| Carbamazepine | | Suppression | Rat | Albright & Burnham (1980) |
| Valproic acid | | Suppression | Rat | Albright & Burnham (1980) |
| Diazepam | | Suppression | Rat | Albright & Burnham (1980) |
| | No effect | No effect | Rat | Racine et al (1975) |
| | | Suppression | Rat | Racine et al (1979) |
| Ethosuximide | | No effect | Rat | Albright & Burnham (1980) |
| Phenacemide | | Suppression[a] | Rat | Babington & Wedeking (1973) |

[a] Only in toxic doses.

reveals clear, age-related differences in seizure susceptibility and in the behavioral expression of convulsions that parallel the age-related changes reported in epidemiological studies of children (Moshé, in press). Furthermore, in both the model and the clinical condition there is evidence that transsynaptic changes take place including enhancement of evoked potentials (Buser & Bancaud 1983, Racine et al 1975) and of excitability at distant sites (Goddard et al 1969, Engel et al 1983). Spontaneous interictal spikes are also present in both (McNamara et al 1986), and most antiepileptic drugs that are effective against partial seizures suppress kindling (Table 2.8). The most notable exception is phenytoin which is ineffective against amygdala kindled seizures. The efficacy of valproate in kindling is somewhat surprising, since this drug is not considered to be particularly effective in patients with partial seizures (Aird et al 1984).

To date, the available clinical data do not support the notion that kindling mechanisms are responsible for the establishment of epileptogenic foci in humans (Engel & Cahan 1986). Nor is it appropriate to propose kindling-like mechanisms as justification for early surgical intervention in patients with intractable seizures. However, some progressive changes that occur in human epileptics are reminiscent of kindling phenomena. Continued study of kindling may eventually shed some light into these mechanisms and lead to the development of new treatments that are etiologically related to the pathophysiology of the human condition.

## ACKNOWLEDGEMENTS

Supported by NIH grant NS-20253 from the NINCDS and R-36986 from the United Cerebral Palsy Associations. The authors thank Drs R. F. Ackermann, M. C. Cornblath and E. S. Goldensohn for their thoughtful comments and suggestions and Ms Donna Platyan for her secretarial assistance.

## REFERENCES

Ackermann R F, Chugani H T, Handforth A et al 1986 Autoradiographic studies of cerebral metabolism and blood flow in rat amygdala kindling. In: Wada J A (ed) Kindling 3. Raven Press, New York, p 73–87

Aihara H, Araki H, Ohzeki M 1982 Hippocampal kindling and effects of antiepileptic drugs. Japanese Journal of Pharmacology 32: 37–45

Aird R B, Masland R L, Woodbury D M 1984 The epilepsies. A critical review. Raven Press, New York

Albala B J, Moshé S L, Okada R 1984 Kainic-acid-induced seizures: A developmental study. Developmental Brain Research 13: 139–148

Albala B J, Moshé S L, Cubells J F et al 1986 Unilateral peri-substantia nigra catecholaminergic lesion and amygdala kindling. Brain Research 370: 388–392

Albright P S, Burnham W M. 1980 Development of a new pharmacological seizure model: Effects of anticonvulsants on cortical- and amygdala-kindled seizures in the rat. Epilepsia 21: 681–689

Albright P, Burham W M, Okazaki M 1979 Effect of atropine sulfate on amygdaloid kindling. Experimental Neurology 66: 409–412

Albertson T E, Peterson S L, Stark L G 1980 Anticonvulsant drugs and their antagonism of kindled amygdaloid seizures in rats. Neuropharmacology 19: 643–652

Albertson T E, Peterson S L, Stark L G et al 1981 Valproic acid serum levels and protection against amygdala kindled seizures in the rat. Neuropharmacology 20: 95–97

Albertson T E, Joy R M, Stark L G 1984 Carbamazepine: A pharmacological study in the kindling model of epilepsy. Neuropharmacology 23: 1117–1123

Araki H, Aihara H, Watanabe S, Yamamoto T, Ueki S 1985 Role of the amygdala in the hippocampal kindling effect of rats. Japanese Journal of Pharmacology 37: 173–179

Arnold P S, Racine R J, Wise R A 1973 Effects of atropine, reserpine, 6-hydroxydopamine and handling on seizure development in the rat. Experimental Neurology 40: 457–470

Ashton D, Leysen J. E, Wauquier A 1980 Neurotransmitters and receptor binding in amygdaloid kindled rats: serotonergic and noradrenergic modulatory effects. Life Sciences 27: 1547–1556

Babb T, Brown W J, Pretorius J et al 1984 Temporal lobe volumetric cell densities in temporal lobe epilepsy. Epilepsia 25: 729–740

Babbington R G, Wedeking P W 1973 The pharmacology of seizures induced by sensitization with low intensity brain stimulation. Pharmacology Biochemistry and Behavior 1: 461–467

Ben-Ari Y, Tremblay E, Riche D et al 1981 Electrographic, clinical and pathological alterations following systemic administration of kainic acid, bicuculline or pentylenetrazol: Metabolic mapping using the deoxyglucose method with special reference to the pathology of epilepsy. Neuroscience 6: 1361–1391.

Ben-Attia M, Lerner-Natoli M, Rondouin G et al 1984 Changes in benzodiazepine receptors in the limbic system following kindling of the olfactory bulb in rats. Transactions of the Biological Society [Cr Soc Biol (Paris)] 178: 697–704

Bliss T V P, Lømo T 1973 Long-lasting potentiation of synaptic transmission in the dentate area of the anaesthetized rabbit following stimulation of the perforant path. Journal of Physiology 232: 331–356

Bonhaus D W, Walters J. R, McNamara J O 1986 Activation of substantia nigra neurons: role in the propagation of seizures in kindled rats. Journal of Neuroscience 6: 3024–3030

Brown W J 1973 Structural substrates of seizure foci in the human temporal lobe. In: Brazier A B (ed) Epilepsy: its clinical phenomena in man. Academic Press, New York, p 339–374

Burchfiel J L, Duchowny M S, Duffy F H 1979 Neuronal supersensitivity to acetylcholine induced by kindling in the rat hippocampus. Science 204: 1096–1098

Burnham W M 1978 Cortical and limbic kindling: similarities and differences. In: Livingston K E, Hornykiewicz O (eds) Limbic mechanisms. The continuing evolution of the limbic system concept. Plenum Press, New York, p 507–519

Burnham W M, Niznik H B, Okazaki M M et al 1983 Binding of [3H] flunitrazepam and [3H] Ro5-4864 to crude homogenates of amygdala-kindled rat brain: two months post seizure. Brain Research 279: 359–362

Buser P, Bancaud J 1983 Unilateral connections between amygdala and hippocampus in man. A study of epileptic patients with depth electrodes. Electroencephalography and Clinical Neurophysiology 55: 1–12

Byrne M C, Gottlieb R, McNamara J O 1980 Amygdala kindling induced muscarinic cholinergic receptor declines in a highly specific distribution within the limbic system. Experimental Neurology 69: 85–98

Cain D P 1977 Seizure development following repeated electrical stimulation of central olfactory structures. Annals of New York Academy of Science 290: 200–216

Cain D P 1983 Bidirectional transfer of electrical and carbachol kindling. Brain Research 260: 135–138

Cain D P, Corcoran M E 1978 Kindling in olfactory-lesioned rats. Behavioral Biology 22: 264–268

Cain D P, Corcoran M E 1980 Kindling in the seizure-prone and seizure-resistant mongolian gerbil. Electroencephalography and Clinical Neurophysiology 49: 360–365

Cain D P, Corcoran M E 1981 Kindling with low frequency stimulation: generality, transfer, and recruiting effects. Experimental Neurology 73: 219–232

Cain D P, Corcoran M E 1984 Intracerebral beta-endorphin, met-enkephalin and morphine: kindling of seizures and handling-induced potentiation of epileptiform effects. Life Sciences 34: 2535–2542

Callaghan D A, Schwark W S 1979 Involvement of catecholamines in kindled amygdaloid convulsions. Neuropharmacology 18: 541–545

Callaghan D A, Schwark W S 1980 Pharmacological modification of amygdaloid-kindled seizures. Neuropharmacology 19: 1131–1136

Caspers H, Speckmann E J 1972 Cerebral $PO_2$, $PCO_2$ and pH: changes during convulsive activity and their significance for spontaneous arrest of seizures. Epilepsia 13: 699–725

Collins R C 1978 Kindling of neuroanatomic pathways during recurrent focal penicillin seizures. Brain Research 150: 503–517

Corcoran M E, Cain D P 1980 Kindling of seizures with low-frequency electrical stimulation. Brain Research 196: 262–265

Corcoran M E, Mason S T 1980 Role of forebrain catecholamines in amygdaloid kindling. Brain Research 190: 473–484

Chiu P, Lipnowski S, Bruni J et al 1982 The effect of cinromide on 'kindled' seizures in the rat. Neuropharmacology 21: 273–276

Cullen N, Goddard G V 1975 Kindling in the hypothalamus and transfer to the ipsilateral amygdala. Behavioral Biology 15: 119–131

Dasheiff R M, McNamara J O 1980 Evidence for an agonist independent down regulation of hippocampal muscarinic receptor in kindling. Brain Research 195: 345–53

Dasheiff R M, Byrne M C, Patrone V et al 1981 Biochemical evidence of decreased muscarinic cholinergic neuronal communication following amygdala kindled seizures. Brain Research 106: 233–238
Diehl R G, Smialowski A, Gotwo T 1984 Development and persistence of kindled seizures after repeated injections of pentylenetetrazol in rats and guinea pigs. Epilepsia 25: 506–510
Dray A 1980 The physiology and pharmacology of mammalian basal ganglia. Progress in Neurobiology 14: 221–335
Ehle A L 1980 Effects of phenytoin on amygdaloid kindled seizures in the rat. Electroencephalography and Clinical Neurophysiology 48: 102–105
Ehlers C L, Clifton D K, Sawyer C B 1980 Facilitation of amygdala kindling in the rat by transecting ascending noradrenergic pathways. Brain Research 189: 274–278
Engel J Jr, Ackermann R F 1980 Interictal EEG spikes correlate with decreased, rather than increased, epileptogenicity in amygdaloid kindled rats. Brain Research 190: 543–548
Engel J Jr, Cahan L 1986 Potential relevance of kindling to human partial epilepsy. In: Wada J A (ed) Kindling 3. Raven Press, New York, p. 37–51
Engel J Jr, Wolfson L, Brown L 1978 Anatomical correlates of electrical and behavioral events related to amygdaloid kindling. Annals of of Neurology 3: 538–544
Engel J Jr, Ackermann R F, Caldecott-Hazard S et al 1981 Epileptic activation of antagonistic systems may explain paradoxical features of experimental and human epilepsy: a review and hypothesis. In: Wada J A (ed) Kindling 2. Raven Press, New York, p. 193–217
Engel J Jr, Kuhl D E, Phelps M E et al 1983 Local cerebral metabolism during partial seizures. Neurology 33: 400–413
Fabisiak J P, Schwark W S 1982 Aspects of the pentylenetetrazol kindling model of epileptogenesis in the rat. Experimental Neurology 78: 7–14
Fanelli R J, McNamara J O 1986 Effects of age on kindling and kindled seizure — induced increase of benzodiazepine receptor binding. Brain Research 362: 17–32
Farjo I B, Blackwood D H 1978 Reduction in tyrosine hydroxylase activity in the rat amygdala induced by kindling stimulation. Brain Research 153: 423–426
Frenk H, Yitzhaky J 1981 Effects of amygdaloid kindling on the pain threshold of the rat. Experimental Neurology 71: 487–496
Frenk H, Engel J Jr, Ackermann R F et al 1979 Endogeneous opioids may mediate postictal behavioral depression in amygdaloid-kindled rats. Brain Research 167: 435–440
Gale K 1985 Mechanisms of seizure control mediated by gamma-aminobutyric acid: role of the substantia nigra. Federation Proceedings Federation American Societies Experimental Biology 44: 2414–2424
Garant D, Gale K 1983 Lesions of substantia nigra protect against experimentally induced seizures. Brain Research 273: 156–161
Garant D, Gale K 1986 Nigrotectal protection is essential to the anticonvulsant action of GABA transmission in substantia nigra. Neuroscience Abstracts p 80
Gastaut H, Gastaut J L, Concalves e Silva G E, Fernandez Sanchez G R 1975 Relative frequency of different types of epilepsy. A study employing the classification of the International League against Epilepsy. Epilepsia 16: 457–461
Gilbert M E Cain D P 1982 A developmental study of kindling in the rat. Developmental Brain Research 2: 321–328
Girgis M 1980 Participation of muscarinic cholinergic receptors may be an important requirement of the kindling process. Experimental Neurology 70: 458–461
Girgis M 1981 Electrical versus cholinergic kindling. Electroencephalography and Clinical Neurophysiology 51: 417–425
Goddard G V 1967 Development of epileptic seizures through brain stimulation at low intensity. Nature 204: 1020–1021
Goddard G V 1983 The kindling model of epilepsy. Trends in Neuroscience 7: 275–279
Goddard G V, Douglas R M 1975 Does the engram of kindling model the engram of long-term memory? Canadian Journal of Neurological Sciences 2: 385–394
Goddard G V, McIntyre D C, Leech C K 1969 A permanent change in brain function resulting from daily electrical stimulation. Experimental Neurology 25: 295–330
Goldensohn E S 1984 The relevance of secondary epileptogenesis to the treatment of epilepsy: Kindling and the mirror focus. Epilepsia 25 (suppl 2): S156–S168
Gonzalez L P, Hettinger M K 1984 Intranigral muscimol suppresses ethanol withdrawal seizures. Brain Research 298: 163–166
Higushi T, Kato N, Noguchi T et al 1986 Kindling and somatostatin. In: Wada J A (ed) Kindling 3. Raven Press, New York, p. 349–359
Holmes G L Weber D A 1986 Effects of ACTH on seizure susceptibility in the developing brain. Annals of Neurology 20: 82–88

Iadarola M J, Gale K 1982 Substantia nigra: site of anticonvulsant activity mediated by gamma-aminobutryic acid. Science 218: 1237–1240
Iadarola M J, Shin C, McNamara J O et al 1986 Changes in dynorphin, enkephalin and cholecystokinin content of hippocampus and substantia nigra after amygdala kindling. Brain Research 365: 185–191
Joy R M, Albertson T E Stark L G 1984 An analysis of the action of progabide, a specific GABA receptor agonist, on kindling and kindled seizures. Experimental Neurology 83: 144–154
Kairiss E W, Racine R J, Smith G K 1984 The development of the interictal spike during kindling in the rat. Brain Research 322: 101–110
Kamphuis W, Wadman W J, Buijs R M et al 1986 Decrease in number of hippocampal gamma-aminobutyric acid (GABA) immunoreactive cells in the rat kindling model of epilepsy. Experimental Brain Research 64: 491–495
Kato N, Sundmark V C, Van Middlesworth L et al 1982 Immunoreactive somatostatin and $\beta$-endorphin content in the brain of mature rats after neonatal exposure to propylthiouracil. Endocrinology 110: 1851–1855
Kato N, Higuchi T, Friesen H G et al 1983 Changes of immunoreactive somatostatin and beta-endorphin content in rat brain after amygdaloid kindling. Life Science 32: 2415–2422
Kelsey J E, Belluzzi J D 1982 Endorphin mediation of post-ictal effects of kindled seizures in rats. Brain Research 253: 337–340
King G L, Dingledine R, Giacchino J L et al 1985 Abnormal neuronal excitability in hippocampal slices from kindled rats. Journal of Neurophysiology 54: 1295–1304
Leach M J, Marden C N, Miller A A et al 1985 Changes in cortical amino acids during electrical kindling in rats. Neuropharmacology 24: 937–940
Leach M J, O'Donnell R A, Collins K J et al 1987 Effect of cortical kindling on [3H] D-aspartate uptake and glutamate metabolism in rats. Epilepsy Research 1: 145–148
Lee S, Kawawaki H, Matsuoka O et al 1986 Effect of Ca-antagonist (flunarizine) on kindling seizures in suckling rats. No To Hattatsu 18: 292–298
Leech C K, McIntyre D C 1976 Kindling rates in inbred mice: an analog to learning? Behavioral Biology 16: 439–452
Le Gal La Salle G 1979 Kindling of motor seizures from the bed nucleus of the stria terminalis. Experimental Neurology 66: 309–318
Le Gal La Salle G 1982 Amygdaloid organization related to the kinding effect. Electroencephalography and Clinical Neurophysiology (Suppl) 36: 239–248
Le Gal La Salle G, Kaijima M, Feldblum S 1983 Abortive amygdaloid kindled seizures following microinjection of gamma-vinyl-GABA in the vicinity of substantia nigra in rats. Neuroscience Letter 36: 69–74
Leviel V, Naquet R 1977 A study of the action of valproic acid on the kindling effect. Epilepsia 18: 229–234
Löscher W, Schwark W S 1985 Evidence for impaired GABA-ergic activity in the substantia nigra of amygdaloid kindled rats. Brain Research 339: 146–150
Lothman E W, Collins R C 1981 Kainic acid induced limbic seizures: metabolic, behavioral, electroencephalographic and neuropathological correlates. Brain Research 218: 299–318
Lothman E W, Hatlelid J M, Zorumski C F et al 1985 Kindling with rapidly recurring hippocampal seizures. Brain Research 360: 83–91
Ludvig N, Moshé S L 1988 Deep prepiriform cortex lesion and the development of amygdala kindling. Epilepsia. In press
Mason S T, Corcoran M E 1979 Catecholamines and convulsions. Brain Research 170: 497–507
McCaughran J A Jr, Corcoran M E, Wada J A 1977 Facilitation of secondary-site amygdaloid kindling following bisection of the corpus callosum and hippocampal commissure in rats. Experimental Neurology 57: 132–141
McCaughran J A Jr, Corcoran M E, Wada J A 1978 Role of the forebrain commissures in amygdaloid kindling in rats. Epilepsia 19: 19–33
McIntyre D C 1975 Split-brain rat: transfer and interference of kindled amygdala convulsions. Canadian Journal of Neurology Science 2: 429–437
McIntyre D C 1980 Amygdala kindling in rats: facilitation after local amygdala norepinephrine depletion with 6-hydroxydopamine. Experimental Neurology 69: 395–407
McIntyre D C, Goddard G V 1973 Transfer, interference and spontaneous recovery of convulsions kindled from the rat amygdala. Electroencephalography and Clinical Neurophysiology 35: 533–543
McIntyre D C, Roberts D C 1983 Long-term reduction in beta-adrenergic receptor binding after amygdala kindling in rats. Experimental Neurology 82: 17–24
McIntyre D C, Wong R K S 1985 Modification of local neuronal interactions by amygdala kindling in vitro. Experimental Neurology 88: 529–537

McIntrye D C, Racine R J 1986 Kindling mechanisms: Current progress on an experimental epilepsy model. Progress in Neurobiology 27: 1–12
McIntyre D C, Saari M, Pappas B A 1979 Potentiation of amygdala kindling in adult or infant rats by injection of 6-hydroxydopamine. Experimental Neurology 63: 527–544
McIntyre D C, Nathanson D, Edson N 1982a A new model of partial status epilepticus based on kindling. Brain Research 250: 53–63
McIntyre D C, Stuckey G N, Stokes K A 1982b Effects of amygdala lesions on dorsal hippocampus kindling in rats. Experimental Neurology 75: 184–190
McIntyre D C, Rajalla J, Edson N 1987 Suppression of amygdala kindling with short interstimulus intervals: effect of norepinephrine depletion. Experimental Neurology 95: 391–402s
McNamara J O 1978a Selective alterations of regional b-adrenergic receptor binding in the kindling model of epilepsy. Brain Research 154: 415–420
McNamara J O 1978b Muscarinic cholinergic receptors participate in the kindling model of epilepsy. Brain Research 154: 415–420
McNamara J O, Peper A M, Patrone V 1980 Repeated seizures induce long-term increase in hippocampal benzodiazepine receptors. Proceedings National Academy of Science 77: 3029–32
McNamara J O, Galloway M T, Rigsbee L C et al 1984 Evidence implicating substantia nigra in regulation of kindled seizure threshold. Journal of Neuroscience 4: 2410–2417
McNamara J O, Bonhaus D W, Shin C et al 1986 The kindling model of epilepsy: a critical review. Critical Reviews in Clinical Neurobiology 1: 341–391
Miller J J, Baimbridge K G, Mody I 1986 Calcium regulation in kindling-induced epilepsy. In: Wada J A (ed) Kindling 3. Raven Press, New York, p 301–304
Mason S T, Corcoran M E 1979 Catecholamines and convulsions. Brain Research 170: 497–507
Minabe Y, Tanii Y, Kadono Y et al 1986 Low-frequency kindling as a new experimental model of epilepsy. Experimental Neurology 94: 317–323
Mody I, Heinemann U 1987 NMDA receptors of dentate gyrus granule cells participate in synaptic transmission following kindling. Nature 326: 701–704
Monroe R R 1970 Episodic behavioral disorders: a psychodynamic and neurophysiological analysis. Haravard University Press, Cambridge, p 76–77
Morimoto K, Goddard G V 1986 Kindling induced changes in EEG recorded during stimulation from the site of stimulation: collapse of GABA-mediated inhibition and onset of rhythmic synchronous burst. Experimental Neurology 94: 571–584
Morimoto K, Goddard G V 1987 The substantia nigra is an important site for the containment of seizure generalization in the kindling model of epilepsy. Epilepsia 28: 1–10
Morimoto K, Dragunow M, Goddard G V 1986 Deep prepiriform cortex kindling and its relation to amygdale kindling in the rat. Experimental Neurology 94: 637–648
Morrell F 1985 Secondary epileptogenesis in man. Archives of Neurology 42: 318–355
Morrell F 1969 Physiology and histochemistry of the mirror focus. In: Jasper H H, Ward A A, Pope A (ed) Basic mechanisms of the epilepsies. Little Brown, Boston, p 357–370
Morrell F, de Toledo-Morrell L 1986 Kindling as a model of neuronal plasticity. In: Wada J A (ed) Kindling 3. Raven Press, New York, p 17–33
Morrell F, Tsuru N 1976 Kindling in the frog: development of spontaneous epileptiform activity. Electroencephalography Clinical Neurophysiolgy 40: 1–11
Moshé S L 1981a The effects of age on the kindling phenomenon. Developmental Psychobiology 14: 75–81
Moshé S L 1981b The kindling phenomenon and its possible relevance to febrile seizures. In: Nelson K B, Ellenberg J H (eds), Febrile seizures. Raven Press, New York, p 59–63
Moshé S L Ontogeny of seizures and substantia nigra modulation. In: Kellaway P (ed) Neurophysiology of the newborn. Johns Hopkins Press, Baltimore. In press
Moshé S L, Albala B J 1982 Kindling in developing rats: persitence of seizures into adulthood. Developmental Brain Research 4: 67–71
Moshé S L, Albala B J 1983 Maturational changes in postictal refractoriness and seizure susceptibility in developing rats. Annals of Neurology 13: 552–557
Moshé S L, Albala B J 1984 Nigral muscimol infusions facilitate the development of seizures in immature rats. Developmental Brain Research 13: 305–308
Moshé S L, Sharpless N S, Kaplan J 1981 Kindling in developing rats: Variability of afterdischarge thresholds with age. Brain Research 211: 190–195
Moshé S L, Albala B J, Ackermann R F et al 1983 Increased seizure susceptibility of the immature brain. Developmental Brain Research 7: 81–85
Moshé S L, Ackermann R F, Albala B J et al 1986 The role of substantia nigra in seizures of developing animals. In: Wada J A (ed) Kindling 3. Raven Press, New York, p 91–105
Nelson K B, Ellenberg J H 1978 Prognosis in children with febrile convulsions. Pediatrics 61: 720–727

Niznik H B, Burnham W M, Kish S J 1984 Benzodiazepine receptor binding following amygdala-kindled convulsions: differing results in washed and unwashed brain membranes. Journal of Neurochemistry 43: 1732–1736
Nobrega J N, Gaito J 1978 Long term induction of kindled seizures in rats: interhemispheric factors. Canadian Journal of Neurological Sciences 5: 223–230
Noda Y, Wada J A, McGeer E G 1982 Lasting influence of amygdaloid kindling on cholinergic neurotransmission. Experimental Neurology 78: 91–98
Okada R, Moshé S L, Wong B Y et al 1986 Age-related substantia nigra-mediated seizures facilitation. Experimental Neurology 93: 180–187
Oliver M W, Miller J J 1985 Alterations of inhibitory processes in the dentate gyrus following kindling-induced epilepsy. Experimental Brain Research 57: 443–447
Oliver A P, Hoffer B J, Wyatt R J 1980 Kindling induces long-lasting alterations in response of hippocampal neurons to elevated potassium levels in vitro. Science 208: 1264–1265
Peterson S L, Albertson T E, Stark L G 1981 Internal intervals and kindled seizures. Experimental Neurology 71: 144–153
Pinel J P J, Rovner L I 1978 Electrode placement and kindling-induced experimental epilepsy. Experimental Neurology 58: 335–346
Pinel J P J, Van Oot P H 1975 Generality of kindling phenomenon: some clinical implications. Canadian Journal of Neurology Science 2: 467–475
Piredda S, Gale K 1985 A crucial epileptogenic site in the deep prepiriform cortex. Nature 317: 623–625
Piredda S, Gale K 1986a Anticonvulsant action of 2-amino-7-phosphonoheptanoic acid and muscimol in the deep prepiriform cortex. European Journal of Pharmacology 120: 115–118
Piredda S, Gale K 1986b Role of excitatory aminoacid transmission in the genesis of seizures elicited from the deep prepiriform cortex. Brain Research 377: 205–210
Post R M 1977 Progressive changes in behavior and seizures following chronic cocaine administration relationship to kindling and psychosis. Advances in Behavioral Biology 21: 353–372
Post R M, Kopanda R T, Lee A 1975 Progressive behavioral changes during chronic lidocaine administration: relationship to kindling. Life Science 17: 943–950
Post R M, Davenport S, Pert A 1979 Lack of effect of an opiate agonist and antagonist on the development of amygdala kindling in the rat. Communications in Psychopharmacology 3: 185–190
Post R M, Weiss S R B, Pert A 1984 Differential effects of carbamazepine and lithium on sensitization and kindling. Progress in Neuro-psychopharmacology and Biological Psychiatry 8: 425–434
Przewlocki R, Lason W, Stach R et al 1983 Opioid peptides, particularly dynorphin after amygdaloid-kindled seizures. Regulatory Peptides 6: 385–392
Racine R J 1972a Modification of seizures activity by electrical stimulation: I. after-discharge threshold. Electroencephalography and Clinical Neurophysiology 32: 269–279
Racine R J 1972b Modification of seizure activity by electrical stimulation: II. motor seizures. Electroencephalography and Clinical Neurophysiology 32: 281–294
Racine R 1978 Kindling: the first decade. Neurosurgery 3: 234–252
Racine R J, Milgram N W 1983 Short-term potentiation phenomena in the rat limbic forebrain. Brain Research 260: 201–216
Racine R J, Burnham M W, Gartner J G et al 1973 Rates of motor seizure development in rats subjected to electrical brain stimulation: strain and interstimulation interval effects. Electroencephalography and Clinical Neurophysiology 55: 553–556
Racine R J, Livingston K, Joaquin A 1975a Effects of procaine hydrochloride, diazepam, and diphenylhydantoin on seizure development in cortical and subcortical structures in rats. Electroencephalography and Clinical Neurophysiology 38: 355–365
Racine R J, Neuberry F, Burnham W M 1975b Post-activation potentiation and the kindling phenomenon. Electroencephalography and Clinical Neurophysiology 39: 261–271
Racine R, Rose P A, Burnham W M 1977 Afterdischarge thresholds and kindling rates in dorsal and ventral hippocampus and dentate gyrus. Canmadian Journal of Neurological Sciences 4: 273–278
Racine R J, Migram N W, Hafner S 1983. Long-term poentiation phenomena in the rat limbic forebrain. Brain Research 260: 217–231
Ramer D, Pinel J P J 1976 Progressive intensification of motor seizures produced by periodic electroconvulsive shock. Experimental Neurology 51: 421–433
Rial R V, Gonzalez J 1978 Kindling effect in the reptilian brain: motor and electrographic manifestations. Epilepsia 19: 581–589.
Schwartzkroin P A, Wyler A R 1980 Mechanisms underlying epileptiform burst discharge. Annals of Neurology 7: 95–107
Seidel W T, Seidel W T, Corcoran M E 1986 Relations between amygdaloid and anterior neocortical kindling. Brain Research 385: 375–378

Shin C, Pedersen H B, McNamara J O 1985 Gamma-aminobutyric acid and benzodiazepine receptors in the kindling model of epilepsy: a quantitative radiohistochemical study. Journal of Neuroscience 5: 2696–2701

Sircar R, Ludvig N, Moshé S L et al 1987 Amygdala kindled seizures lower the density of phencyclidine receptors in the hippocampus. Epilepsia 28: 594

Spehlmann R, Norcross K 1984 Decreased sensitivity of neurons in the basolateral amygdala to dopamine and noradrenaline iontophoresis after a kindling stimulus. Experimental Neurology 83: 204–210

Sramka M, Sedlak P, Nadvornik P 1977 Observation of the kindling phenomenon in treatment of pain by stimulation in thalamus. In: Sweet W H (ed) Neurosurgical treatment in psychiatry, pain, and epilepsy. University Park Press, Baltimore, p 651–654

Stelzer A, Slater N T, ten Bruggencate G 1987 Activation of NMDA receptors blocks GABergic inhibition in an in vitro model of epilepsy. Nature 326: 698–701

Stripling J S, Ellinwood E H Jr 1977 Augmentation of the behavioural and electrophysiologic responses to cocaine by chronic administration in the rat. Experimental Neurology 54: 546–564

Tanaka A 1972 Progressive changes of behavioral and electroencephalographic responses to daily amygdaloid stimulation in rabbits. Fukuoka Acta Medicine 63: 152–163

Tietz E I, Gomex F, Berman R F 1985 Amygdala kindled seizure stage is related to altered benzodiazepine binding site density. Life Science 36: 183–190

Torres F, Jacome D 1982 Secondary epileptogenesis in the human. In: Mayersdord A, Schmidt R P (eds). Secondary epileptogenesis. New York, Raven Press, p 15–26

Tuff L P, Racine R F, Mishra R K 1983 The effects of kindling on GABA-mediated inhibition in the dentate gyrus of the rat. II. Receptor binding. Brain Research 277: 91–98

Tulloch I F, Walter D S, Howe G M et al 1982 The relationship between plasma concentration of valproic acid and its anticonvulsant and behavioral effects in the rat. Neuropharmacology 555–562

Turner I M, Newman S M, Louis S et al 1977 Pharmacological prophylaxis against the development of kindled amygdaloid seizures. Annals of Neurology 2: 221–224

Vindrola O, Briones R, Asai M et al 1981a Brain content of leu$^5$- and met$^5$enkephalin changes independently during the development of kindling in the rat. Neuroscience Letters 26: 125–130

Vindrola O, Briones R, Asai M et al 1981b Amygdaloid kindling enhances the enkephalin content in the rat brain. Neuroscience Letters 2: 39–43

Vosu H, Wise R A 1975 Cholinergic seizure kindling in the rat: Comparison of caudate, amygdala and hippocampus. Behavioral Biology 13: 491–495

Wada J A 1977 Pharmacological prophylaxis in the kindling model of epilepsy. Archives of Neurology 34: 389–395

Wada J A 1986 Preface. In: Wada J A (ed) Kindling 3. Raven Press, New York, p v–vi

Wada J A, Osawa T 1976 Spontaneous recurrent seizure state induced by daily electric amygdaloid stimulation in Senegalese baboons (Papio Papio). Neurology 26: 273–286

Wada J A, Sato M, Corcoran M E 1974 Persistent seizure susceptibility and recurrent spontaneous seizures in kindled cats. Epilepsia 15: 465–478

Wada J A, Sato M, McCaughran J A Jr 1975 Cortical electrographic correlates on convulsive seizure development induced by daily electrical stimulation of the amygdala in rats and cats. Folia Psychiatrica Neurologica Japonica 29: 329–339

Wada J A, Osawa T, Sato M et al 1976a Acute anticonvulsant effects of diphenylhydantoin, phenobarbital and carbamazepine: a combined electroclinical and serum level study in amygdaloid kindled cats and baboon. Epilepsia 17: 77–88

Wada J A, Sato M, Wake A et al 1976b Prophylactic effects of phenytoin, phenobarbital and carbamazepine examined in kindling cat preparations. Archives of Neurology 33: 426–34

Wada J A, Mizoguchi, Osawa T 1978 Secondarily generalized convulsive seizures induced by daily amygdaloid stimulation in rhesus monkeys. Neurology 28: 1026–1036

Wasterlain C G, Jonec V 1983 Chemical kindling by muscarinic amygdaloid stimulation in the rat. Brain Research 271: 311–323

Wasterlain C G, Fairchild M D, Bronstein J M et al 1986 Molecular changes in the synaptic apparatus associated with septal kindling. In Wada J A (ed) Kindling 3. Raven Press, New York, p 55–69

Watson R E Jr, Troiano R, Poulakos J, et al 1983 A $C_{14}$ 2-deoxyglucose analysis of the functional neural pathways of the limbic forebrain in the rat. I. The amygdala. Brain Research Reviews 5: 1–44

Waszczak B L, Eng N, Walters J R 1980 Effects of muscimol and picrotoxin on single unit activity of substantia nigra neurons. Brain Research 188: 185

Wauquier A, Ashton D, Melis W 1979 Behavioral analysis of amygdaloid kindling in beagle dogs and the effects of clonazepam, diazepam, phenobarbital, diphenylhydantoin, and flunarizine on seizure manifestation. Experimental Neurology 64: 579–586

Westerberg V, Corcoran M E 1987 Antagonism of central but not peripheral cholinegic receptors retards amygdala kindling in rats. Experimental Neurology 95: 194–206

Westerberg V, Lewis J, Corcoran M E 1984 Depletion of noradrenaline fails to affect kindled seizures. Experimental Neurology 84: 237–240
Wise R A, Chinerman J 1974 Effects of diazepam and phenobarbital on electrically induced amygdaloid seizures and seizure development. Experimental Neurology 45: 355–363
Wong B Y, Moshé S L 1987 Mutual interactions between repeated flurothyl convulsions and electrical kindling. Epilepsy Research 1: 159–164
Zaide J 1974 Differences between Tryon Bright and Dull rats in seizure activity evoked by amygdala stimulation. Physiology and Behavior 12: 527–534
Zhao D Y, Moshé S L 1987 Deep prepiriform cortex and amygdala interactions. Epilepsy Research 1: 94–101

# 3. Amino acid abnormalities in plasma, CSF and brain in epilepsy

*A. G. Chapman*

## INTRODUCTION

The etiology of seizure-susceptibility in epileptic individuals is generally unknown.

The search for possible metabolic abnormalities that might account for epileptiform activity has frequently focused on the inhibitory (mainly GABA, but also glycine and taurine) or excitatory (glutamate, aspartate and sulfur-containing amino acids) transmitter systems, since these amino acid transmitter systems have been firmly implicated in the modulation of seizure activity. Pharmacological manipulations that enhance GABAergic or antagonize excitatory amino acid transmission protect against spontaneous or induced seizure activity. Conversely, excitatory amino acid agonists or compounds that impair GABAergic transmission have direct proconvulsant or convulsant action. The interplay between excitatory and inhibitory amino acid transmitter systems in controlling the seizure threshold has been extensively documented and reviewed (Meldrum 1982, Meldrum & Chapman 1983, Meldrum 1985).

In light of the required homeostasis of these inhibitory and excitatory transmitter systems in a normally functioning brain, it is reasonable to suspect that an abnormality (impaired inhibitory transmission; excessive excitatory transmission) in the amino acid transmitter systems could be one of the mechanisms responsible for seizure-susceptibility in epilepsy-prone animals or man.

This chapter will examine the evidence for amino acid neurotransmitter abnormalities (release, regional transmitter concentration) in brain tissue and CSF and plasma from patients with epilepsy and compare these findings with changes reported in spontaneously epileptic animal species.

## NEUROPATHOLOGY AND EPILEPSY

Before considering the regional distribution of metabolic abnormalities in clinical or experimental epilepsy, it is useful to briefly summarize the anatomical distribution of gross and microscopic pathological changes found associated with epilepsy. The related topic of anatomical involvement in the spread of seizure activity is dealt with in another chapter in this volume (Meldrum 1988).

'Epileptic brain damage' is characterized by selective neuronal loss and by glial proliferation and is observed to a varying degree both in patients with primary or idiopathic epilepsy or in those where the epilepsy is secondary to a focal disorder. It is believed to be both a consequence of prolonged seizures and to contribute to subsequent seizure activity (Meldrum 1976, Meldrum 1981, Meldrum & Corsellis 1984).

The neuronal loss predominates in the hippocampus (pyramidal neurons in the endfolium and the Sommer sector), neocortex (pyramidal neurons, especially in the third cortical lamina) and cerebellum (Purkinje and basket cells), while groups of neurons in the thalamus and amygdala are occasionally affected. Very similar neuropathological changes are observed in animals following drug-induced focal or generalized sustained seizures.

Any relationship between cerebral metabolic abnormalities in epilepsy and the observed seizure-related neuropathology remains conjectural. If the neuronal loss reflects loss of inhibitory interneurons, a facilitation of epileptiform activity would be expected. So far there has been no direct and unequivocal demonstration of such a mechanism being responsible for epilepsy in humans, although some animal studies indicate an association between the loss of inhibitory synapses and the development of seizure activity (see Ribak 1986).

## PATHOPHYSIOLOGY AND EPILEPSY

The paroxysmal activity characteristic of an epileptic focus can be reproduced by applying excitatory amino acid agonists to different regions (e.g. the hippocampus) of a normal brain. Activation of the N-methyl-D-aspartate (NMDA) receptor is particularly effective in inducing burst discharges. Physiological evidence for an upregulation of NMDA receptors has recently been obtained in the hippocampus of amygdala kindled rats (Mody & Heinemann 1987).

Such a mechanism for generating epileptiform activity is not necessarily associated with overt neuropathology at early stages, although excessive firing of neurons would eventually lead to 'excitotoxic' neuronal loss akin to that observed following experimental seizures induced by the administration of excitatory agonists such as quinolinate or kainate. Indeed, the sequence of events initiated at the excitatory synapse may play a key role in the selective neuronal loss observed following seizure activity (Schwarcz & Meldrum 1985, Sloviter & Dempster 1985, Greenamyre 1986, Collins 1986).

## AMINO ACID CHANGES IN GENETICALLY SEIZURE-SUSCEPTIBLE ANIMALS

### Baboons

There is a high incidence of seizures in response to light stimulation in the Senegalese baboon, *Papio papio*, (see Killam & Killam 1984). The cortical levels of inhibitory and excitatory amino acids (GABA, taurine, glycine, glutamate and aspartate) in seizure-susceptible baboons are unchanged from those in seizure-resistant animals (Hansen et al 1973). The cortical density and affinity of benzodiazepine receptors are also unaltered in a seizure-susceptible baboon (Squires et al 1979). There is, however, a reduced level of GABA in the CSF of seizure-susceptible *Papio papio* compared to the CSF GABA level in non-responders (Lloyd et al 1986a,b).

### Dogs

Spontaneously epileptic dogs have a similar cortical and CSF amino acid pattern to the above baboons with photically-induced epilepsy. There is no alteration in the cortical levels of excitatory and inhibitory amino acids (nor in the plasma and CSF levels of taurine, glycine, aspartate or glutamate; Van Gelder et al 1980b). There is however a lower GABA level in the CSF of spontaneously epileptic or seizure-prone dogs than in resistant dogs (Löscher 1982b, Löscher & Schwartz-Porsche 1986).

**Gerbils**

In a strain of gerbils sensitive to stimulus evoked seizures, there is a decrease in the benzodiazepine binding in the substantia nigra and the midbrain tectum relative to seizure-resistant gerbils (Olsen et al 1984, Olsen et al 1986). The activity of the GABA synthesizing enzyme, glutamate decarboxylase, GAD, is unchanged in many brain regions of seizure-prone gerbils despite reports of a markedly increased number of hippocampal GAD positive cells (by immunocytochemistry) in the seizure-prone strain compared to the resistant strain (see Löscher 1987).

**Mice**

There are a number of mouse strains susceptible to spontaneous or evoked seizures, including the audiogenic DBA/2 mice. The excitatory and inhibitory amino acid levels in the whole brain, the cortex or other gross anatomical regions are, on the whole, unaltered from those in seizure-resistant strains, or they show no consistent alterations (see Chapman & Meldrum 1987). The benzodiazepine binding (receptor density) is reduced in the pons-medulla, midbrain, substantia nigra, and in the inferior colliculus of DBA/2 mice relative to seizure-resistant mice (Horton et al 1984, Olsen et al 1986). GABA release is reduced in brain slices from DBA/2 mice (Hertz et al 1974). GABA receptors in DBA/2 mice have been reported to be unchanged or decreased (see Frandsen et al 1987). There is an increased density of glutamate receptors (AMPA binding at the quisqualate-preferring glutamate receptor) in most brain regions in the DBA/2 mice compared to seizure-resistant mice (Frandsen et al 1987).

**Rats**

A number of different abnormalities have been described for genetically epilepsy-prone rats susceptible to sound-induced seizures, including a defect in taurine metabolism (see Laird et al 1984, Huxtable et al 1986). Regional brain levels of endogenous amino acids have been reported as unaltered (see Huxtable et al 1986) or changed in the inferior colliculus and other regions (Chapman et al 1986, Reiffenstein et al 1987). There is an increased number of GAD positive neurons in the inferior colliculus of audiogenic rats (Roberts et al 1985), an unaltered in vivo release of GABA from the hippocampus, but an increased hippocampal in vivo release of aspartate in the seizure-susceptible rats (Huxtable et al 1986). The enhanced release of aspartate is similar to the enhanced release of excitatory amino acids observed in fully responsive amygdala-kindled rats (Leach et al 1985) or in animals with an epileptogenic cobalt lesion (Dodd et al 1980).

## AMINO ACID CHANGES IN HUMAN EPILEPTIC TISSUE

**Endogenous amino acid levels**

Analysis of brain tissue for possible amino acid abnormalities associated with epilepsy is necessarily restricted to tissue removed from patients undergoing neurosurgery (usually anterior temporal lobectomy) for intractable focal epilepsy. 'Epileptic tissue' is identified by the paroxysmal EEG activity recorded from the tissue (by stereotaxically implanted depth electrodes or by scalp electrodes, after reducing anti-epileptic medication in order to enhance focal discharge). Subsequent histopathological assessment (astroglial proliferation; neuronal loss) is used to characterize the tissue further (Lloyd et al 1981, 1985, Sherwin & Van Gelder 1986).

Table 3.1 summarizes amino acid changes observed in epileptic cortical foci. The

**Table 3.1** Levels of excitatory and inhibitory amino acids in human epileptic foci

| | n | % of control[a] | | | | |
|---|---|---|---|---|---|---|
| Reference | (E/C)[b] | GLU | ASP | GABA | TAU | GLY |
| Van Gelder et al (1972) | 18/18 | 91* | 94 | 100 | 87* | 157* |
| Rougier et al (1987) | 23/9 | 81 | 77 | 96 | 146* | 183* |
| Perry & Hansen (1981) | 34/14 | 125* | 99 | 130* | 106 | 141* |
| Sherwin et al (1986a) | 12/9 | 126* | 125* | 108 | 119 | 155* |

[a] Controls in top two studies: distal, 'normal' zones from same brain; controls in Perry & Hansen (1981): temporal or frontal cortex of tumor patients; controls in Sherwin et al (1986a): 'non-spiking cortex' of epileptic patients (see text).
[b] Number of epileptic (E) and control (C) subjects in each study.
* Values significantly different from control values.

availability of suitable control tissue presents a problem in such studies. Studies by Van Gelder et al (1972) and by Rougier et al (1987) in Table 3.1 both compare amino acid levels in the epileptic focus to levels in the surrounding tissue from the same brains. Except for a discrepancy in the taurine results, these two studies are in good agreement regarding reduced levels of aspartate and glutamate, elevated glycine levels and unchanged GABA levels in the epileptic focus relative to the surrounding area.

It has subsequently been established however, that the amino acid alterations extend beyond the epileptic focus (Sherwin, personal communication). Therefore, a different picture emerges when amino acid levels in the 'spiking' cortical epileptic focus are compared to 'control' levels in a separate group of patients: (cortical material from non-epileptic tumor patients in the case of Perry & Hansen (1981), or cortical samples from a group of epileptic surgical patients with a 'non-spiking' cortex in the case of Sherwin et al (1986a)). Again, these two latter studies show reasonably good internal consistency (Table 3.1). Both studies report significant elevations in glutamate and glycine levels in the epileptic groups, but differ re the significance of the aspartate and GABA elevations. GABA levels are also found to be similar in brain tumors from epileptic and non-epileptic patients (Schmidt et al 1984).

In summary, there appears to be an elevation of the excitatory amino acids, glutamate and perhaps aspartate, in actively spiking epileptic cortex which extends beyond the actual focus. The levels in the (necrotic?) focus itself appear to be lower than in the surrounding tissue, in agreement with the focal decrease in the levels of these amino acids observed in experimentally induced cobalt- or penicillin-seizures (see Bradford & Dodd 1976, Sherwin & Van Gelder 1986).

The levels of the inhibitory transmitters, GABA and taurine, appear to remain unchanged in the epileptic focus or show no consistent alteration. There is probably a metabolic basis for the apparently paradoxical increase in the level of glycine. Folate deficiency (Perry et al 1975) or abnormal protein synthesis (Van Gelder et al 1972) have been suggested as possible reasons for the glycine increase. Glycine metabolism is closely linked to serine and alanine metabolism through equilibrium reactions, and consequently the levels of these amino acids commonly change in parallel (Chapman et al 1987). The glycine increase in the epileptic tissue, therefore, could merely reflect a seizure-induced alanine increase (Bradford & Dodd 1976, Janjua et al 1982, Sherwin & Van Gelder 1986), which again is a direct consequence of the pyruvate and lactate increases usually observed during seizures in experimental studies (Bradford & Dodd 1976, Chapman 1985). Lactate levels in plasma and CSF are also increased postictally in humans (Brooks 1980).

The absolute cortical amino acid levels in the 'control' tissue for the studies presented in Table 3.1 are given as part of Table 3.2 There is good consistency concerning

**Table 3.2** Control levels of excitatory and inhibitory amino acids in human tissue

| | CORTEX[a] (μmol/g) | PLASMA[b] (mmol/ml) | CSF[c] (mmol/ml) |
|---|---|---|---|
| Glutamate | 6.7–8.7 | 34–104 | 11.3–45.4 |
| Aspartate | 1.08–1.49 | 6–14 | 0.4–2.8 |
| Taurine | 1.16–1.34 | 53–78 | 4.5–8.4 |
| Glycine | 0.35–0.74 | 212–283 | 3.4–8.2 |
| GABA | 0.63–6.27 | 0.31–0.43 | 0.08–0.25 |

[a] Range of mean cortical control values ('normal zone' or 'non-spiking cortex' from Perry et al 1975, Perry & Hansen 1981, Sherwin et al 1986a, Rougier et al 1987).
[b] Range of mean plasma control values (glu, asp, tau and gly) from 9 studies (Perry & Hansen 1969, Plum 1975, Monaco et al 1975, McGale et al 1977, Van Gelder et al 1980a, Janjua et al 1982, Huxtable et al 1983, Hagenfeldt et al 1984, Haines et al 1985); and range of 3 plasma control values for GABA (Löscher & Schmidt 1980, Schmidt & Löscher 1981, 1982).
[c] Range of mean CSF control values (glu, asp, tau and gly) from 7 studies (Gjessing et al 1974, Mutani et al 1974, Plum 1974, McGale et al 1977, Engelsen & Elsayed 1984, Hagenfeldt et al 1984, Crawford & Chadwick 1987); and range of control CSF GABA levels (Wood et al 1979, Manyam et al 1980, Hare et al 1980, 1981, Löscher et al 1981, Schmidt & Löscher 1981, 1982, Grove et al 1982a,b, Hare et al 1982, Perry et al 1982, Kuroda et al 1982, Ferraro et al 1983, Rating et al 1983, Manyam & Tremblay 1984, Ito et al 1984, Löscher & Siemes 1985, 1987, Crawford & Chadwick 1987).

control cortical levels of glutamate (6.7–8.7 μmol/g), aspartate (1.1–1.5 μmol/g), taurine (1.2–1.3 μmol/g), and to a lesser extent glycine (0.4–0.7 μmol/g). One of the GABA control values (6.3 μmol/g) from Rougier et al (1987) falls outside of the remaining range of values (0.5–1.4 μmol/g). Control (peripheral cortical tissue of epileptic patients) values for aspartate (approximately 2 μmol/g) and glutamate (approximately 12 μmol/g) estimated from the figure in Van Gelder et al (1972) are somewhat higher than those in the other studies.

## Receptor density and enzyme activity

Studies have focused on the determination of the activities of the GABA synthesizing enzyme, glutamate decarboxylase (GAD) and the GABA metabolizing enzyme, GABA-transaminase (GABA-T) in human cortical samples from patients undergoing surgery for refractory epilepsy.

There is general agreement that GABA-T activity is relatively unaltered in epileptic brains (Lloyd et al 1984, Schmidt et al 1984, Sherwin et al 1984). However there are conflicting data concerning the activity of GAD in epileptic brains. Lloyd and coworkers have reported a significant decrease in GAD activity in the epileptic focus in approximately half of their patient population (Lloyd et al 1981, 1984). The decrease in GAD activity was observed by this group both when distal, apparently normal tissue from the same brains, or when cortical samples from a different patient group served as control tissue (Lloyd et al 1984). Other studies have failed to detect any difference in GAD activity in actively spiking cortical areas of epileptic patients (Sherwin et al 1984, Schmidt et al 1984). Nor is there a selective loss of GAD positive neurons (using GAD immunocytochemistry) in different hippocampal areas of human epileptic brains (Babb 1986).

A decrease in the density of GABA receptors ($^{3}$H-GABA binding) has been reported in the cortical tissue from about half of the epileptic patients undergoing surgery (Lloyd et al 1981), whereas the benzodiazepine receptor density ($^{3}$-H-flunitrazepam binding) is unaltered in human epileptogenic cortical foci (Sherwin et al 1986b).

Therefore, the majority of patients undergoing surgery for intractable focal epilepsy appear to have no gross metabolic manifestation of an abnormal GABAergic transmitter system. However, there appears to be a sub-population of epileptic patients with a reduced GAD activity. Whether this GAD reduction represents a selective GABAergic degeneration, or reflects a general neuronal loss remains to be established.

Information relating to excitatory receptors or related enzyme activities in human epileptic brain is very sparse at the present. There is no systematic pattern of change in $^{3}$-H-kainic acid binding in cortical samples from epileptic patients (Lloyd et al 1981). A recent study has reported an increase in the activity of aspartate aminotransferase in actively spiking human epileptic cortex (Dixon et al 1987).

## RELATIONSHIP BETWEEN BRAIN AMINO ACID METABOLISM AND AMINO ACID LEVELS IN CSF OR PLASMA

Are the CSF or plasma levels of amino acids a reflection of the brain concentrations of these compounds, and would abnormalities in brain amino acid metabolism be reflected in changes in the CSF and plasma?

Table 3.2 shows endogenous levels of transmitter amino acids in human cortex, plasma and CSF in a control population. Not only are the absolute levels drastically different in the three tissues (note that concentrations in brain are given as μmol/g, whereas the concentrations for plasma and CSF are given as nmol/ml; i.e. a 1000 fold difference), but their concentration ranking orders are also different, evoking the need for separate and selective exchange systems for the different compounds at the blood/brain or blood/CSF barriers. A brief outline of the metabolite exchange between the three compartments is therefore merited before discussing epilepsy-related changes in these compartments.

### Blood/brain exchange

The tight junctions of the cerebral capillary endothelium ensure a highly selective, restrictive uptake of molecules into the brain. The bidirectional movement of amino acids through the blood brain barrier is mediated by three separate carrier systems for basic, neutral and acidic amino acids (Pardridge & Oldendorf 1977). The rate of facilitated transport from plasma to brain differs greatly for the different amino acids, with the non-essential amino acids, glutamate, aspartate and glycine penetrating most poorly (Oldendorf 1971). Systemically administered aspartate is only taken up into the circumventricular organs and causes no aspartate elevation in any other mouse brain region (Price et al 1984). The rate of taurine influx from plasma to brain is also very low (see Davson et al 1987).

The rate of cerebral circulation in man is approximately 0.5 ml/min/g brain, or around 800 ml/min for the average 1500 g brain (see Siesjö 1978). Cerebral circulation is the major route for removing products of cerebral metabolism. The venous outflow contains metabolites derived both from brain tissue and from the CSF (see Fishman 1980).

**CSF/blood exchange**

The volume of total CSF in man is around 140 ml. The rate of CSF formation is given as 0.35 ml/min or 500 ml/day; in other words, there is a complete turnover of the CSF about every 8 hours. The principle site of CSF formation is the choroid plexus, where a serum filtration process across the choroidal capillary wall is followed by an active transport-dependent secretion of the newly formed CSF by the choroidal epithelium. The drainage of the CSF into the venous system from the subarachnoid space occurs via the arachnoid villi and is essentially a unidirectional flow into the venous blood. The choroidal epithelium therefore represents the CSF/plasma barrier (Fishman 1980, Davson et al 1987).

The composition of the CSF is similar to, but not identical with, filtered plasma. On the average, the CSF amino acid concentration in man is approximately one third that of the plasma concentration (Davson et al 1987). But CSF/plasma ratios for individual amino acids vary between 0.8 for glutamine to 0.02 for glycine (McGale et al 1977, Hagenfeldt et al 1984). The blood/CSF barrier is relatively impermeable to GABA, glycine and aspartate, with little or no increase observed in the ventricular concentrations of these amino acids following their intravenous administration (Davson et al 1987).

**Brain/CSF exchange**

There is free exchange between brain interstitial fluid and the CSF (ventricular, cisternal, subarachnoid and lumbar fluids) and their compositions are very similar (allowing for rostro-caudal gradients; Fishman 1980, Davson et al 1987). Brain metabolites can therefore freely enter the CSF following their release or facilitated transport into the extracellular fluid. This route, in combination with the blood/brain barrier, also constitutes an alternative path for the transport of compounds from blood to the CSF. Conversely, amino acids perfused into the ventricles are readily taken up both by blood and brain tissue (Davson et al 1982). There are both glial and neuronal high affinity uptake systems for amino acids neurotransmitters (see Fagg & Foster 1983).

There is an increased in vivo release of transmitter amino acid, especially taurine and glutamate, from different brain regions during experimentally induced seizures in animals (Dodd et al 1980, Lehmann et al 1983, Jacobson & Hamberger 1985, Young & Bradford 1986, Wade et al 1987). Such an increased release could presumably subsequently be reflected in an increased CSF level of these compounds.

**Extracellular brain space**

Estimates of extracellular brain volume based on electron microscopic assessment, or distribution of extracellular markers following ventriculo-cisternal perfusion, have ranged from 5–25% of total brain volume. Recent estimates of extracellular space of mammalian brain cluster around 15–20% (Davson et al 1987). For instance, the extracellular volume (inulin or sucrose space) for cerebral cortex or caudate nucleus of rhesus monkey is 18–20% (Levin et al 1970).

The relative distribution of metabolites between brain and CSF would therefore be influenced by pathophysiological situations where extracellular space is affected (e.g. post-traumatic edema).

**Correlation between GABA levels in brain, CSF and plasma**

There is no correlation between plasma and CSF GABA levels in individual patients in a population with various neurological disorders who have a spontaneous variation in CSF GABA (four fold range) and plasma GABA (three fold range) levels (Schmidt & Löscher 1982, Enna et al 1980). However, when CNS GABA levels increase following pharmacological intervention, the GABA increases are observed in plasma and CSF, as well as in brain of animals, but usually only after a given time interval. This is best illustrated following the acute administration of GABA-transaminase inhibitors (γ-vinyl-GABA or γ-acetylenic-GABA) to animals. A progressive increase in brain GABA levels is observed during the following 2–3 h, as well as a delayed (1–2 h) GABA increase in CSF and plasma (Böhlen et al 1979, Ferkany et al 1979, Löscher 1982a). There is also a marked increase in release of GABA from the cortex following γ-vinyl-GABA administration to rats (Abdul-Ghani et al 1980). At steady state conditions (18 h after γ-vinyl-GABA administration) there is a linear correlation between total GABA in CSF and brain GABA levels (Böhlen et al 1979). An increased CSF GABA level is also observed in humans following chronic antiepileptic administration of γ-vinyl-GABA (Grove et al 1981, Schechter et al 1984, Halonen et al 1987).

In summary, changes in amino acid levels in plasma and CSF probably reflect a change in the release (or reuptake) of transmitter amino acids, rather than changes in the brain endogenous transmitter amino acid levels per se. Such changes would only be manifested during chronic alteration of brain metabolism, or following a substantial lag period after acute alterations. Impaired blood/brain barrier or pathological changes in the extracellular space would also affect the amino acid levels in CSF of plasma.

## FACTORS AFFECTING AMINO ACID LEVELS IN CSF AND PLASMA

Several authors have pointed out potential pitfalls in the determination of amino acid levels in the plasma or CSF of epileptic patients (Perry & Hansen 1969, Perry et al 1976, Löscher & Schmidt 1980, Hare 1981, Grove et al 1982a,b, Ferraro et al 1983, Huxtable et al 1983, Schecter et al 1984, Haines et al 1985, Löscher & Schmidt 1987). Summarized below are general and epilepsy-related factors influencing the levels of transmitter amino acids in biological fluids.

**Age and sex**

With advancing age in females there is a progressive, significant decrease in the CSF GABA concentration, whereas the CSF GABA concentration in males is much less influenced by age (Hare 1981, Hare et al 1982). The CSF glycine levels show a progressive, significant increase with age (as do CSF alanine and glutamine levels) both in male and female subjects (Gjessing et al 1974, McGale et al 1977). The CSF taurine level in adults appears to be unaffected by age. CSF aspartate level is reported to be reduced with age, while an apparent CSF glutamate increase in the old age group is not statistically significant (Gjessing et al 1974).

Conflicting results have been reported concerning possible differences in CSF and plasma amino acid levels between fasted males and females. McGale et al (1977) (excluding from the study females taking oestrogen-progestogen compounds, which are known to influence plasma amino acid levels) find no difference between males and females in the levels of taurine, glutamate and glycine in either CSF or plasma, whereas Hagenfeldt et al (1984), (including females on contraceptives in the study) find significantly lower values of taurine, aspartate and glutamate in plasma of females, and lower values of taurine, aspartate and glycine in CSF of females.

**Diet**

The plasma concentrations of several amino acids in humans and rats are markedly affected by the protein content of the diet and by time interval since the last feed (Wurtman et al 1968, Glaeser et al 1983, Huxtable et al 1983). However, the plasma levels of the transmitter amino acids considered in this review are all relatively resistant to variations caused by daily rhythms and nutritional composition (Wurtman et al 1968, Huxtable et al 1983). Nonetheless, most of the recent studies on plasma and CSF composition in epileptic patients have been conducted using fasted subjects.

**Antiepileptic therapy**

Some anticonvulsant drugs, such as the GABA-transaminase inhibitor $\gamma$-vinyl-GABA (vigabatrin) have been designed to elevate the synaptic concentration of GABA. It is therefore no surprise that CSF and plasma concentrations of GABA are elevated in epileptic patients receiving such drugs. $\gamma$-vinyl-GABA administration markedly elevates GABA levels in brain, CSF and plasma of animals and humans (Böhlen et al 1979, Grove et al 1981, Schechter 1986). The $\gamma$-vinyl-GABA-induced increase in total CSF GABA levels may be higher in patients with complex partial epilepsy that respond favorably to $\gamma$-vinyl-GABA therapy than in the poor responders (Riekkinen et al 1987). Other GABA-transaminase inhibitors have similar effects on GABA levels (Ferkany et al 1979, Butler et al 1980).

GABA levels are significantly elevated in the CSF and plasma of patients receiving valproate therapy (Löscher & Schmidt 1980, Schmidt & Löscher 1981, Löscher & Siemes 1985). Valproate administration also elevates glycine levels in plasma and urine of epileptic patients (Jaeken et al 1977, Mortensen et al 1980, Haines et al 1985). There is a rapid (2–8 min after i.v. injection) elevation of GABA levels in human CSF following the administration of diazepam (Löscher & Schmidt 1987).

Increased plasma aspartate and glutamate levels in patients with generalized tonic-clonic seizures correlate strongly with the prescription of phenytoin in one study (Huxtable et al 1983), whereas in another study the administration of phenytoin has no effect on plasma amino acid concentration (Haines et al 1985).

**Sampling and storage**

A rostro-caudal gradient for GABA results in higher GABA concentrations in subоccipital samples than in lumbar samples (Grove et al 1982a, Schechter et al 1984). A similar rostro-caudal gradient exists for glycine. The remaining amino acids have similar levels in the ventricular and lumbar spaces (Fishman 1980).

Post-sampling treatment and storage conditions of the CSF samples can easily cause artifactual elevation of free GABA levels by hydrolysis of conjugated GABA present in much higher concentrations in the CSF (Hare 1981, Grove et al 1982b, Perry et al 1982, Ferraro et al 1983). Minor technical variations in the sampling and post-sampling treatment of plasma samples can be a source of major errors in the plasma levels of taurine, aspartate and glutamate (Perry & Hansen 1969).

**Damaged blood/brain barrier**

Animal experiments have shown that the arterial hypertension frequently associated with the onset of seizure activity (see Meldrum 1976) can be sufficient to damage the blood/brain barrier and make it permeable to macromolecules (Johansson & Lund 1978, Westergaard et al 1978). It is therefore possible that alterations in CSF amino acid levels could be a consequence of impaired amino acid transport occurring during seizures.

## PLASMA AMINO ACIDS AND EPILEPSY

Plasma amino acid levels in patients with epilepsy (expressed as percentage of corresponding values in control groups) are listed in Table 3.3. The control values for

**Table 3.3** Plasma levels of excitatory and inhibitory amino acids in epilepsy

| | n | % of control | | | | |
|---|---|---|---|---|---|---|
| | (E/C) | GABA | Taurine | Glycine | Aspartate | Glutamate |
| Plum (1975) | 25/75 | — | 103 | 91 | 100 | 86 |
| Monaco et al (1975) | 10/50 | — | 239* | 88 | 71 | 86 |
| Van Gelder et al (1980a) | 44/22 | — | 83* | 110 | 45* | 119* |
| Janjua et al (1982) | 11/22 | — | 78 | 99 | 39* | 143 |
| Huxtable et al (1983) | 11/12 | — | 96 | 134* | 200* | 382* |
| Haines et al (1985) | 43/20 | — | 92 | 135* | 77 | 107 |
| Janjua et al (1986) | 22/32 | — | — | — | — | 167* |
| Schmidt & Löscher (1981) | 30/22 | 119 | — | — | — | — |

E, number of epileptic patients; C, number of control subjects in study.
* Statistically significant differences between epileptic and corresponding control values.

taurine (53–78 μmol/l) and glycine (212–249 μmol/l) are very consistent in all the studies. The plasma aspartate level (14 μmol/l) is somewhat higher in the studies of Van Gelder and coworkers (Van Gelder et al 1980a, Janjua et al 1982) than in the other studies listed in the table (6–10 μmol/l). The variation in the control glutamate levels in plasma (37–104 μmol/l) is greater than for the other amino acids. The plasma level of GABA is below detection using the automatic amino acid analyzer method employed in the top 6 studies of Table 3.3. However, using a radioreceptor assay, a control plasma GABA level of around 430 pmol/ml is determined (Schmidt & Löscher 1981).

The epileptic patients listed in Table 3.3 were all on continued antiepileptic medication. In some of the studies (Plum 1975, Huxtable et al 1983, Haines et al 1985) it is specified that plasma was obtained from fasted subjects. The patient populations differ in the studies. A homogeneous group of patients with 3/sec spike-wave epilepsy is used in one study (Van Gelder et al 1980a); patients with generalized tonic-clonic seizures constitute another study (Huxtable et al 1983), while the majority of the studies involve a mixed group of epileptic patients.

Effects of antiepileptic medication on plasma amino acid levels probably account for many of the apparent plasma abnormalities tabulated for the epileptic groups (Table 3.3). If patients receiving valproate therapy had been included in the study of Schmidt & Löscher (1981), the plasma GABA level would have been significantly higher than the control value. Likewise, the increase in plasma glycine level in epileptic patients reported by Haines et al (1985) is fully accounted for by the large number of patients in this group receiving valproate therapy. A similar explanation cannot account for the plasma glycine rise reported by Huxtable et al (1983) as only one patient in this group received valproate. The increase reported by Huxtable et al (1983) in plasma aspartate level in epileptic patients is completely removed, and the apparent glutamate increase severely reduced (but still elevated) when patients receiving phentyoin are eliminated from the study.

The most consistent finding in Table 3.3 which persists after correcting for the effects of antiepileptic medication, is an elevated plasma glutamate level in 4 out of 7 studies. The Montreal group also reports that the plasma glutamate level is raised (and the aspartate level lowered) in the first-degree relatives (who, of course, are not receiving antiepileptic medication) of the patients with 3/sec spike-wave epilepsy (Van Gelder et al 1980a, Janjua et al 1982) or with primary generalized epilepsy (Janjua et al 1986). These changes in plasma levels of excitatory amino acids were not confirmed by Haines et al (1985) either in the epileptic patient group or in their relatives. The reason for this discrepancy is not known.

The increased plasma taurine level reported by Monaco et al (1975) in patients with epilepsy is not observed in any of the other studies in Table 3.3. However, an increased urinary excretion of taurine in epileptic patients (Plum 1975, Rao et al 1983) may be relevant in this connection.

It is not possible from these studies to assess whether the different clinical types of epilepsy affect the plasma amino acids differently. Another variable that might affect the plasma amino acid levels is seizure frequency and time interval since last ictal episode, since it is known from animal studies that endogenous levels, synthesis and release of transmitter amino acid are markedly affected by seizure activity (Chapman et al 1977, Ciesielski et al 1981, Chapman et al 1984, 1985, Green & Vincent 1987). Corresponding information is lacking in humans.

## CSF AMINO ACIDS AND EPILEPSY

Cerebrospinal GABA levels have been measured in a number of studies (Table 3.4). Except for one study with anomalously high GABA values (Knight et al 1985), the studies in infants with either febrile convulsions or infantile spasms show significantly reduced CSF GABA levels compared to age-matched controls (Löscher et al 1981, Rating et al 1983, Ito et al 1984, Löscher & Siemes 1985). The CSF may thus reflect a decreased extracellular fluid GABA content in seizure susceptible infants. Somewhat older children with epilepsy of mixed etiology have normal GABA levels in the CSF

**Table 3.4** CSF GABA levels in epilepsy

| Seizure type | n (E/C) | GABA (pmol/ml) control | epilepsy | % of control | References |
|---|---|---|---|---|---|
| Febrile convulsions | 23/16 | 210 | 134* | 64 | Löscher et al (1981) |
| | 51/32 | 148 | 103* | 70 | Rating et al (1983) |
| | 14/13 | 471 | 554 | 118 | Knight et al, 1985 |
| Infantile spasms | 9/41 | 174 | 109* | 63 | Löscher & Siemes (1985) |
| | 22/35 | 244 | 86* | 35 | Ito et al (1984) |
| Myoclonic | 10/14 | 251 | 116* | 46 | Enna et al (1980) |
| | 8/10 | 135 | 89* | 66 | Ohisalo et al (1983) |
| Gen tonic clonic | 5/20 | 239 | 118* | 49 | Wood & Brooks (1980) |
| | 16/41 | 174 | 137 | 79 | Löscher & Siemes (1985) |
| | 15/15 | 159 | 156 | 98 | Crawford & Chadwick (1987) |
| Mixed (children) | 14/32 | 148 | 144 | 97 | Rating et al (1983) |
| | 31/41 | 174 | 141 | 81 | Löscher & Siemes (1985) |
| Mixed | 21/20 | 239 | 139* | 58 | Wood et al (1979) |
| | 8/19 | 239 | 162* | 68 | Manyam et al (1980) |
| | 3/6 | 131 | 128 | 98 | Schmidt & Löscher (1982) |
| | 9/16 | 143 | 143 | 100 | Kuroda et al (1982) |
| | 7/15 | 208 | 159 | 76 | Manyam & Tremblay (1984) |
| Mixed, untreated | 43/51 | 106 | 130 | 123 | Crawford & Chadwick (1987) |
| Mixed, treated | 26/51 | 106 | 120 | 113 | Crawford & Chadwick (1987) |

E, number of epileptic patients; C, number of control subjects in study.
* Statistically significant differences between epileptic and corresponding control values.

(Rating et al 1983, Löscher & Siemes 1985). CSF GABA levels are also reduced in patients with myoclonic epilepsy (Enna et al 1980, Ohisalo et al 1983). This condition is associated with a marked loss of Purkinje cells (see Ohisalo et al 1983).

One study (Wood & Brooks 1980) reports a reduced GABA level in the CSF in patients with generalized tonic clonic seizures, whereas two other studies (Löscher & Siemes 1985, Crawford & Chadwick 1987) detect no CSF GABA changes in these patients.

GABA levels in the CSF of patient groups with different types of epilepsy would presumably depend on the composition of the groups and their antiepileptic therapy. It is known that two commonly used antiepileptic drugs, valproate (Löscher & Schmidt 1980, Schmidt & Löscher 1981, Löscher & Siemes 1985) and diazepam (Löscher & Schmidt 1987) can elevate CSF GABA levels, which would counteract any trend toward a reduction in CSF GABA levels in patients with epilepsy. Two of the studies on mixed patient populations report a significant decrease in CSF GABA levels (Wood et al 1979, Manyam et al 1980), while the CSF GABA levels are unaltered in remaining studies in Table 3.4 (Schmidt & Löscher 1982, Kuroda et al 1982, Manyam & Tremblay 1984, Crawford & Chadwick 1987). There is no difference in CSF GABA values between untreated patients or patients treated with antiepileptic drugs (Crawford & Chadwick 1987). An exceptionally low CSF GABA level (13 pmol/ml) has recently been reported for an infant with seizures due to pyridoxine deficiency. Following the administration of vitamin $B_6$ the seizures were blocked and the CSF GABA level restored to within normal control range (Kurlemann et al 1987).

Concerning the levels of other transmitter amino acids in the CSF: Mutani et al (1974) observe a dramatic decrease in the CSF glutamate level in a group with severe refractory epilepsy, detecting only trace levels of glutamate in their epileptic group, while their control glutamate level is the highest of the control glutamate levels reported above in Table 3.2. Plum (1974) reports *increased* aspartate and glutamate levels in the CSF of the epileptic patients; Engelsen & Elsayed (1984) also report increased CSF aspartate levels in epileptic patients. A case study of a single infant with severe intractable neonatal seizures likewise reports very high aspartate levels in the CSF (compared to controls in the literature, Weitz et al 1981). An increased level of excitatory amino acids in the CSF might reflect an increased release of these transmitters as discussed above.

## SUMMARY

Analysis of brain tissue, CSF and plasma from epileptic patients yields no unequivocal biochemical 'marker' for epilepsy. Despite the strong pharmacological and electrophysiological case for an imbalance between excitatory and inhibitory amino acid transmitter systems in epileptic disorders, there are few metabolic clues as to the nature of the defect(s) giving rise to the epileptiform activity.

Many of the biochemical changes in brain or fluid from epileptic patients are probably a secondary consequence of physiological changes associated with epilepsy or of the antiepileptic therapy. However, some observations persist in a number of studies. A reduced CSF GABA level is associated with certain types of seizures and has a counterpart in animal species with genetically determined seizure susceptibility. A reduced synaptic release of GABA could underly both the epilepsy and the CSF abnormality. The reports of increased levels of excitatory amino acids in plasma, brain tissue and perhaps in the CSF of epileptic patients, combined with the evidence for upregulation of excitatory receptors and increased release of excitatory amino acid transmitters in experimental seizures, suggest that enhanced excitatory transmission may also contribute to some epileptic syndromes.

## REFERENCES


Abdul-Ghani A-S, Coutinho-Netto J, Bradford H F 1980 The action of γ-vinyl-GABA and γ-acetylenic-GABA on the resting and stimulated release of GABA in vivo. Brain Research 191: 471–481

Babb T L 1986 GABA-mediated inhibition in the ammon's horn and pre-subiculum in human temporal lobe epilepsy. In: Nisticò G, Morselli P L, Lloyd K G, Fariello R G, Engel Jr J (eds) Neurotransmitters, seizures and epilepsy, III. Raven Press, New York, p 293–299

Böhlen P, Huot S, Palfreyman M G 1979 The relationship between GABA concentrations in the brain and cerebrospinal fluid. Brain Research 167: 297–305

Bradford H F, Dodd P R 1976 Biochemistry and basic mechanisms in epilepsy. In: Davison A N (ed) Biochemical basis for neurological disease. Blackwell Scientific, London, p 114–167

Brooks B R 1980 Seizure-induced metabolic alterations in human cerebrospinal fluid. In: Wood J H (ed) Neurobiology of cerebrospinal fluid, vol I. Plenum Press, New York, p 237–257

Butler I J, Seifert W E, Ferkany J W, Vernon N L, Enna S J 1980 Neurochemical analysis of rat cisternal cerebrospinal fluid. In: Wood J H (ed) Neurobiology of cerebrospinal fluid, vol II. Plenum Press, New York, p 157–162

Chapman A G 1985 Cerebral energy metabolism and seizures. In: Pedley T A, Meldrum B S (eds) Recent advances in epilepsy, vol 2. Churchill Livingstone, Edinburgh, p 19–63

Chapman A G, Meldrum B S 1987 Epilepsy-prone mice. Genetically determined sound-induced seizures. In: Jobe P C, Laird H E (eds) Neurotransmitters and epilepsy. Humana Press, Clifton, New Jersey, p 9–40

Chapman A G, Meldrum B S, Siesjö B K 1977 Cerebral metabolic changes during prolonged epileptic seizures in rats. Journal of Neurochemistry 28: 1025–1035

Chapman A G, Westerberg E, Premachandra M, Meldrum B S 1984 Changes in regional neurotransmitter amino acid levels in rat brain during seizures induced by L-allylglycine, bicuculline, and kainic acid. Journal of Neurochemistry 43: 62–70
Chapman A G, Cheetham S C, Hart G P, Meldrum B S, Westerberg E 1985 Effects of two convulsant $\beta$-carboline derivatives, DMCM and $\beta$-CCM, on regional neurotransmitter amino acid levels and on in vitro D-[$^3$H]aspartate release in rodents. Journal of Neurochemistry 45: 370–381
Chapman A G, Faingold C L, Hart G P, Bowker H M, Meldrum B S 1986 Brain regional amino acid levels in seizure susceptible rats: changes related to sound-induced seizures. Neurochemistry International 8: 273–279
Chapman A G, Meldrum B S, Nanji N, Watkins J C 1987 Anticonvulsant action and biochemical effects in DBA/2 mice of CPP (3-(($\pm$)-2-carboxypiperazin-4-yl)-propyl-1-phosphonate) a novel N-methyl-D-aspartate antagonist. European Journal of Pharmacology 139: 91–96
Ciesielski L, Simler S, Mandel P 1981 Effect of repeated convulsive seizures on brain GABA levels. Neurochemical Research 6: 267–273
Collins R C 1986 Selective vulnerability of brain: new insight from the excitatory synapse. Metabolic Brain Disease 1: 231–240
Crawford P M, Chadwick D W 1987 GABA and amino acid concentrations in lumbar CSF in patients with treated and untreated epilepsy. Epilepsy Research 328–338
Davson H, Hollingsworth J G, Carey M B, Fernstermacher J D 1982 Ventriculo-cisternal perfusion of 12 amino acids in the rabbit. Journal of Neurobiology 13: 293–318
Davson H, Welch K, Segal M B 1987 The physiology and pathophysiology of the cerebrospinal fluid. Churchill Livingstone, Edinburgh
Dixon L M, Sherwin A, Olivier A, Andermann F, Quesney F, Andermann E, Robitaille Y, Kish S J 1987 Aspartate aminotransferase activity in actively spiking vs. non spiking human epileptic cerebral cortex. Neuroscience 22 Supplement: p S68
Dodd P R, Bradford H F, Abdul-Ghani A S, Cox D W G, Continho-Netto J 1980 Release of amino acids from chronic epileptic and subepileptic foci in vivo. Brain Research 193: 505–517
Engelsen B, Elsayed S 1984 Increased concentrations of aspartic acid in the cerebrospinal fluid of patients with epilepsy and trigeminal: an effect of medication? Acta Neurologica Scandinavica 70: 70–76
Enna S J, Ziegler M G, Lake C R, Wood J H, Brooks B R, Butler I J 1980 Cerebrospinal fluid $\gamma$-aminobutytic acid. In: Wood J H (ed) Neurobiology of cerebrospinal fluid, vol I. Plenum Press, New York, p 189–196
Fagg G E, Foster A C 1983 Amino acid neurotransmitters and their pathways in the mammalian central nervous system. Neuroscience 9: 701–719
Ferkany J W, Butler I J, Enna S J 1979 Effect of drugs on rat brain, cerebrospinal fluid and blood GABA content. Journal of Neurochemistry 33: 29–33
Ferraro T N, Manyam B V, Hare T A 1983 Further characterization of in vitro conditions appropriate for GABA determination in human CSF: Impact of acid deproteinization and freeze/thaw. Journal of Neurochemistry 41: 1057–1064
Fishman R A 1980 Cerebrospinal fluid in diseases of the nervous system. Saunders, Philadelphia
Frandsen A, Belhage B, Schousboe A 1987 Differences between seizure-prone and non-seizure-prone mice with regard to glutamate and GABA receptor binding in the hippocampus and other regions of the brain. Epilepsy Research 1: 107–113
Gjessing L R, Gjesdahl P, Dietrichson P, Presthus J 1974 Free amino acids in the cerebrospinal fluid in old age and in Parkinson's disease. European Neurology 12: 33–37
Glaeser B S, Mahler T J, Wurtman R J 1983 Changes in brain levels of acidic, basic, and neutral amino acids after consumption of single meals containing various proportions of protein. Journal of Neurochemistry 41: 1016–1021
Green A R, Vincent N D 1987 The effect of repeated electroconvulsive shock on GABA synthesis and release in regions of rat brain. British Journal of Pharmacology 92: 19–24
Greenamyre J T 1986 The role of glutamate in neurotransmission and in neurologic disease. Archives of Neurology 43: 1058–1063
Grove J, Schechter P J, Tell G, Koch-Weser J, Sjoerdsma A, Warter J-M, Marescaux C, Rumbach L 1981 Increased gamma-aminobutyric acid (GABA), homocarnosine and $\beta$-alanine in cerebrospinal fluid of patients treated with $\gamma$-vinyl GABA (4-amino-hex-5-enoic acid). Life Science 28: 2431–2439
Grove J, Schechter P J, Tell G, Rumbach L, Marescaux C, Warter J-M, Koch-Weser J 1982a Artifactual increases in the concentration of free GABA in samples of human cerebrospinal fluid are due to degradation of homocarnosine. Journal of Neurochemistry 39: 1061–1065
Grove J, Schechter P J, Hanke N F J, de Smet Y, Agid Y, Tell G, Koch-Weser J 1982b Concentration gradients of free and total $\gamma$-aminobutyric acid and homocarnosine in human CSF: comparison of suboccipital and lumbar sampling. Journal of Neurochemistry 39: 1618–1622

Hagenfeldt L, Bjerkenstedt L, Edman G, Sedvall G, Wiesel F-A 1984 Amino acids in plasma and CSF and monoamine metabolites in CSF: interrelationship in healthy subjects. Journal of Neurochemistry 42: 833–837

Haines J L, Rich S S, Tsai M Y, Anderson V E 1985 Altered amino acid levels in multiply affected sibships with seizures. Epilepsia 26: 642–648

Halonen T O, Pitkänen A, Lehtinen M, Ylinen A, Riekkinen P J 1987 The effect of γ-vinyl GABA treatment on cholinergic and aminergic neurotransmission and on cyclic nucleotides in human complex partial epilepsy. Neuroscience 22 Supplement: S665

Hansen S, Perry T L, Wada J A, Sokol M 1973 Brain amino acids in baboon with light-induced epilepsy. Brain Research 50: 480–483

Hare T A 1981 Alterations of central GABAergic activity in neurologic and psychiatric disorders: evaluation through measurements of GABA and GAD activity in cerebrospinal fluid. Molecular and Cellular Biochemistry 39: 297–304

Hare T A, Manyam N V B, Glaeser B S 1980 Evaluation of cerebrospinal fluid γ-aminobutyric acid content in neurological and psychiatric disorders. In: Wood J H (ed) Neurobiology of cerebrospinal fluid, vol I. Plenum Press, New York, p 171–187

Hare T A, Wood J H, Manyam B V 1981 Clinical implications of enzyme-mediated alterations of γ-aminobutyric acid content of human CSF. Archives of Neurology 38: 491–494

Hare T A, Wood J H, Manyam B V, Gerner R H, Ballenger J C, Post R M 1982 Central nervous system γ-aminobutyric acid activity in man. Relationship to age and sex as reflected in CSF. Archives of Neurology 39: 247–249

Hertz L, Schousboe A, Formby L, Lennox-Buchthal M 1974 Some age-dependent biochemical changes in mice susceptible to seizures. Epilepsia 15: 619–631

Horton R W, Prestwich S A, Jazrawi S P 1984 Neurotransmitter binding in genetically seizure susceptible mice. In: Fariello R G, Morselli P L V, Lloyd K G, Quesney L F, Engel J Jr (eds) Neurotransmitters, seizures, and epilepsy, II. Raven Press, New York, p 191–199

Huxtable R J, Laird H, Lippincott S E, Walson P 1983 Epilepsy and the concentrations of plasma amino acids in humans. Neurochemistry International 5: 125–135

Huxtable R J, Bonhaus B, Lehmann A 1986 Excitatory and inhibitory amino acids in the genetically seizure-susceptible rat. In: Nisticò G, Morselli P L, Lloyd K G, Fariello R G, Engel Jr J (eds) Neurotransmitters, seizures and epilepsy, III. Raven Press, New York, p 369–383

Ito M, Mikawa H, Taniguchi T 1984 Cerebrospinal fluid GABA levels in children with infantile spasms. Neurology 34: 235–238

Jacobson, I, Hamberger A 1985 Kainic acid induced changes of extracellular amino acid levels, evoked potentials and EEG activity in rabbit olfactory bulb. Brain Research 348: 289–296

Jaeken J, Corbeal L, Casaer P, Carchon H, Eggermont E, Eeckels R 1977 Dipropylacetate (valproate) and glycine metabolism. Lancet II: 617

Janjua N J, Metrakos J D, van Gelder N M 1982 Plasma amino acids in epilepsy. In: Anderson V E, Hauser W A, Penry J K, Sing C F (eds) Genetic basis of the epilepsies. Raven Press, New York, p 181–197

Janjua N A, Andermann E, Eeg-Olofsson O, Metrakos K, Palmour R, Lemieux B, Giguère R 1986 Plasma glutamic acid elevation in epileptic patients and their relatives. Epilepsia 27: 615

Johansson B B, Lund S 1978 Effect of sympathetic stimulation on the blood-brain barrier dysfunction induced by amphetamines and by epileptic seizures. Acta Physiologica Scandinavica 104: 281–285

Killam E K, Killam K F Jr 1984 Evidence for neurotransmitter abnormalities related to seizure activity in the epileptic baboon. Federation Proceedings 43: 2510–2515

Knight M, Ebert J, Parish R A, Berry H, Fogelson M H 1985 γ-aminobutyric acid in CSF of children with febrile seizures. Archives of Neurology 42: 474–475

Kurlemann G, Löscher W, Dominick H C, Palm G D 1987 Disappearance of neonatal seizures and low CSF GABA levels after treatment with vitamine $B_6$. Epilepsy Research 1: 152–154

Kuroda H, Ogawa N, Yamawaki Y, Nukina I, Ofuji T, Yamamoto M, Otsuki S 1982 Cerebrospinal fluid GABA levels in various neurological and psychiatric diseases. Journal of Neurology, Neurosurgery, and Psychiatry 45: 257–260

Leach M J, Marden C M, Miller A A, O'Donnell R A, Weston S B 1985 Changes in cortical amino acids during electrical kindling in rats. Neuropharmacology 24: 937–940

Lehmann A, Isacsson H, Hamberger A 1983 Effects of in vivo administration of kainic acid on the extracellular amino acid pool in the rat hippocampus. Journal of Neurochemistry 40: 1314–1320

Levin V A, Fernstermacher J D, Patlak C S 1970 Sucrose and inulin space measurements of cerebral cortex in four mammalian species. American Journal of Physiology 219: 1528–1533

Lloyd K G, Munari C, Bossi L, Stoeffels C, Talairach J 1981 Biochemical evidence for the alterations of GABA-mediated synaptic transmission in pathological brain tissue (stereo EEG or morphological definition) from epileptic patients. In: Morselli P L, Lloyd K G, Löscher W, Meldrum B, Reynolds E H (eds) Neurotransmitters, seizures, and epilepsy. Raven Press, New York, p 325–334

Lloyd K G, Zivkovic B, Scatton B, Bartholini G 1984 Evidence for functional roles for GABA pathways in the mammalian brain. In: Bowery N G (ed) Actions and interactions of GABA and benzodiazepines. Raven Press, New York, p 59–79

Lloyd K G, Bossi L, Morselli P L, Rougier M, Loiseau P, Munari C 1985 Biochemical evidence for dysfunction of GABA neurons in human epilepsy. In: Bartholini G (ed) LERS, vol 3. Raven Press, New York, p 43–51

Lloyd K G, Scatton B, Voltz C, Bryere P, Valin A, Naquet R 1986a Cerebrospinal fluid amino acid and monoamine metabolite levels of *Papio papio*: correlation with photosensitivity. Brain Research 363: 390–394

Lloyd K G, Scatton B, Voltz C, Bryere P, Valin A, Naquet R 1986b Amino acid and monoamine metabolite levels in the CSF of Papio papio: correlation with photosensitive response. In: Nisticò G, Morselli P L, Lloyd K G, Fariello R G, Engel Jr J (eds) Neurotransmitters, seizures and epilepsy, III. Raven Press, New York, p 151–162

Löscher W 1982a GABA in plasma, CSF and brain of dogs during acute and chronic treatment with γ-acetylenic GABA and valproic acid. In: Okada Y, Roberts E (eds) Problems in GABA research from brain to bacteria. Excerpta Medica, Amsterdam, p 102–109

Löscher W 1982b Relationship between GABA concentrations in cerebrospinal fluid and seizure excitability. Journal of Neurochemistry 38: 293–295

Löscher W 1987 Hippocampal glutamate decarboxylase activity is not altered in gerbils with high seizure susceptibility. Biochemical Pharmacology 36: 979–982

Löscher W, Frey H-H 1984 Kinetics of penetration of common antiepileptic drugs into cerebrospinal fluid. Epilepsia 25: 346–352

Löscher W, Schmidt D 1980 Increase of human plasma GABA by sodium valproate. Epilepsia 21: 611–615

Löscher W, Schmidt D 1987 Diazepam increases γ-aminobutyric acid in human cerebrospinal fluid. Journal of Neurochemistry 49: 152–157

Löscher W, Schwartz-Porsche D 1986 Low levels of γ-aminobutyric acid in cerebrospinal fluid of dogs with epilepsy. Journal of Neurochemistry 46: 1322–1325

Löscher W, Siemes H 1985 Cerebrospinal fluid γ-aminobutyric acid levels in children with different types of epilepsy: effect of anticonvulsant treatment. Epilepsia 26: 314–319

Löscher W, Rating D, Siemes H 1981 GABA in cerebrospinal fluid of children with febrile convulsions. Epilepsia 22: 697–702

McGale E H F, Pye I F, Stonier C, Hutchinson E C, Aber G M 1977 Studies of the inter-relationship between cerebrospinal fluid and plasma amino acid concentrations in normal individuals. Journal of Neurochemistry 29: 291–297

Manyam B V, Tremblay R D 1984 Free and conjugated GABA in human cerebrospinal fluid: effect of degenerative neurologic diseases and isoniazid. Brain Research 307: 217–223

Manyam N V B, Katz L, Hare T A, Gerber J C, Grossman M H 1980 Levels of γ-aminobutyric acid in cerebrospinal fluid in various neurologic disorders. Archives of Neurology 37: 352–355

Meldrum B S 1976 Neuropathology and neurophysiology. In: Laidlaw J, Richens A (eds) A textbook of epilepsy. Churchill Livingstone, Edinburgh, p 314–354

Meldrum B S 1981 Epilepsy. In: Davison A N, Thompson R H S (eds) The molecular basis of neuropathology. Edward Arnold, London, p 265–301

Meldrum B S 1982 Epilepsy. In: Crow T (ed) Disorders of neurohumoral transmission. Academic Press, New York, p 183–254

Meldrum B S 1985 GABA and other amino acids. In: Frey H H, Janz D (eds) Handbook of experimental pharmacology, vol 74. Springer, Berlin, p 153–188

Meldrum B S 1988 Initiation and neuroanatomical spread of seizure activity. In: Pedley T A, Meldrum B S (eds) Recent advances in epilepsy 4. Churchill Livingstone, Edinburgh, this volume

Meldrum B S, Chapman A G 1983 Excitatory amino acids and anticonvulsant drug action. In: Hertz L, Kvamme E, McGeer E G, Schousboe A (eds) Glutamine, glutamate, and GABA in the central nervous system. Liss, New York, p 625–641

Meldrum B S, Corsellis J A N 1984 Epilepsy. In: Adams J H, Corsellis J A N, Duchen L W (eds) Greenfield's Neuropathology, 4th edn. Edward Arnold, London, p 921–950

Mody I, Heinemann U 1987 NMDA receptors of dentate gyrus granulate cells participate in synaptic transmission following kindling. Science 326: 701–704

Monaco F, Mutani R, Durelli L, Delsedime M 1975 Free amino acids in serum of patients with epilepsy: significant increase in taurine. Epilepsia 16: 245–249

Mortensen P B, Kølvraa S, Christensen E 1980 Inbition of the glycine cleavage system: hyperglycinaemia and hyperglycinuria caused by valproic acid. Epilepsia 21: 563–569

Mutani R, Monaco F, Durelli L, Delsedime M 1974 Free amino acids in the cerebrospinal fluid of epileptic subjects. Epilepsia 15: 593–597

Ohisalo J J, Murros K, Fredholm B B, Hare T A 1983 Concentrations of γ-aminobutyric acid and adenosine in the CSF in progressive myoclonus epilepsy without Lafora's bodies. Archives of Neurology 40: 623–625

Oldendorf W H 1971 Brain uptake of radiolabeled amino acids, amines, and hexoses after arterial injection. American Journal of Physiology 221: 1629–1639

Olsen R W, Snowman A M, Lee R, Lomax P, Wamsley J K 1984 Role of the γ-aminobutyric acid receptor-ionophore complex in seizure disorders. Annals of Neurology 16 (suppl): s90–97

Olsen R W, Wamsley J K, McCabe R T, Lee R J, Lomax P, Seyfried T N 1986 Midbrain GABA receptor deficit in genetic animal models of epilepsy. In: Nisticò G, Morselli P L, Lloyd K G, Fariello R G, Engel Jr J (eds) Neurotransmitters, seizures and epilepsy, III. Raven Press, New York, p 279–291

Pardridge W M, Oldendorf W H 1977 Transport of metabolic substrates through the blood-brain barrier. Journal of Neurochemistry 28: 5–12

Perry T L, Hansen S 1969 Technical pitfalls leading to errors in the quantitation of plasma amino acids. Clinica Chimica Acta 25: 53–58

Perry T L, Hansen S 1981 Amino acid abnormalities in epileptogenic foci. Neurology 31: 872–876

Perry T L, Hansen S, Kennedy J, Wada J A, Thompson G B 1975 Amino acids in human epileptogenic foci. Archives of Neurology 32: 752–754

Perry T L, Hansen S, MacLean J 1976 Cerebrospinal fluid and plasma glutamine elevation by anticonvulsant drugs: a potential diagnostic and therapeutic trap. Clinica Chimica Acta 69: 441–445

Perry T L, Hansen S, Wall R A, Gauthier S G 1982 Human CSF GABA concentrations: revised downward for controls, but not decreased in Huntington's chorea. Journal of Neurochemistry 38: 766–773

Plum C M 1974 Free amino acid levels in the cerebrospinal fluid of normal humans and their variation in cases of epilepsy and Spielmeyer–Vogt–Batten disease. Journal of Neurochemistry 23: 595–600

Plum C M 1975 Renal handling of free amino acids in normal adults, in patients with epilepsy, and in patients with Spielmeyer–Vogt–Batten disease. Danish Medical Bulletin 22: 194–201

Price M T, Pusateri M E, Crow S E, Buchsbaum S, Olney J W, Lowry O H 1984 Uptake of oxogenous aspartate into circumventricular organs but not other regions of adult mouse brain. Journal of Neurochemistry 42: 740–744

Rao A, Baliga L, Raja A, Rao S N 1983 Urinary excretion of taurine in epilepsy. Acta Neurologica Scandinavia 68: 421–423

Rating D, Siemes H, Löscher W 1983 Low CSF GABA concentration in children with febrile convulsions, untreated epilepsy, and meningitis. Journal of Neurology 230: 217–225

Reiffenstein R J, Ruiz G T, Dyun M, Mele F, Ribak C E 1987 Amino acid increases in inferior colliculus of genetically epilepsy-prone rats (GEPR). Neuroscience 22 Supplement: S69

Ribak C E 1986 Neurocytology and chemistry of focal epilepsy. In: Pedley T A, Meldrum B S (eds) Recent advances in epilepsy, 3. Churchill Livingstone, Edinburgh, p 1–20

Riekkinen P J, Ylinen A, Halonen T, Silvenius J, Pitkänen A 1987 Relationship of GABA levels in CSF to clinical improvement during γ-vinyl-GABA treatment in complex partial epilepsy. Neuroscience 22 Supplement: p S68

Roberts R C, Ribak C, Oertel W H 1985 Increased number of GABAergic neurons occur in the inferior colliculus of an audiogenic model of genetic epilepsy. Brain Research 361: 324–338

Rougier A, LLoyd K G, Loiseau H, Morselli P L, Loiseau P 1987 Amino acids in human epileptic foci. Abstract, 17th Epilepsy International Congress, Jerusalem, September 6–11

Schechter P J 1986 Vigabatrin. In: Meldrum B S, Porter R J (eds) New anticonvulsant drugs. Libbey, London, p 265–275

Schechter P J, Hanke N F J, Grove J, Huebert N, Sjoerdsma A 1984 Biochemical and clinical effects of γ-vinyl-GABA in patients with epilepsy. Neurology 34: 182–186

Schmidt D, Löscher W 1981 GABA concentrations in cerebrospinal fluid and plasma of patients with epileptic seizures. In: Morselli P L, Lloyd K G, Löscher W, Meldrum B, Reynolds E H (eds) Neurotransmitters, seizures, and epilepsy. Raven Press, New York, p 315–322

Schmidt D, Löscher W 1982 Plasma and cerebrospinal fluid γ-aminobutryic acid in neurological disorders. Journal of Neurology, Neurosurgery, and Psychiatry 45: 931–935

Schmidt D, Cornaggia C, Löscher W 1984 Comparative studies of the GABA system in neurosurgical brain specimens of epileptic and non-epileptic patients. In: Fariello R G, Morselli P L, Lloyd K G, Quesney L F, Engel Jr J (eds) Neurotransmitters, seizures and epilepsy, II. Raven Press, New York, p 275–282

Schwarcz R, Meldrum B 1985 Excitatory amino acid antagonists provide a therapeutic approach to neurological disorders. Lancet, July 20, p 140–143

Sherwin A L, van Gelder N M 1986 Amino acid and catecholamine markers of metabolic abnormalities in human focal epilepsy. In: Delgado-Escueta A V, Ward Jr A A, Woodbury D M (eds) Advances in neurology, 44. Raven Press, New York, p 1011–1032

Sherwin A, Quesney F, Gauthier S et al 1984 Enzyme changes in actively spiking areas of human epileptic cerebral cortex. Neurology 34: 927–933
Sherwin A, Olivier A, Quesney F et al 1986a Glutamate and aspartate but not GABA or taurine concentrations are elevated in actively spiking versus nonspiking human epileptic cerebral cortex. Neurology 37 (Suppl 1): 247
Sherwin A, Matthew E, Blain M, Guévremont D 1986b Benzodiazepine receptor binding is not altered in human epileptogenic cortical foci. Neurology 36: 1380–1382
Siesjö B K 1978 Brain energy metabolism. Wiley, Chichester
Sloviter R S, Dempster D W 1985 'Epileptic' brain damage is replicated qualitatively in rat hippocampus by central injection of glutamate or aspartate but not by GABA or acetylcholine. Brain Research Bulletin 15: 39–60
Squires R, Naquet R, Riche D, Braestrup C 1979 Increased thermolability of benzodiazepine receptors in cerebral cortex of a baboon with spontaneous seizures: a case report. Epilepsia 20: 215–221
Van Gelder N M, Sherwin A L, Rasmussen T 1972 Amino acid content of epileptogenic human brain: focal versus surrounding regions. Brain Research 40: 385–393
Van Gelder N M, Janjua N A, Metrakos K, MacGibbon B, Metrakos J D 1980a Plasma amino acids in 3/sec spike-wave epilepsy. Neurochemical Research 5: 659–671
Van Gelder N M, Edmonds H J Jr, Hegreberg G A, Chatburn C C, Clemmons R M, Sylvester D M 1980b Amino acid changes in a genetic strain of epileptic beagle dogs. Journal of Neurochemistry 35: 1087–1091
Wade J V, Samson F E, Nelson S R, Pazdernik T L 1987 Changes in extra-cellular amino acids during soman- and kainic acid-induced seizures. Journal of Neurochemistry 49: 645–650
Weitz R, Merlob P, Amir J, Reisner S H 1981 A possible role for aspartic acid in neonatal seizures. Archives of Neurology 38: 258–259
Westergaard E, Hertz M M, Bolwig T G 1978 Increased permeability to horseradish peroxidase across cerebral vessels, evoked by electrically induced seizures in the rat. Acta Neuropathologica Berlin 41: 73–80
Wood J H, Brooks B R 1980 Neurotransmitter, metabolite, and cyclic nucleotide alterations in cerebrospinal fluid of seizure patients. In: Wood J H (ed) Neurobiology of cerebrospinal fluid, vol I. Plenum Press, New York, p 259–278
Wood J H, Hare T A, Glaeser B S, Ballenger J C, Post R M 1979 Low cerebrospinal fluid $\gamma$-aminobutyric acid content in seizure patients. Neurology 29: 1203–1208
Wurtman R J, Rose C M, Chou C, Larin F F 1968 Daily rhythms in the concentrations of various amino acids in human plasma. New England Journal of Medicine 279: 171–175
Young A M J, Bradford H F 1986 Excitatory amino acid neurotransmitters in the corticostriatal pathway: studies using intracerebral microdialysis in vivo. Journal of Neurochemistry 47: 1399–1404

# 4. The role of the electroencephalogram in the diagnosis and management of epilepsy

*A. J. Rowan J. A. French*

Since its earliest days, the electroencephalogram (EEG) has been the most important diagnostic test in epilepsy. It was quickly realized that the recorded paroxysms in epileptic patients confirmed Jackson's concept, put forward in 1873, that epilepsy is 'the name for occasional, sudden, excessive, rapid and local discharges of grey matter.' In recent years, owing largely to the efforts of The Epilepsy Branch of the NINCDS, intense research efforts into the nature and phenomenology of epilepsy, as well as new approaches to therapeutics, have been undertaken. In most of these efforts, the EEG has played a central role.

This chapter will explore some of the major areas in which the EEG has furthered our understanding of epilepsy and allowed new concepts to be applied to everyday management. In particular, we will discuss how maximum information can be obtained from a routine study in the EEG laboratory. We will give guidelines of what can be expected from the EEG in terms of sensitivity and specificity in the diagnosis of epilepsy. Prognosis will be explored, as well as the role of the EEG in treating and following an epileptic patient. Finally, we will discuss applications of newer EEG technology such as ambulatory monitoring, intensive monitoring, and depth studies.

## THE STANDARD EEG: OBTAINING MAXIMUM YIELD

As in any laboratory test, the value of the EEG depends on an understanding of its limits as well as methods of maximizing the probability of obtaining useful information. Of critical importance is the quality of the recording, and this is largely dependent on the training and competence of the EEG technologist. EEG technology is a highly specialized field and requires not only in-depth training but also considerable experience in order to produce interpretable tracings. For example, the head must be accurately measured and electrodes carefully applied. Moreover, a clear understanding of the machine controls, the clinical question to be answered, and the ability to obtain maximum patient cooperation and relaxation are factors associated with excellence of the EEG write-out. Only under such circumstances can an electroencephalographer render an accurate interpretation.

Several activation techniques may be used to increase the likelihood of obtaining positive results in the standard laboratory. Hyperventilation and photic stimulation are routine procedures. If the EEG is unrevealing despite the use of these techniques, special studies may be done utilizing sleep deprivation or special electrodes. Below is a discussion of these various methods.

### Duration of recording

Theoretically, if one records for an indefinite period of time, the EEG would be abnormal in all patients with epilepsy. It has been shown that the yield of epileptiform discharges improves with increased recording time, as for example in long-term telemetric or ambulatory EEG monitoring (vide infra). In the EEG laboratory, however, routine studies do not last longer than 1 h, and in many laboratories 20 min EEGs are commonplace. We recommend that a routine waking EEG has a duration of not less than 30 min, and preferably 60 min.

**Hyperventilation**

Hyperventilation (HV) is routine in most EEG laboratories, and for good reason. It is particularly valuable for producing de novo activation of epileptiform activity, especially in the generalized epilepsies, and may enhance pre-existing abnormalities in generalized as well as partial epilepsies. HV should be performed with deep, regular respirations, exaggerating the phase of expiration, at a rate of about 20/min (Takahashi et al 1982). This produces a rapid reduction in blood $CO_2$, leading to progressive cerebral arterial constriction, and a parallel decrease in cortical blood flow (Meyer & Gotoh 1960).

In most healthy adults, HV produces either no change, or diffuse background slowing, which may last up to 3 min after HV has ceased. In children, the reponse usually consists of high voltage delta activity, maximal in the frontal regions. This may appear quite paroxysmal and must not be mistaken for epileptiform activity. The magnitude of change during HV may also be influenced by metabolic disturbances such as hypoglycemia, which may exaggerate or prolong the response. If changes persist in an adult for longer than 5 min after cessation of HV, blood sugar levels should be obtained.

The most significant activation occurs in patients with absence seizures (petit mal epilepsy). The vast majority of untreated patients will have typical 3 Hz spike-wave paroxysms during adequately performed HV. This can be diagnostic in patients with normal baseline records.

The partial epilepsies do not show as much effect. Miley & Forster (1977) reported that 11% of patients with complex partial seizures had activation of the EEG during HV. Clinical seizures occurred in 4%, over one third of whom had no paroxysmal discharges in the resting record. In a varied group of patients with clinical seizures other than absence, Morgan & Scott (1970) found new paroxysmal abnormalities in 7% of patients with no such activity prior to activation.

In general, great care must be used not to over-read responses to HV. Only spike-wave, sharp-slow wave complexes, or clear focal or lateralizing changes should be taken as unequivocally abnormal (Kellaway 1979).

The hyperventilation response depends on reactive cerebral arteries and good effort, and little additional information will be obtained in the elderly. We therefore do not recommend HV in patients over the age of 65. Although it is a generally safe procedure, it should not be attempted in patients with subarachnoid hemorrhage, intracerebral hemorrhage or cardiopulmonary disease (Klass & Daly 1979).

**Photic stimulation**

During photic stimulation, an intense intermittent light stimulus is delivered to a patient's visual field. This usually produces low voltage waves in the occipital regions, linked to flash rate, termed the following (or driving) response. Although photic stimulation is usually performed on all patients during a routine EEG, it may not be useful in non-epileptic patients (Coull & Pedley 1978). In patients with known epilepsy, however, the procedure may add important information.

Several types of responses to photic stimulation are possible (Newmark & Penry 1979, Jeavons 1982).

1. *Photomyoclonic response:* seen only in the anterior head regions. Spikes occur at the flash frequency, associated with twitching and jerking about the eyes.

2. *Occipital spikes:* seen only in the posterior head regions. These occur at flash frequency, or as a subharmonic response (one-half flash frequency).

3. *Photoconvulsive responsive:* generalized spike-wave discharges, usually at about 3 Hz, maximal in the fronto-central regions and at the vertex. This response usually outlasts the stimulus and is more common with eyes open than closed. However, it is often seen at the time of eye closure. Patterned stimuli and red color also enhance the response. The photoconvulsive response may be accompanied by a myoclonic jerk, and may proceed to a clinical convulsion.

The first two responses may be seen in patients with and without epilepsy, and are of uncertain diagnostic significance. The photoconvulsive response, however, has a high correlation with clinical epilepsy. It does occur in some normal subjects, but frequently there is a family history of generalized epilepsy. In fact, the photoconvulsive response appears to be a marker of genetic lowering of the convulsive threshold, and is usually associated with the primary generalized epilepsies including absence epilepsy, myoclonic epilepsy of Janz (juvenile myoclonic epilepsy), and primarily generalized tonic-clonic convulsions. Patients with other types of epilepsy may also show this response, but this is presumed to be due to secondary factors superimposed on a lower seizure threshold. A photoconvulsive response has been found in about 25% of patients with primary generalized epilepsy, and in 1.4–4% of non-epileptic subjects (Jeavons & Harding 1975). The response is most commonly seen in children between the ages of 6 and 15 years old (Doose et al 1969).

Findings that invariably are associated with clinical epilepsy are polyspike-wave discharges and clinical absence attacks induced by photic stimulation. Also highly correlated with epilepsy is a photo-convulsive response accompanied by a myoclonic jerk (Jeavons 1982). If the photoconvulsive response outlasts the stimulus, the patient has a 90% chance of having a history of epilepsy (Reilly & Peters 1973). Only 51% of patients with responses that end during a stimulus train, or at the termination of the stimulus, have such a history.

If a photoconvulsive response is associated with a history of seizures after exposure to flickering light, the patient has photosensitive epilepsy. This condition is age-specific, frequently occuring after puberty, and abating by the age of 30. The diagnosis may be suspected by a history of seizures at discotheques, when driving along a tree-lined highway during times when the sun is low, or while riding on trains or subways. It is important to confirm this diagnosis, as photosensitive epilepsy is effectively treated with valproate.

Photic stimulation should be carried out over a wide range of frequencies. Although 96% of photosensitive patients will show a response to flash rates between 15–20 Hz (Jeavons & Harding 1975), others may be sensitive at higher or lower frequencies.

An attempt should be made to locate the frequency range in which the patient is sensitive, and each frequency should be tested with eyes open and closed. If a photoconvulsive response is elicited, the stimulus should be discontinued immediately to reduce the risk of seizure provocation.

## Sleep

If natural sleep can be obtained during a routine EEG, it may be valuable for uncovering epileptiform activity. Usually during a routine record the patient will only attain non-REM sleep stages. Fortunately, these frequently are the most fruitful in a search for abnormalities (Niedermeyer 1982). An increase in discharges may occur in patients with generalized as well as partial epilepsies. It is important to recognize that the morphology of epileptiform discharges may be altered during drowsiness and sleep. For example, a patient who has classical 3/sec spike-wave during wakefulness will frequently have irregular polyspike-wave bursts during sleep (Sato et al 1973). The distribution of discharges may also change. An example of this would be a patient with a focal spike abnormality on the waking record, but bilateral, independent or multifocal spikes during sleep (Gabor & Seyal 1986).

### *Sleep deprivation and sedated sleep*

It has long been known that sleep deprivation may lead to activation of seizures and may occasionally induce seizures in otherwise healthy adults (Bennett 1963). Most investigators have found sleep deprivation to be of value in activating epileptiform discharges in patients whose routine EEG studies were either normal or questionably abnormal. Mattson et al (1965) found the EEGs were activated in 34% of patients with normal resting records who had unequivocal histories of epilepsy. In patients with previously abnormal EEGs, 56% became qualitatively or quantitatively more abnormal after sleep deprivation. Similar results were reported by Pratt et al (1968), Geller et al (1969) and Scollo-Lavizzari et al (1975). Arne-Bes et al (1982) found new localizing information after sleep deprivation in 32% of adults and 28% of children, and Rowan et al (1982) found either a new type of discharge or an additional focus in 7%. In some instances activation occurred only during wakefulness (Pratt et al 1968, Spadetta 1971), although usually the most prominent activation occurred during sleep stages I and II (Veldhuizen et al 1983, Bechinger & Kornhuber 1973, Degen & Degen 1984). A history of seizures related to sleep deprivation does not appear to be necessary to see activation of the EEG (Pratt et al 1968), and age does not play a role (Pratt et al 1968, Arne-Bes et al 1982). In addition, antiepileptic drugs do not appear to interfere with the effect (Degen & Degen 1984).

Sleep deprivation appears to be effective in activating discharges in patients with all seizure types, both generalized and partial (Ellingson et al 1984).

Sleep deprivation for 24 h or more is considered by most patients to be a difficult and disrupting task, and alternatives have been proposed. Some authors feel that sleep deprivation provides no advantage over natural sleep (Veldhuizen et al 1983, Degen & Degen 1984). Other centers use the 'forced nap' as an activation technique, in which a hypnotic drug is administered to patients who have not slept more than 4–5 h the previous night, followed by a sleep recording of 40–60 min. With this technique activation was observed in 62% of patients (Gastaut et al 1984), a figure that compares favourably with studies of 24-h sleep deprivation. Sedated sleep is another alternative, but it has not proved as effective. Rowan et al (1982) found new or additional information in only 14% of patients after sedated sleep, compared with 44% after sleep deprivation. Sedated sleep, however, provided useful information in 12% when sleep deprivation did not. In children, partial sleep deprivation is usually employed, and has been found to be effective (Ellingson et al 1984). Few studies have been done in adults, but Kubicki et al (1984) found activation in 54% of patients using this technique.

In summary, sleep deprivation is a useful technique to increase diagnostic yield in patients with known or suspected epilepsy. If sleep deprivation is difficult for a given patient, or if both routine and sleep deprived studies have been normal, a sedated sleep record may add further information. If all these techniques are used, success in recording discharges may be expected in up to 90% of patients with epilepsy.

**Additional electrodes**

We have discussed several methods to increase the yield of epileptiform activity in the EEG. There are, however, areas of the cerebral cortex from which it is difficult to record with the standard array of electrodes used in the 10–20 international system, most notably the basal portion of the temporal lobe. Several methods have been devised to demonstrate epileptiform discharges from this area.

*Nasopharyngeal electrodes*

Nasopharyngeal (NP) electrodes were first introduced in the late 1940's. Although initially constructed as rigid, curved rods, they now are available as fine, flexible coated wires. NP electrodes are introduced through the nostrils and come to rest against the mucous membrane of the nasopharynx, in close proximity to the middle fossa. This places the recording tip near the basal portion of the temporal lobe. This, and the fact that there is an increase in inter-electrode distance, may play a role in their effectiveness. Several studies have shown that NP leads have detected infero-mesial spike foci that were not appreciated on surface recording. De Jesus & Masland (1970), for example, found crucial abnormalities during NP recording in 7 of 1100 patients, none of whom had clear epileptiform activity on the routine EEG. An additional 28 had a more definitive abnormality during NP recording than on routine EEG. On the other hand, Dinner & Lüders (1985) noted that it was unusual to see epileptiform discharges *only* at the NP electrodes, although frequently the abnormality was better defined. There are drawbacks to NP recording. Many patients experience discomfort during and after introduction. Also, they are difficult if not impossible to introduce in patients with nasal septal irregularities, and are susceptible to pulse (from the carotid arteries), muscle, respiration and swallowing artifacts.

*Sphenoidal electrodes*

Sphenoidal electrodes have been in use since the late 1940's and, due to technical improvements, are relatively easy to insert. They may remain in place for up to 3 weeks during long-term EEG recording (Ives & Gloor 1977). The electrodes consist of multi-stranded wires which are inserted through the lumen of a spinal needle. The needle is advanced beneath the zygomatic arch until the tip lies at a point near the foramen ovale. The needle is then withdrawn, leaving the fine wire in place (King et al 1986). If properly inserted, artifacts are few, and the electrodes are well tolerated.

Complications are rare. There is one report of a broken wire, but this occurred before the technique of silver/silver chloriding the electrodes came into use (Ives & Gloor 1977). Local bleeding has been observed, but this also is rare.

Sphenoidal electrodes have proved useful for evaluation of patients with a history suspicious of complex partial seizures without a clear EEG abnormality. Several studies indicate that 30–50% of these patients may have abnormalities during sphenoidal recording that do not appear on the simultaneous surface recording (Pampiglione & Kerridge 1956, Christodoulou 1967, Kristensen & Sindrup 1978). Sphenoidal recordings are superior to those made using nasopharyngeal electrodes. In a study by Marcus et al (1984), 3 of 11 patients with simultaneous NP and sphenoidal electrodes had epileptiform discharges exclusively from the sphenoidal leads.

Patients evaluated for temporal lobectomy require more precise localization of discharges than can be obtained with surface electrodes alone (Rovit et al 1961, Christodoulou 1967). In some centers, information derived from sphenoidal electrodes may obviate the need for depth electrode studies (King et al 1986).

*Low anterior temporal electrodes*

Recently there has been renewed interest in the utilization of low anterior temporal electrodes, first described by Silverman in 1960. These electrodes, termed $T_1$ and $T_2$, are placed inferior and posterior to the $F_7$ and $F_8$ (anterior temporal) electrodes of the 10–20 international system. Sperling & Engel (1985), believe that these electrodes precisely overlie the anterior and inferior aspect of the temporal lobe. In a recent study by these authors, $T_1$ and $T_2$ electrodes were found, in combination with ear electrodes, to be equivalent in sensitivity to NP electrodes, and superior for purposes of localization.

In summary, it is unlikely that NP electrodes provide a clear advantage over less invasive techniques for recording from the mesial-basal surfaces of the temporal lobes. Low anterior temporal electrodes are easily applied and will record mesial temporal spikes in most patients. Sphenoidal electrodes may be required, but their use should be reserved for patients in whom there is a strong suspicion of a temporal lobe focus in spite of repeatedly normal routine and sleep deprivation recordings. They are also useful for localization in patients being evaluated for temporal lobe surgery.

## SENSITIVITY AND SPECIFICITY OF THE EEG IN EPILEPSY

The physician is often confronted with the problem of diagnosing single or recurrent episodes of altered consciousness, falling, motor activity, or subjective symptoms which could be manifestations of seizure activity. Such symptoms are distressing becaue of their sudden and unexpected onset. The patient fears loss of control, and may worry that something is wrong with his brain or mind. In some instances, the reported events may be well described and recognizable, leading to a relatively confident diagnosis on clinical grounds alone. More often, episodes are vaguely or incompletely reported due to the patient's lack of awareness of what has happened, or the inability of observers to describe accurately what they have seen. The same applies to experienced physicians. One of our favorite teaching techniques is to show a videotape of various clinical seizures to a group of neurologists, having them write down everything they saw after a single viewing. It should come as no surpirse that their descriptions not only vary widely, but are usually inaccurate with respect to details of phenomenology and duration of events. Moreover, when shown a series of seizures, some of which are epileptic while others are psychogenic, their ability to differentiate the two is often poor. This results not so much from lack of ability as it does from the wide variety of overlapping manifestations and the rapidity with which seizures progress. This highlights the problem faced by the physician in the consulting room. Thus, reliance on descriptive material alone is full of pitfalls and invites misdiagnosis. It is true that a typical *grand mal* convulsion may be suspected from the description of any reasonable observer. On the other hand, the complex partial seizure is extremely difficult to describe and may simulate a variety of non-epileptic events.

Although the laboratory evaluation of these patients will include a number of tests including blood and imaging studies, in most cases the EEG is the most important study. However, the diagnosis of epilepsy cannot be established on the basis of EEG findings alone unless a clinical event occurs during EEG recording, a so-called ictal EEG. In this case, the presence of electrographic seizure activity during the event is diagnostic. Conversely, the absence of electrographic seizure activity during a recorded event excludes with a reasonable degree of certainty the diagnosis of epilepsy. Unfortunately, in the majority of clinical situations only an EEG recorded between seizures, the interictal EEG, is available. The findings from such a record will not be diagnostic, but may provide convincing support for the clinical suspicion.

EEG support for a diagnosis of epilepsy depends primarily on the demonstration of epileptiform activity. In its strict definition, epileptiform activity consists of spike or spike-wave discharges, although in many cases this may be extended to the presence of sharp waves, episodic rhythmic slow or fast frequencies, and other clearly episodic phenomena. Studies which report the occurrence of epileptiform activity in groups or populations should indicate what definition is employed. For example, those reporting only the incidence of spike discharges may not be comparable to those reporting the incidence of 'paroxysmal activity'.

**EEG abnormalities in the non-epileptic population**

The presence of epileptiform activity cannot be assumed to support a clinical diagnosis of epilepsy without knowledge of the incidence of such activity in persons without epilepsy. This incidence has been reported to be between 0.0 and 3.8% (Gastaut & Tassinari 1975, Iida et al 1985). Variation among studies depends largely on two factors. The first is the definition of epileptiform activity. In addition to issues already mentioned, studies vary in their reporting of non-epileptogenic patterns. These are defined as patterns that resemble epileptiform discharges, but are frequently found in normal subjects and are not thought to have clinical significance. They include small sharp spikes, wicket spikes, 14 and 6/sec positive spikes, and 6 Hz spike-wave pattern (phantom spike-wave). Although some authors have considered one or more of these patterns to be related in some way to epilepsy, no convincing evidence exists of such an association. An excellent discussion of this subject can be found in a review by Klass & Westmoreland (1985). Studies that include these patterns as epileptiform will tend to overestimate the incidence of abnormalities in normal subjects.

A second factor in the evaluation of incidence studies is the nature of the population. Ideally, a population should be chosen that is free of any past or present illness or condition affecting the brain. The subjects of the study should have careful histories and neurological examinations including inquiry into factors surrounding pregnancy, delivery, perinatal factors, growth and development, and the like. Any deviation of what is recognized as normal would be reason for exclusion. The same would apply to a family history of epilepsy. To our knowledge, such a study has not been done. Instead, studies usually involve review of EEG records of inpatients or outpatients who do not have epilepsy, but who were referred to the laboratory because of other suspected cerebral pathology, thus placing the label 'normal' in doubt.

With this as backgound, the following series are of interest. Iida et al (1985) studied an outpatient population referred for EEG because of various complaints including headache, dizziness and fainting spells. After exclusion of small sharp spikes and positive spikes, they found a 5.8% incidence of epileptiform activity. In a follow-up period of 1 to 13 years, 3 of 202 subjects (1.5%) developed epilepsy, a figure close to the prevalence of epilepsy in large populations. Gibbs & Gibbs (1964) reported a 1.4% incidence of epileptiform discharges in adult patients without epilepsy. Zivin & Ajmone-Marsan (1968) studied an inpatient medical population and found a 2.2% incidence of epileptiform discharges. Even in these patients, many of whom had progressive illnesses involving the central nervous system, only 14% subsequently developed clinical seizures. Cavazzuti et al (1980) performed EEGs on 3726 normal school children and found epileptiform patterns in 3.5%, a figure nearly equal to the number of children in the same area with epilepsy; of the 3.5%, only 6.4% subsequently had clinical seizures. Thus, the available data, while imperfect, suggest that the incidence of epileptiform activity in normals is very low. However, the risk of developing epilepsy when such patterns are present is correspondingly low, perhaps little different than the general prevalence of epilepsy itself.

Although it is true that nearly every type of epileptiform discharge may be seen in persons without epilepsy, some patterns correlate more clearly with clinical disease. For example, the pattern of hypsarrhythmia, a continuous, high voltage admixture of spikes and slow waves, has a nearly 100% correlation with clinical seizures. In contrast, the central-midtemporal spike discharge, found in patients with Rolandic seizures, and the occipital spike discharge, have only a 50% correlation with epilepsy (Westmoreland 1985). Similarly, 37% of siblings of children with absence attacks (*petit mal* epilepsy) demonstrate 3 Hz spike-wave discharges, whereas only 13% have clinical evidence of epilepsy (Metrakos & Metrakos 1961).

Patterns resembling ictal discharges may occur rarely in patients without clinical epilepsy. Westmoreland & Klass (1981) described a subclinical rhythmic EEG discharge of adults (SREDA). The pattern was seen in patients not suspected of having epilepsy. Close observation during the discharge failed to reveal clinical signs of seizure activity. Although morphologically impressive, SREDA is not known to have specific diagnostic significance.

## Epilepsy and the normal EEG

In a retrospective study of patients with undoubted epilepsy, Ajmone-Marsan & Zivin (1970) found that 55% of initial EEG tracings showed no epileptiform activity. However, repeated tracings performed over the ensuing year reduced the figure to 8%. Negative tracings were associated with older age at the time of study, older age of seizure onset, and a history of head trauma. Patients with temporal lobe epilepsy were more likely to have at least one tracing containing epileptiform discharges. Of interest was the observation that seizure frequency bore little relationship to the chance of having a negative tracing.

A more recent study by Salinsky et al (1987) studied the probability of finding interictal epileptiform discharges in patients with a clinical diagnosis of epilepsy if serial EEGs were performed. Sleep was achieved in 67% of first EEGs and in all subsequent EEGs. In 50% of patients, epileptiform activity was present on the first EEG, in 84% by the third and in 92% by the fourth EEG. It would thus seem that while about half of patients with epilepsy may have a normal first EEG, multiple EEGs substantially increase the yield of 'positive' tracings. However, Salinsky et al (1987) found that the probability of discovering new epileptiform activity, while initially high, decreased continuously with subsequent recordings, and that if 4 consecutive routine EEGs were normal, more were unlikely to be productive.

## RISK OF EPILEPSY AFTER FIRST SEIZURE—PREDICTIVE VALUE OF THE EEG

Epilepsy may be defined as a chronic, non-progressive condition characterized by one major symptom—recurrent seizures. A single seizure, therefore, is insufficient for a diagnosis of epilepsy. Over 50% of adults and 40–50% of children will never experience another attack (Johnson et al 1972, Blom et al 1978, Hauser et al 1982, Hirtz et al 1984, Camfield et al 1985). The occurrence of a second seizure is dependent on a number of factors including the presence of cerebral damage, age at seizure onset, and family history. Many studies have tried to evaluate the role of the EEG as a predictive factor. Unfortunately, there is no consistency among the studies which makes comparison of data difficult. For example, the age of the population studied is an important variable. Different EEG prognostic factors were found in studies that evaluated children and adults separately (Johnson et al 1972, Blom et al 1978, Camfield et al 1985) than in those that studied patients of all ages and evaluated EEG data as a whole (Hauser et al 1982, Annegers et al 1986). Other variables include the interval betweent the EEG study and the last seizure, and whether or not activation procedures such as sleep or hyperventilation were used routinely.

### Children

In children, EEG abnormalities seem to be somewhat predictive of seizure recurrence. Aass et al (1956) found that 31% of children with normal EEGs had recurrent seizures, compared with 75% whose EEGs were abnormal. However, 31% of these children had febrile seizures, a group more likely to have normal EEGs with no seizure recurrence (vide infra). Aass et al (1956) also noted that 23 of 24 children with organic cerebral disorders had abnormal EEGs and a correspondingly high incidence of recurrent seizures.

Blom et al (1978) found no definitive EEG criteria for predicting which patients might develop epilepsy after a single seizure; however, some specific factors were of interest. Patients with vaguely described seizures were more likely to have normal EEGs and were less likely to develop epilepsy, whereas those with typical 3 Hz spike-wave discharges or central-midtemporal spikes were more likely to have further seizures as compared to the group as a whole.

Camfield et al (1985), in a retrospective study that excluded children with febrile seizures, acute infections and absence attacks, found seizure recurrence in 41% of children with non-epileptiform EEGs. Recurrence rate increased to 60% in those with generalized spike-wave discharges, and to 68% in those with focal discharges.

## Adults

In studies of adults or populations of mixed ages, the EEG also appears to have predictive value. Hauser et al (1982) found a significantly higher recurrence rate in patients with generalized spike-wave discharges than in those with normal or non-specific findings. Focal spikes and focal slowing, however, failed to predict a higher rate of recurrence. Similar findings were reported by Johnson et al (1972). Annegers et al (1986) and Cleland et al (1981) reported that an abnormal EEG, regardless of the type of abnormality, was associated with 100% increase in risk of seizure recurrence. Saunders & Marshall (1975), however, found no difference in the EEGs of patients with and without recurrence, but this study involved only a small number of subjects.

In summary, children with first seizures and abnormal EEGs are at greater risk of seizure recurrence than their counterparts with normal EEGs. This is particularly true in children with focal EEG abnormalities. In adults, seizure recurrence is more likely if the EEG is abnormal, with possibly a higher risk for those with generalized epileptiform abnormalities. However, the differences are relatively small, and many patients with epileptiform EEGs will never have a second seizure. The EEG, therefore, provides some useful data after a first seizure, but cannot substitute for careful analysis of all factors in a particular case before a treatment decision is made.

## Febrile seizures

Febrile seizures (a semantically imperfect term) are defined as seizures in association with fever but not due to acute neurological or neurosurgical disease or directly causative medical disorders. This is a common condition, occurring in 2–5% of all children under the age of 6 (Rose et al 1973). Febrile seizures represent a special category when discussing isolated events. Several studies indicate that paroxysmal activity in the EEG, although more common in children with febrile seizures, is not predictive of the development of subsequent febrile or afebrile seizures (Frantzen et al 1968, Lennox-Buchthal, 1973).

If an EEG is performed within the first several days after a febrile seizure, it has a high likelihood of being abnormal: 88% after 1 day (Laplane & Salbreaux 1963), and 33% after 7 days (Frantzen et al 1968). The abnormality usually consists of marked slowing, usually posterior and often asymmetric. Marked asymmetric slowing within the first week may be associated with the subsequent development of a spike focus, but is not predictive of subsequent epilepsy (Frantzen et al 1968).

Paroxysmal spike-wave activity is rarely seen at the time of the initial febrile convulsion (Frantzen et al 1968, Lennox-Buchthal 1973). This may be due to the fact that this pattern is rare in the age group in which the risk of febrile convulsions is greatest. The subsequent development of paroxysmal activity seems to be related to a family history of convulsions and the age at which febrile convulsions occurred.

## EEG FINDINGS IN SPECIFIC EPILEPTIC SYNDROMES: IMPLICATIONS FOR THERAPY

Although the diagnosis of epilepsy is primarily a clinical one, the EEG has always played an important supportive role. The utility of the EEG for planning therapy, however, was felt in the past to be limited. Indeed, with the exception of absence attacks, the majority of patients were treated similarly irrespective of EEG results. Recently, the value of the EEG in designing therapeutic programs has been recognized owing to the development of a more accurate classification of the epilepsies and seizures, and the introduction of new antiepileptic drugs which show relative specificity for certain seizure types and syndromes.

A new Proposal for Classification (1985) defines the term epileptic syndrome as an epileptic disorder characterized by a cluster of signs and symptoms customarily occurring together. The signs and symptoms may be clinical, or findings detected by ancillary studies such as the EEG. Broadly speaking, this system of classification divides the epilepsies into two groups—generalized, and localization-related (focal or partial). In each group, there is further subdivision into idiopathic (no known cause other than possible hereditary factors) and symptomatic (the cause is known or suspected) types. Described below are several syndromes for which the EEG provides an important element in the definition, along with implications for therapy. A more detailed discussion of specific epileptiform patterns and their clinical significance, along with representative illustrations, may be found in Pedley (1987).

### Generalized epilepsies and syndromes

*Benign myoclonic epilepsy in infancy*

These patients have brief episodes of generalized myoclonus which occur during the first or second years of life. The EEG shows generalized spike-wave discharges occurring in brief bursts during early stages of sleep. Such patients may respond to treatment with ethosuximide, valproate or clonazepam (Erba & Brown 1983).

*Childhood absence epilepsy*

Also called *petit mal*, this syndrome has a strong genetic predisposition. Characteristically there are very frequent brief absences, and minor automatisms may be observed. The EEG contains bilaterally synchronous, symmetrical spike-wave complexes at 3 Hz, arising from a normal background. Generalized tonic-clonic convulsions may develop during adolescence. If the patient has only absence attacks, an excellent reponse to ethosuximide may be expected (Browne et al 1975). If there are co-existing generalized tonic-clonic seizures, ethosuximide must be used in conjunction with another drug, e.g. phenytoin or carbamazepine. Valproate, on the other hand, is effective in both seizure types (Simon & Penry 1975, Pinder et al 1977, Villarreal et al 1978).

*Juvenile absence epilepsy*

Its onset is about the time of puberty. Absence attacks are less frequent than with childhood absence epilepsy, and associated generalized tonic-clonic convulsions are more common. The EEG shows generalized spike-wave discharges which often are faster than 3 Hz. Treatment is similar to that of childhood absence epilepsy.

*Juvenile myoclonic epilepsy*
This also appears around puberty and is characterized by seizures with bilateral myoclonic jerks, mainly in the arms. Some patients fall suddently without apparent loss of consciousness. Generalized tonic-clonic seizures occur frequently, and there may be infrequent absence attacks. The EEG shows generalized, often irregular spike-wave and polyspike-wave discharges. Treatment with valproate is highly effective (Delgado-Escueta & Enrile-Bascal 1984).

*West syndrome*
This represents a generalized epilepsy which usually has a poor prognosis. The clinical picture is characterized by infantile spasms and retarded psychomotor development, and the EEG shows a chaotic, continuous generalized abnormality known as hypsarrhythmia. Treatment consists of ACTH or oral corticosteroids which may favorably influence the seizures and degree of EEG abnormality but not the mental retardation.

*Lennox-Gastaut syndrome*
This occurs in children of mainly pre-school age. Multiple seizure types are the rule including tonic, atonic and absence seizures. The EEG usually shows generalized slow spike-wave discharges at less than 3 Hz, and often there are multifocal discharges. Response to treatment is usually poor. In some case, atypical absence attacks with slow generalized spike-wave bursts may respond to a combination of valproate and ethosuximide (Rowan et al 1983).

## Localization-related epilepsies and syndromes

*Benign childhood epilepsy with central-midtemporal spikes*
It is of importance because of its favorable outcome. This idiopathic syndrome consists of brief hemifacial motor seizures with associated somatosensory symptoms which may evolve into generalized tonic-clonic seizures. Onset may be in early or late childhood. The EEG shows blunt, high voltage spikes, maximal in the central and midtemporal regions, which are markedly accentuated during sleep. Response to treatment with carbamazepine or phenytoin is excellent.

*Symptomatic localization-related epilepsies*
In these disorders the seizure characteristics and investigative studies point to a localized origin for the seizures. Many different seizure subtypes are recognized, some deriving from depth electrode studies (q.v.). In general, the EEG demonstrates focal or localized epileptiform activity occurring in cerebral regions which may correlate with clinical manifestations. As an example, a focal abnormality in the frontal lobe over the motor cortex may be associated with unilateral motor activity without loss of consciousness. The most common focal seizure type in adults, the complex partial seizure, usually originates in the hippocampal structures or amygdala. The seizures themselves are characterized by alteration of consciousness and a variety of other manifestations including staring, automatisms, and autonomic changes. Classically the interictal EEG shows a spike or sharp wave focus in the anterior temporal region. In the symptomatic localization-related epilepsies, carbamazepine and phenytoin are regarded as the most effective drugs (Gamstorp 1975, Mattson et al 1985). It should be noted that occasional patients with clinical attacks resembling complex partial

seizures have generalized spike-wave paroxysms in the EEG. In such cases, consideration should be given to a trial of valproate.

**Non-convulsive status epilepticus**

The EEG is of critical value in the diagnosis of non-convulsive status epilepticus. There are two main types: absence status and complex partial status. In the former, the patient displays a continuous state of altered consciousness, sometimes with myoclonic phenomena or automatisms (Porter & Penry 1983). The EEG shows generalized spike-wave discharges, either regular at 3 Hz or more irregular at 2–4 Hz. In many cases the episode can be interrupted with intravenous acetazolamide or diazepam. The patient should then be treated with ethosuximide or valproate.

Complex partial status is characterized by repeated complex partial seizures without full recovery between attacks. A prolonged twilight state may also be observed. The EEG shows repeated episodes of focal epileptiform activity beginning in the temporal region with characteristics similar to those of the single complex partial seizure. The acute episode may be terminated with intravenous phenytoin, phenobarbital or diazepam (Treiman & Delgado-Escueta 1982). Long-term treatment is the same as for complex partial seizures.

The importance of the EEG in the definition of the aforementioned syndromes should be emphasized. The clinical presentation alone is often insufficient for accurate diagnosis. For example, tonic-clonic convulsions may be a manifestation of an idiopathic generalized epilepsy, or a localization-related (focal) epilepsy. In the former case, the EEG will demonstrate generalized spike-wave bursts, and treatment with valproate would be appropriate. In the latter, the EEG may contain focal epileptiform activity, and after investigation for a possible mass lesion, treatment with carbamazepine or phenytoin would be indicated. Similarly, staring spells may be a symptom of one of the idiopathic absence epilepsies, or of complex partial seizures. Again, the EEG findings of generalized spike-wave activity or a focal epileptiform abnormality in the temporal lobe will lead to the correct diagnosis and appropriate therapy. The clinician, therefore, should not institute treatment on clinical grounds alone. A thorough search for an EEG abnormality should be carried out along lines discussed previously.

## LONG-TERM FOLLOW-UP: ROLE OF THE EEG

It is common clinical practice to obtain repeated EEG studies as a guide to managing patients with epilepsy. This often is done on a yearly basis, although more frequent follow-up EEGs are not uncommonly ordered. We recently encountered a patient who, in the space of 4 months, had eight EEG studies, apparently for the purpose of determining the effects of alterations in drug therapy. It is not unreasonable to presume that electrophysiological abnormalities bear some relationship to the occurrence of seizures. We will discuss the EEG as it pertains to the everyday management of epilepsy.

Possible information to be gained from repeated EEG studies might include changes in morphology or distribution of epileptiform discharges, discharge frequency and background activity, and the development of focal slowing. Several well understood factors that are not directly related to a change in the epileptic condition might produce such alterations. Age, for example, is associated with profound EEG changes, particularly in the young and elderly (Takahashi et al 1965). Other influences include the temporal relationship of the EEG to the patient's most recent seizure. Epileptiform activity may either be increased or decreased in the post-seizure period. Background slowing may be increased, and the posterior dominant rhythm disrupted. Pharmacotherapy may influence epileptiform activity or the background, depending on the drug used (vide infra). Still other factors known to influence the EEG include the patient's emotional state, state of awareness, sleep deprivation, and a variety of other external and internal events.

Hughes (1967) discussed the types of epileptiform abnormalities found at different ages. Hypsarrhythmia (associated with infantile spasms) had a peak incidence at 2 years of age, whereas the probability of finding a temporal lobe spike focus was maximal between the ages of 30 and 39. The 3 Hz spike-wave discharge had a maximum incidence in the second decade as did occipital spikes, whereas temporal and frontal spikes peaked in the fourth decade. When he considered the probability of encountering a particular abnormality at a given age, the temporal lobe spike showed the highest probability of occurrence in all decades of life, linearly increasing with age. Hughes (1985) later studied long term changes in EEG paroxysms (over 10–40 years) and concluded that changes in epileptogenic foci occur in nearly 90% of epileptic patients. For example, hypsarrhythmia changes to the slow (2 Hz) spike-wave pattern, with later evolution to focal discharges and irregular spike-wave complexes. Hughes argued that age is an important variable, and concluded that nearly all paroxysmal EEG patterns eventually result in a temporal lobe focus. He also noted that the development of bilateral temporal foci from a unilateral focus was associated with new or increased seizures in one-third, but stable or decreased seizure frequency in the majority. It is possible that discharging foci become less epileptogenic over time, arguing for the development of intrinsic protective mechanisms with advancing age.

Strobos & Kavallinis (1968) studied the characteristics of serial EEGs in 123 patients, including 26 with bilaterally synchronous discharges (centrencephalic group) and 50 with focal temporal abnormalities. In the centrencephalic group, patients with the same or minimally reduced seizure frequency showed no change in follow-up EEGs, whereas those who had reduced seizure frequency or complete seizure control usually showed improvement in their EEGs. In the focal temporal group, lack of seizure control was associated with no EEG improvement and, in a few cases, the development of either secondary bilaterally synchronous discharges, or emergence of a focal discharge in the opposite temporal lobe. Seizure control was associated with normalization of the EEG in half and improvement in the majority, although the authors state that secondary bilaterally synchronous discharges were observed in two patients in this group.

Although this study makes it tempting to regard the EEG as a reflection of the clinical status of the patient, there is considerable evidence that routine serial EEGs provide less information of value than might be supposed. In a study by Hosokawa et al (1979) of 66 patients, each of whom had serial EEGs performed over a period of at least 6 years, there was no statistical correlation between attainment of seizure control and disappearance rate of spike discharges. Moreover, they were unable to find any difference in spike incidence in those with and those without continuing seizures, regardless of whether the patients had primary generalized or focal epilepsy.

Theodore et al (1984) reported on serial EEGs in 70 patients with intractable epilepsy who underwent intensive monitoring studies. EEGs were obtained on admission, at discharge, and at a follow-up interval varying from 5–57 months (mean 25). No statistically significant correlation was found between any EEG feature and any clinical measure of seizure frequency or drug toxicity. They comment on the 'capricious and bewildering' variability of clinical EEGs. In a study of long-stay patients in an epilepsy center, Rowan et al (1980b) found the initial EEG to be a significant predictor of seizure prognosis, whereas serial EEGs provided no additional significant prognostic information.

The foregoing illustrates many of the variables that confound interpretation of serial EEGs and tend to reduce their clinical utility. Another important consideration is the short term variability of EEG discharges. In a study by Binnie et al (1984) of the time relationship of epileptiform discharges in 48 hour EEGs, there was strong evidence of non-stationarity of discharges reflecting, in their opinion, the changing internal and external 'milieu' of the patient. They comment that the only feature common to all their studies was lack of any correlation between successive interdischarge intervals. A further study from this group (Martins da Silva et al 1984) confirmed in long-term EEGs that the discharge rate was extremely variable from epoch to epoch, and indeed between successive days of recording. It therefore appears to be wishful thinking that a brief EEG window of 20–30 min can accurately depict the on-going physiological state of the brain.

A recent report by Frost et al (1986) offers preliminary evidence that analysis of computer-derived parameters of interictal spike waveform measured on serial EEGs may provide a quantitative estimate of seizure risk. Patients who had achieved seizure control had interictal spikes that differed significantly in spike amplitude, duration and sharpness and in a mathematically-derived composite expression of these three parameters compared to baseline values.

In summary, the evidence suggests that serial EEGs are of limited value in the assessment of a patient's clinical progress. Whether repeated quantitative measurement of specific components of an EEG as proposed by Frost et al (1986) will be valuable remains to be demonstrated by controlled prospective studies. In terms of development of certain EEG patterns over time, as in the case of hypsarrhythmia, the findings are certainly of interest and possibly of therapeutic value. In the case of adults with changing EEG discharge patterns, e.g. the development of bilaterial temporal foci, the practical implications are less clear. It should be emphasized, however, that repeat EEG studies are indicated in patients who experience a change in seizure pattern or a marked change in seizure frequency without apparent reason. In these instances, the development of progressive cerebral disease, such as a brain tumor, may underlie the change in clinical status. The EEG may then reveal a new slow wave focus not previously apparent. For the most part, serial EEG studies should be reserved for such occasions and not simply to check on the patient's progress.

## EEG CHANGES DUE TO ANTIEPILEPTIC DRUGS

The ideal antiepileptic drug (AED) selectively suppresses seizures without affecting general cerebral function. Some currently available AEDs approach this ideal, whereas others achieve seizure control but at the expense of cerebral side-effects. At therapeutic concentrations, an AED may completely suppress seizures in one patient and produce an incomplete response in another. At toxic levels, all AEDs cause diffuse cerebral symptoms with a variable effect on seizure frequency. Two features of the EEG might be expected to reflect these clinical results of AED treatment: ongoing background activity and epileptiform discharges. Presumably, changes in EEG background should relate to the development of diffuse cerebral symptoms, and the abundance of epileptiform discharges to seizure frequency. In the former case the relationship is reliable, but in the latter it is questionable. This section discusses these issues and explores the possible practical consequences of EEG changes secondary to AED therapy.

Background activity is influenced by AEDs in two major ways. The first is slowing, which includes slowing of the posterior dominant rhythmic activity as well as irregular, diffuse slowing in theta and/or delta frequency bands. In some instances slowing is an expected result of therapeutic AED levels, while in others it is a sign of toxicity. The other background change is an increase in low voltage fast (beta) activity. This is observed only with AEDs of certain classes, mainly the barbiturates and benzodiazepines.

The influence of AEDs on interictal spike discharges has proved difficult to study. A major problem is the temporal fluctuation in their frequency of occurrence. The presence of interictal spikes may vary from day to day, even from minute to minute as discussed in the previous section. Apparent changes of spike frequency due to AEDs must therefore be interpreted in this light. Further, there is an unclear relationship between the number of interictal discharges and seizure control. Some patients continue to have epileptiform activity in the EEG after they have become seizure-free, and long-term monitoring studies have shown that seizure occurrence is not related to interictal spike frequency in a given patient (Gotman & Marciani 1985).

Generalized spike-wave discharges represent a different situation. There is evidence that these discharges, even when brief, are associated with alteration of awareness as determined by decreased reaction time (Goode et al 1970, Browne et al 1974). In general, therefore, a decrease in generalized spike-wave discharges is associated with a decline in clinical seizures.

**Valproate**

Valproate is highly effective in the treatment of simple absence attacks (petit mal) and myoclonic seizures. There is convincing evidence that it is also effective in primarily generalized tonic-clonic convulsions. Its efficacy in focal seizures is less clearly defined. Valproate in therapeutic doses will produce a substantial reduction in the number and duration of generalized spike-wave paroxysms (Bruni et al 1980). Of 22 patients followed for 1 year, only 2 who had good to excellent improvement failed to demonstrate an improved EEG. Similarly, it is unusual to see an EEG improvement without clinical improvement (Maheshwari & Jeavons 1975, Villarreal et al 1978). The time of maximum reduction in spike-wave paroxysms does not correlate with maximum serum levels (Villarreal et al 1978, Rowan et al 1979, Sato et al 1982, Burr et al 1986). Rowan et al (1979) found that the maximal reduction of the photoconvulsive response after a single dose of sodium valproate occurred several hours after peak serum levels had been obtained. The effect was observed as long as 5 days after valproate was no longer detectable in the blood.

In most studies, therapeutic levels of valproate have not produced slowing of background rhythms (Adams et al 1978, Bruni et al 1980, Benninger et al 1986). Background slowing has been noted, however, in patients with clinical evidence of toxicity (Adams et al 1978, Villarreal et al 1978). In some cases, consideration must be given to the possibility that slowing is due to the presence of co-medication, particularly phenobarbital.

**Carbamazepine**

Carbamazepine is effective for focal and generalized tonic-clonic seizures but is ineffective in absence attacks. It is, therefore, an expected finding that generalized spike-wave paroxysms show no change, or even an increase, after treatment with carbamazepine (Pryse-Phillips & Jeavons 1970, Scheffner & Schiefer 1972, Wilkus et al 1978). The unexpected finding is that other types of EEG abnormalities, such as focal spikes and generalized spikes, also do not change, and in fact may also increase (Pryse-Phillips & Jeavons 1970, Wilkus et al 1978). In addition, there does not appear to be a relationship between EEG findings and seizure control, or a correlation between paroxysmal activity and serum levels of carbamazepine. Background slowing may occur with therapeutic levels. This is manifested by a decrease in the frequency of the posterior dominant rhythm, as well as diffuse theta activity which increases with rising serum levels (Wilkus et al 1978).

**Phenytoin**

Phenytoin is effective in a variety of focal and generalized seizures with the exception of absence attacks. In contrast to carbamazepine, there is good evidence that phenytoin decreases the number of epileptiform discharges in the EEG, both chronically (Buchthal et al 1960, Wilkus & Green 1974) and after an acute intravenous dose (Milligan et al). Buchthal et al (1960) found that this effect was dependent on the serum level. Patients with levels above 10 μg/ml had 50% fewer paroxysms, whereas those with lower levels tended to have increased discharges. Mild slowing of the background may occur with therapeutic levels (Wilkus & Green 1974), but background changes may not be as marked as with carbamazepine (Wilkus et al 1978). As serum levels increase, slowing becomes more marked, and with severe toxicity the EEG resembles a diffuse encephalopathy. In this case, high voltage delta activity dominates the EEG. Resolution of the abnormality may require 1–3 weeks, lagging behind clinical improvement (Roseman 1961). There are reports of increased spike-wave activity with phenytoin (Levy & Fenichel 1965, Zwarts & Sie 1985), which may relate to an increase in seizure frequency.

**Clonazepam**

Clonazepam is effective in the treatment of absence attacks, myoclonic seizures and photosensitive epilepsy. There is clear evidence that it suppresses spike-wave and polyspike-wave complexes in the EEG (Martin & Hirt 1973, Gregonades & Frangos 1977). Nanda et al (1977) found complete resolution of polyspike-wave complexes in 7/10 patients with myoclonic epilepsy after introduction of clonazepam. Three Hz spike-wave complexes and photoconvulsive responses may also be completely suppresed (Nanda et al 1977). Hypsarrhythmic patterns show a variable response (Martin & Hirt 1973). As with other benzodiazepines, clonazepam at therapeutic levels produces slowing of the EEG background. At toxic concentrations the slowing is even more pronounced. In addition, beta activity is markedly increased, especially in the frontocentral regions.

**Ethosuximide**

Ethosuximide is used specifically for the treatment of absence seizures. It is ineffective against tonic-clonic and partial seizures and indeed has been reported to increase the incidence of these seizure types when used alone. Ethosuximide significantly reduces generalized spike-wave bursts (Penry et al 1972). Kellaway et al (1979) showed that increasing ethosuximide levels led first to decreased discharges during REM sleep, followed by those in wakefulness, and finally those during slow wave sleep. Of interest was the observation of increasing seizure control as each level of discharge suppression was reached. Ethosuximide has little effect on background activity at therapeutic doses (Saunders & Westmoreland 1979).

**Phenobarbital**

Phenobarital has long been used in the treatment of both focal and generalized motor seizures (Buchthal & Svensmark 1968). Antiepileptic effect is related to drug levels, and there is also evidence that reduction in EEG epileptiform activity may be correlated with effectiveness against seizures. Kellaway et al (1978) found that 6 patients with partial seizures who attained complete seizure control after treatment with phenobarbital had 100% reduction in spike activity, whereas in 5 patients with poorer clinical response, there was only a 20–30% reduction. It should be noted that phenobarbital is not effective against 3 Hz spike-wave paroxysms, and indeed may increase their occurrence (Buchthal & Svensmark 1968).

Phenobarbital increases beta activity at therapeutic levels (Saunders & Westmoreland 1979). In patients with partial seizures of focal pathology, the abnormal side may not show the expected increase in these faster frequencies. This, therefore, may be useful as a diagnostic procedure.

As phenobarbital levels increase, there is a progressive increase in slower frequencies, first theta, and ultimately delta activity. With high toxic levels, intermittent paroxysmal slow waves are seen (Saunders & Westmoreland 1979).

**Table 4.1** Effects of major AEDs on the EEG

| AED | Slowing with therapeutic dose | Slowing with toxicity | Increased beta | Decreased interictal spike | May cause increased interictal spike | Decreased generalized spike-wave |
|---|---|---|---|---|---|---|
| Valproate | − | + | − | +/− | − | ++ |
| Carbamazepine | + | + | − | − | + | − |
| Phenytoin | +/− | ++ | − | + | − | − |
| Phenobarbital | + | ++ | ++ | + | − | − |
| Ethosuximide | − | ? | − | − | − | ++ |
| Clonazepam | + | ++ | ++ | + | − | ++ |

## WITHDRAWAL OF ANTIEPILEPTIC DRUGS: DOES THE EEG AID IN PREDICTING OUTCOME?

Epilepsy need not be regarded as a life-long disease. In fact, the probability that an epileptic patient will eventually become seizure-free on medication varies from

30–40% (Rodin 1968, Currie et al 1971) to 70% (Hauser & Kurland 1975), depending on the type of population studied. If remission does occur, patients are frequently considered for AED withdrawal. After medication has been discontinued, the prognosis for remaining seizure-free has been found to be as low as 6% (Rodin & John 1980), and as high as 60% (Janz et al 1983). A number of investigators have considered whether the EEG before and/or after AED withdrawal is a useful prognostic indicator. Juul-Jensen (1964) studied 200 patients who were seizure-free for two years or more. He did not include patients whose EEGs showed a 'tendency to progression'. After 2 years of follow-up, the relapse rate was 35%. He found that the degree of EEG abnormality before beginning withdrawal was of no prognostic significance (37% relapse with normal EEGs; 33% with moderately abnormal EEGs). After a 5 year follow-up period the recurrence rate was 40% (Juul-Jensen 1968). There was a non-significant association of EEG slow wave foci or bilateral paroxysms with the probability of recurrence.

Overweg et al (1987) studied 62 patients from a specialized epilepsy clinic who had been seizure-free 3 or more years. They found a total relapse rate of 66%, the majority occurring up to the point of complete drug withdrawal.

The only difference in initial EEG findings between the seizure-free and relapse groups approaching statistical significance was the presence of larger numbers of sharp waves in seizure-free patients. Other trends, which failed to reach significance, included more prominent diffuse abnormalities in the seizure-free subjects, and more spikes and spike-wave complexes in the relapse group. The authors also mentioned a weak association of large amounts of epileptiform activity with relapse, but the number of patients was small.

A related problem is the appearance of epileptiform discharges during the withdrawal process. Is this a poor prognostic sign? In a review, Schmidt (1985) suggests that recurrence of paroxysmal discharges during AED reduction should delay further reduction and may require reassessment of individual risk. Overweg et al (1987), however, described three patients who developed focal spike-wave activity during AED withdrawal yet remained seizure-free. No such patients were found in the relapse group. They concluded that emergence of epileptiform activity during AED withdrawal is not predictive of relapse.

There is some evidence that the value of the EEG in predicting the outcome of AED withdrawal in children may differ from that in adults. Emerson et al (1981) studied 68 children who had been seizure free for four years. They found that those with an abnormal EEG prior to medication withdrawal were more likely to relapse. Multivariate analysis indicated that an abnormal EEG and a history of many generalized seizures were the major predictors of seizure recurrence. Similarly, in a study of 473 children, Todt (1984) noted relapse in 26% with normal EEGs, and 59% with paroxysmal EEGs before discontinuation of therapy, and Shinnar et al (1985) also found that the presence of EEG abnormalities such as slowing, spikes, and focality were associated with poor outcome. In contrast, Thurston et al (1982) studied 148 children who had discontinued AED therapy between 15 and 23 years previously. The relapse rate was 28% and there was no correlation with the presence or absence of an abnormal EEG.

In summary, the EEG does not appear to be of predictive value in adults when considering whether to discontinue AEDs in seizure-free patients. A possible exception is the presence of a large amount of epileptiform activity, but this remains to be demonstrated convincingly. On the other hand, the EEG may well be helpful in predicting seizure recurrence in children. It should be emphasized that EEG results must be considered in the context of the clinical features of a patient's epilepsy. Thus, only careful assessment of such data as age of seizure onset, seizure type, genetic factors and seizure severity, together with the EEG, will lead to an informed decision about the advisability of discontinuing AED therapy.

## LONG-TERM NEURODIAGNOSTIC MONITORING

The most important recent advance in electroencephalography has been the development and growth of long-term EEG monitoring. Two types of monitoring are now in use: intensive EEG/video monitoring using radio or cable telemetry, and ambulatory EEG cassette monitoring. Both procedures allow recording from a fully mobile patient in both inpatient and outpatient settings. EEG monitoring was initially a research procedure carried out only in specialized epilepsy centers. Its proved clinical utility has led to its broad acceptance as an important clinical tool in epilepsy diagnosis.

### Intensive EEG/video monitoring

Recording the EEG by means of radiotelemetry was introduced over 20 years ago. The patient carried a miniaturized telemetry unit, connected to standard EEG electrodes, which transmitted the preamplified multiplexed EEG via a radio frequency carrier to a distant location. The signal was decoded, further amplified, and written out on a standard EEG machine. The development of cable telemetry obviated the need for a system of antennae and produced more stable recordings, although patient movement was limited by the length of the coaxial cable. At first, only a few channels of EEG could be recorded, but later developments allowed recording of 16 and even 32 channels of information. It was also realized that concurrent observation of the patient would increase the power of the ictal EEG. Early attempts to film the patient simultaneously with the on-going EEG met with some success (Schwab et al 1954), but the development of closed circuit television greatly increased the quality and flexibility of behavioral observation. Further electronic advances led to simultaneous display of the patient and the EEG on the video screen, and the video tape recorder allowed careful study of patient behavior and any recorded epileptic events.

Early work in intensive monitoring was concerned with description of seizure phenomenology and correlation with EEG findings. Key advances were made in understanding the detailed characteristics of absence attacks (Penry et al 1975) and complex partial seizures (Escueta et al 1977). The high cost of intensive monitoring initially limited expansion of its use, but recently a number of firms have produced intensive monitoring equipment at lower cost, thus placing it within the reach of most large medical centers.

As practiced today, most intensive monitoring systems employ cable telemetry to record 16 channels of EEG information. After decoding, the signal is further amplified and written out on a standard EEG machine, or recorded on tape for later playback. Because of the large amount of paper required during continuous monitoring, systems have been devised which reduce the amount of data to be analyzed. In one, the interictal EEG is temporarily stored in computer memory and periodically written out. If a seizure occurs, the patient or an observer activates the EEG write-out with a push-button. The immediate pre-ictal EEG, stored in memory, is written out, along with the continuing on-line electrographic seizure (Ives et al 1976). Methods also have been developed to count interictal epileptiform discharges and electrical seizures automatically (Gotman & Gloor 1976, Gotman et al 1979, Gotman 1982). Such automatic detection systems are highly effective in analyzing generalized spike-wave discharges, but are somewhat less reliable in the case of focal spike discharges, especially in the presence of artifact. For most clinical purposes, continuous EEG write-out is satisfactory, especially if the object is seizure recording. If the EEG is time-coded, the relevant recording can easily be located and reviewed. Spike counting, of course, is laborious and usually not necessary except for research purposes. If one wishes to count the number of spike-wave trains associated with absence seizures, this is easily done by hand. It is emphasized, therefore, that diagnostically important data may be obtained at relatively low cost using simple apparatus: telemetry transmitter and decoder, video camera and monitor, and an EEG machine.

The value of intensive monitoring in diagnosis and therapy has been confirmed in a number of studies. Porter et al (1977) reported on results in 23 patients with intractable epilepsy. They found that monitoring led to improved seizure control in 70% and decreased drug toxicity in 83%. Mattson (1980) reported on 388 patients undergoing intensive monitoring and antiepileptic drug level determinations. The procedure led to more precise diagnosis with resultant improvement in 68%. Rowan et al (1980a) and Binnie et al (1981) reported overall success rates of 67–72% in answering clinical questions posed by referring physicians. Most other studies of the utility of intensive monitoring have yielded similar results (Stålberg 1976, Aarts et al 1983, Bridgers & Ebersole 1985).

Although intensive monitoring usually is carried out for periods of 24 h or more (up to 11 days in one series), there is evidence that shorter recording times may yield similar results to more prolonged studies. Rowan et al (1987) described a procedure of daytime intensive monitoring carried out over a period of 6–8 hours. Methods used to increase diagnostic yield included sleep deprivation, napping during the procedure, hyperventilation, photic stimulation, and techniques of suggestion. Clinical questions were answered in 67% and attacks recorded in 54%, comparing favorably with results in more prolonged intensive monitoring. Daytime intensive monitoring can be carried out in the context of everyday work in an EEG department, thus making it feasible for many hospital and clinic settings.

**Ambulatory EEG monitoring**

Cardiologists have utilized 24-h ambulatory EKG monitoring for over 25 years, an advance made possible by the development of the miniature tape recorder. It was not until 1975 that Ives & Woods (1975) reported on the feasibility of recording the EEG on a standard audio cassette. This advance was made possible by the development of miniature amplifiers affixed to the scalp, and the modification of the tape recorder's transport mechanism which allowed 24 h of continuous recording on a single cassette. Finally, the development of video playback units obviated the need for writing out 24 h of EEG on a standard EEG machine. Initially, only three channels of EEG could be recorded, although this limitation was addressed by development of montages designed to record from areas most likely to show epileptiform activity

(Ebersole 1985). Today, ambulatory EEG allows 8 channels of EEG recording, along with simultaneous EKG and continuous time display (Ebsersole 1985). An audio channel facilitates recognition of epileptiform activity and sleep phenomena.

Ambulatory EEG recording is easily carried out for periods of 24 h, or several days. In the latter instance, it is necessary to change the cassette at 24-h intervals, and check the electrodes for impedance, re-jellying if necessary. Ambulatory monitoring, while offering the advantage of recording the EEG in the patient's natural environment, e.g. at home, school or in the work place, suffers from the drawback of not including continuous observation of behavior. Recognition of artifact is a recurrent problem, and low voltage abnormal potentials may not be evident.

Trouble-shooting is also difficult, and sources of artifact, such as a defective electrode, will not be evident until the patient returns after 24 h. In spite of these pitfalls, ambulatory EEG has proved to be of considerable clinical value. In reported series of ambulatory EEG monitoring, success rates vary from 11% (Ramsey 1982) to 81% (Declerk et al 1982), reflecting the populations studied as well as duration of recording and individual critera for success (recording interictal epileptiform activity and/or seizures). Success in recording seizures ranges from 7% (Ramsey 1982) to 55% (Ives et al 1981).

**Indications for monitoring studies**

It will be appreciated that intensive EEG/video monitoring and ambulatory cassette EEG monitoring each have advantages and disadvantages. In addition, the problems to be addressed by these procedures are not identical. Intensive monitoring is preferred for documentation and analysis of seizures or suspected seizures, due in part to its greater channel capability, but largely to simultaneous video recording of a patient's behavior. Video recording during ambulatory EEG addresses this problem to some extent but at best is only a partial solution.

Intensive monitoring is superior in the differential diagnosis of epileptic versus non-epileptic events. Here, video recording of the behavioral event is a critical element, as is the availability of a physician for observation and intervention. Provocative testing can be carried out with intensive monitoring, as for example in the investigation of possible reflex factors in seizure occurrence. Finally, with intensive monitoring, patients with known epileptiform activity on the EEG can be tested for subtle clinical manifestations.

Ambulatory EEG monitoring, on the other hand, is excellent at the task of uncovering EEG abnormalities not present on routine EEG testing. It is useful in determining seizure or discharge frequency when such events already have been documented. It may elucidate electrographic features of known spells, thus aiding classification. Finally, ambulatory EEG is of value in distinguishing non-epileptic events such as syncope, transient ischemic attacks, or other cardiogenic events from epileptic seizures. The commercial availability of high quality ambulatory monitoring equipment, while not inexpensive, puts ambulatory monitoring within the reach of practicing neurologists and electroencephalographers. It must be pointed out, however, that interpretation of ambulatory EEG is a specialized skill, and much experience is required before such records reliably can be assessed for artifact and epileptiform activity. In the case of generalized spike-wave discharges, ambulatory EEG is highly effective. In the case of more subtle, or low voltage, focal discharges, however, ambulatory

EEG is often difficult to interpret. In these cases, intensive monitoring offers superior diagnostic potential.

## PRESURGICAL EVALUATION: DEPTH AND SUBDURAL RECORDING

### Depth electrodes

Depth electrodes allow recording from intracerebral locations, and are especially useful in the temporal and frontal lobes. Patients considered for depth electrode studies are potential candidates for surgical treatment of their epilepsy because of failed medical regimens. In such patients there must be reasonable evidence that the seizures have a unilateral focal onset in a surgically resectable region. In many patients, evidence from surface and sphenoidal EEG, clinical ictal onset, radiologic studies and other sources will be sufficient for reliable localization of the epileptogenic focus. In others, there may be conflicting information from the various studies, or information imprecise enough to preclude surgical intervention. In such cases the next logical step is the placement of intracranial electrodes.

Depth electrodes are placed stereotactically and are ideal for evaluation of seizures originating in the mesial temporal structures such as the hippocampus and amygdala (Engel & Crandall 1986). Implantation sites are selected on the basis of prior clinical and EEG information. The electrodes are placed under general anesthesia through hollow guidepins that are screwed to the skull (Spenser 1980). The electrodes are often left in place for several weeks during continuous telemetric EEG monitoring. Eight to 10 seizures must be observed on EEG and videotape to define the site of onset with certainty, and to determine that recorded seizures are the same as those the patient usually experiences. Interictal spikes are not sufficient for localization, as they are more likely to be falsely localizing with depth recording than with sphenoidal or surface electrodes (Engel & Crandall 1986).

Risks of depth electrodes include intracerebral bleeding, movement of electrodes during seizures, infection, and current leakage, but overall morbidity and mortality is low (Engel & Crandall 1986). One disadvantage is the relatively small area of brain that can be sampled.

### Subdural electrodes

Subdural electrodes, another technique of intracranial recording, cover a much larger cerebral area and are ideal for frontal, temporal and parietal convexities. This method involves the implantation of a grid of electrodes on the cortical surface overlying the suspected area of epileptogenicity. As with implanted depth electrodes, the patient with subdural electrodes may be monitored for an extended period. By stimulating individual electrodes in the subdural array and monitoring the results, a map of functional cortical areas surrounding the epileptogenic region can be made. In this way, the risk of resecting a functionally essential cortical area can be minimized (Goldring 1978, Gates 1986). As with depth electrodes, spontaneous seizures are recorded and analyzed.

## SUMMARY

1. The EEG is still the most important test for diagnosis in epilepsy, and can provide important information in planning appropriate therapy.

2. An epileptiform EEG abnormality may be expected in up to 90% of patients with epilepsy if appropriate techniques of activation and special electrode placement are utilized.

3. Not all patients with epilepsy will have an abnormal EEG, nor does the presence of an epileptiform abnormality mean epilepsy. The diagnosis must be made on clinical grounds.

4. Once the diagnosis of epilepsy has been made, serial EEG studies are unlikely to provide further useful information in the stable patient. In a patient who is deteriorating, however, a repeat EEG should be performed to detect a progressive cerebral process, a change in epileptiform activity, or evidence of drug toxicity.

5. If a patient has become seizure free, the presence or absence of an epileptiform abnormality is more helpful in predicting relapse in children than in adults.

6. The EEG can provide useful information for determining appropriate antiepileptic drug therapy. Generalized spike-wave discharges, with certain exceptions, suggest that treatment with valproate or ethosuximide is indicated. The presence of focal epileptiform activity is usually an indication for treatment with carbamazepine or phenytoin in the first instance.

7. A particular type of seizure, such as tonic-clonic or absence, may be associated with either generalized or focal epileptiform activity with implications for therapy as indicated above.

8. Specialized tests such as intensive and ambulatory monitoring should be performed in the patient for whom routine studies have not provided sufficient information.

## ACKNOWLEDGEMENTS

We acknowledge the indispensable assistance of Ms Linda Tuchman and Ms Ruby Hough in preparing this manuscript.

## REFERENCES

Aarts J H P, Van Bentum de Boer P T E, Binnie C D et al 1983 Evaluation of intensive EEG and video monitoring in epilepsy. In: Stott F D, Raftery E B, Goulding L (eds) ISAM (Proceedings of the Fourth International Symposium on Ambulatory Monitoring). Academic Press, London, p 208–214

Aass F, Kaada B R, Torp K H 1956 The diagnostic and prognostic value of the initial electroencephalogram in children with convulsions. Acta Paediatrica 45: 335–342

Adams D J, Lüders H, Pippenger C E 1978 Sodium valproate in the treatment of intractable seizure disorders: a clinical and electroencephalographic study. Neurology (Minneap) 28: 152–157

Ajmone-Marsan C, Zivin L S 1970 Factors related to the occurrence of typical paroxysmal abnormalities in the EEG records of epileptic patients. Epilepsia 11: 361–381

Annegers J F, Hauser W A, Elveback L R 1979 Remission of seizures and relapse in patients with epilepsy. Epilepsia 20: 729–737

Annegers J F, Shirts S B, Hauser W A, Kurland L T 1986 Risk of recurrence after an initial unprovoked seizure. Epilepsia 27: 43–50

Arne-Bes M C, Calvet V, Thiberge M, Arbus L 1982 Effects of sleep deprivation in an EEG study of epileptics. In: Sterman M B, Shouse M N, Passouant P (eds) Sleep and epilepsy. Academic Press, New York, p 441–452

Bamberger P, Matthes A 1959 Anfälle im kindesalter. Lerget, Basel

Bechinger D, Kornhuber H H 1976 The sleep deprivation EEG in childhood. Electroencephalography and Clinical Neurophysiology 41: 654

Bennett D R 1963 Sleep deprivation and major motor convulsions. Neurology (Minneap) 13: 953–958

Benninger C, Matthis P, Scheffner D 1986 Changes of the EEG in children with primary generalized epilepsy during the introduction of antiepileptic therapy with sodium valproate. Epilepsia 27: 587

Binnie C D, Rowan A J, Overweg J et al 1981 Telemetric EEG and video monitoring in epilepsy. Neurology (NY) 31: 298–303

Binnie C D, Aarts J H P, Houtkooper M A et al 1984 Temporal characteristics of seizures and epileptiform discharges. Electroencephalography and Clinical Neurophysiology 58: 498–505

Blom S, Heijbel J, Bergfors P G 1978 Incidence of epilepsy in children: a follow-up study three years after the first seizure. Epilepsia 19: 343–350

Bridgers S L, Ebersole J S 1985 The clinical utility of ambulatory cassette EEG. Neurology 35: 166–173

Browne T R, Penry J K, Porter R J, Dreifuss F E 1974 Responsiveness before, during and after spike-wave paroxysms. Neurology (Minneap) 24: 659–665

Browne T R, Dreifuss F E, Dyken P R et al 1975 Ethosuximide in the treatment of absence (petit mal) seizures. Neurology 25: 515–524

Bruni S, Wilder B S, Bauman A W 1980 Clinical efficacy and long-term effects of valproic acid therapy on spike-and-wave discharges. Neurology 30: 42–46

Buchthal F, Svensmark O 1968 Relation of EEG and seizures to phenobarbital in serum. Archives of Neurology 19: 567–572

Buchthal F, Svensmark O, Schilder P J 1960 Clinical and EEG correlations with serum levels of diphenylhydantoin. Archives of Neurology (Chic) 2: 624–630

Burr W, Froscher W, Kreiten K, Stefan H 1986 Investigations of the relationship between VPA serum level profiles and spike-wave activity in the long-term EEG. Epilepsia 27: 587

Camfield P R, Camfield C S, Dooley J M, Tibbles J A R, Fung T, Garner B 1985 Epilepsy after a first unprovoked seizure in childhood. Neurology 35: 1657–1660

Cavazzuti G B, Cappella L, Nalin A 1980 Longitudinal study of epileptiform EEG patterns in normal children. Epilepsia 21: 43–55

Cereghino J J, Brock J T, Van Meter J C, Penry J K, Smith L D, White B G 1974 Carbamazepine for epilepsy: a controlled prospective evaluation. Neurology 24: 401–410

Christodoulou G 1967 Sphenoidal electrodes: their significance in diagnosing temporal lobe epileptogenic foci. Acta Neurologica Scandanavica 43: 587–593

Cleland P G, Mosquera I, Steward W P, Foster J B 1981 Prognosis of isolated seizures in adult life. British Medical Journal 283: 1364

Coull B M, Pedley T A 1978 Intermittent photic stimulation. Clinical usefulness of non-convulsive responses. Electroencephalography and Clinical Neurophysiology 44: 353–363

Currie S, Heathfield K W G, Henson R A, Scott D F 1971 Clinical course and prognosis of temporal lobe epilepsy. A survey of 666 patients. Brain 94: 173–190

Declerk A C, Martens W L J, Schiltz A M 1982 Evaluation of ambulatory EEG cassette recordings. In: Stefan H, Burr W (eds) Mobile long-term EEG monitoring (Proceedings of the MLE Symposium, Bonn, West Germany, May 1982). Fischer, New York, p 29–36

Degen R, Degen H E 1984 Sleep and sleep deprivation in epileptology. In: Degen R, Niedermeyer E (eds) Epilepsy, sleep and sleep deprivation. Elsevier, Amsterdam, p 273–285

De Jesus P V, Masland W S 1970 The role of nasopharyngeal electrodes in clinical electroencephalography. Neurology 20: 869–878

Delgado-Escueta A V 1979 Epileptogenic paroxysms: modern approaches and clinical correlations. Neurology (Minneap) 29: 1014–1022

Delgado-Escueta A V, Enrile-Bascal F 1984 Juvenile myoclonic epilepsy of Janz. Neurology 34: 285–294

Dinner D S, Lüders H 1985 The electroencephalogram in the routine evaluation of patients with epilepsy. In: Porter R J, Morselli P L (eds) The epilepsies. Butterworths International Medical Reviews, Stoneham, p 142–173

Dinner D S, Lüders H, Rothner A D, Erenberg G E 1984 Complex partial seizures of childhood: a clinical and electroencephalographic study. Cleveland Clinic Quarterly 51: 287–291

Doose H, Giesler K, Völzke E 1989 Observations in photosensitive children with and without epilepsy. Zeitschrift für Kinderheilkunde 107: 26

Ebersole J S 1985 Ambulatory cassette EEG. Journal of Clinical Neurophysiology 2: 397–418

Ellingson R J, Wilken K, Bennett D R 1984 Efficacy of sleep deprivation as an activation procedure in epilepsy patients. Journal of Clinical Neurophysiology 1: 83–101

Emerson R, D'Souza B J, Vining E P, Holden K R, Mellits E D, Freeman J M 1981 Stopping medication in children with epilepsy: predictors of outcome. New England Journal of Medicine 304: 1125–1129

Engel J, Crandall P H 1986 Intensive neurodiagnostic monitoring with intracranial electrodes. In: Gumnit R J (ed) Advances in neurology: intensive neurodiagnostic monitoring. Raven Press, New York 46: 85–106

Erba G, Browne T R 1983 Atypical absence, myoclonic, atonic and tonic seizures, and the 'Lennox-Gastaut syndrome.' In: Browne T R, Feldman R G (eds) Epilepsy: diagnosis and management. Little, Brown, Boston, p 90–91

Escueta A V, Kunze U, Waddell G, Boxley J, Nadel A 1977 Lapse of consciousness and automatisms in temporal lobe epilepsy: a videotape analysis. Neurology 27: 144–155
Frantzen E, Lennox-Buchthal M, Nygard A 1968 Longitudinal EEG and clinical study of children with febrile convulsions. Electroencephalography and Clinical Neurophysiology 24: 197–212
Frost J D, Kellaway P. Hrachovy R A, Glaze D G, Mizrahi E M 1986 Changes in epileptic spike configuration associated with attainment of seizure control. Annals of Neurology 20: 723–726
Gabor A J, Seyal M 1986 Effect of sleep on the electrographic manifestations of epilepsy. Journal of Clinical Neurophysiology 3: 23–38
Gamstorp I 1975 Treatment with carbamazepine: children. In: Penry J K, Daly D D (eds) Advances in neurology vol II, Complex partial seizures and their treatment. Raven Press, New York
Gastaut H, Tassinari C A 1975 EEG in diagnosis, prognosis and treatment of epilepsy. In: Gastaut H (ed) Handbook of electroencephalography and clinical neurophysiology. Elsevier, Amsterdam 13: 65–104
Gastaut H, Gomez-Almanzar M, Taury M 1984 The enforced nap: a simple effective method of inducing sleep activation in epileptics. In: Degen R, Niedermeyer E (eds) Epilepsy, sleep and sleep deprivation. Elsevier, Amsterdam, p 75–83
Gates R J 1986 Epilepsy presurgical evaluation in the era of intensive neurodiagnostic monitoring. In: Gumnit R J (ed) Advances in neurology: intensive neurodiagnostic monitoring. Raven Press, New York, 46: 227–248
Geller M R, Gourdji N, Christoff N, Fox E 1969 The effect of sleep deprivation on the EEGs of epileptic children. Developmental Medicine and Child Neurology 11: 771–776
Gibbs F A, Gibbs E L 1964 Atlas of electroencephalography vol III, Neurological and psychiatric disorders. Addison-Wesley, Reading
Goldring S 1978 A method for surgical management of focal epilepsy, especially as it relates to children. Journal of Neurosurgery 49: 344–356
Goode D J, Penry J K, Dreifuss F E 1970 Effects of paroxysmal spike-wave on continuous visual-motor performance. Epilepsia 11: 241–254
Gotman J 1982 Automatic recognition of epileptic seizures in the EEG. Electroencephalography and Clinical Neurophysiology 54: 530–540
Gotman J, Gloor P 1976 Automatic recognition and quantification of interictal epileptic activity in the human scalp EEG. Electroencephalography and Clinical Neurophysiology 41: 513–529
Gotman J, Marciani M G 1985 Electroencephalographic spiking activity, drug levels and seizure occurrence in epileptic patients. Annals of Neurology 17: 597–603
Gotman J, Ives J R, Gloor P 1979 Automatic recognition of interictal epileptic activity in prolonged EEG recordings. Electroencephalography and Clinical Neurophysiology 46: 510–520
Gregonades A D, Frangos E G 1977 Clinical observations on clonazepam in intractable epilepsy. In: Penry J K (ed) Epilepsy, the Eighth International Symposium. Raven Press, New York, p 169–176
Gumnit R J 1986 Intensive neurodiagnostic monitoring: role in the treatment of seizures. Neurology 36: 1340–1346
Hauser W A, Kurland L T 1975 The epidemiology of epilepsy in Rochester, Minnesota 1935 through 1967. Epilepsia 16: 1–66
Hauser W A, Anderson V E, Loewenson R B, McRoberts S M 1982 Seizure recurrence after a first unprovoked seizure. New England Journal of Medicine 307: 522–528
Hirtz D G, Ellenberg J H, Nelson K B 1984 The risk of recurrence of nonfebrile seizures in children. Neurology (Cleveland) 34: 637–641
Hosokawa K, Kugoh T, Otsuki S 1979 Longitudinal study of EEG spike appearance in long-term follow-up patients with epilepsy. Folia Psychiatrica et Neurologica Japonica 33: 141–146
Hughes J R 1967 EEG epileptiform abnormalities at different ages. Epilepsia 8: 93–104
Hughes J R 1985 Long-term clinical and EEG changes in patients with epilepsy. Archives of Neurology 42: 213–223
Iida N, Okada S, Tsuboi T 1985 EEG abnormalities in nonepileptic patients. Folia Psychiatrica et Neurologica Japonica 39: 43–58
Ives J R, Gloor P 1977 New sphenoidal electrode assembly to permit long-term monitoring of the patients ictal or interictal EEG. Electroencephalography and Clinical Neurophysiology 42: 575–580
Ives J R, Woods J F 1975 Four-channel 24-hour cassette recorder for long-term EEG monitoring of ambulatory patients. Electroencephalography and Clinical Neurophysiology 39: 88–92
Ives J R, Thompson C J, Gloor P 1976 Seizure monitoring: a new tool in electroencephalography. Electroencephalography and Clinical Neurophysiology 41: 422–427
Ives J R, Hausser C, Woods J F, Andermann F 1981 Contributions of 4-channel cassette EEG monitoring to differential diagnosis of paroxysmal attacks. In: Dam M, Gram L, Penry J K (eds) Advances in Epileptology (XII Epilepsy International Symposium). Raven Press, New York p 329–336

Janz D, Kern A, Moessinger H J, Puhlmann H U 1983 Ruckfall—prognose wärend und nach reduktion der medikamente bei epilepsiebehandlung. In: Reinschmidt H, Rentz R, Jungmanz J (eds) Epilepsie 1981. Thieme, Stuttgart p 17–24
Jeavons P M 1982 Photosensitive epilepsy. In: Laidlaw J, Richens A (eds) A textbook of epilepsy 2nd edn. Churchill Livingstone, Edinburgh, p 195–211
Jeavons P M, Harding G F A 1975 Photosensitive epilepsy. A review of the literature and a study of 460 patients. Heinemann, London
Johnson L C, DeBolt W L, Long M T et al 1972 Diagnostic factors in adult males following initial seizures: a three year follow-up. Archives of Neurology 27: 193–197
Juul-Jensen P 1964 Frequency of recurrence after discontinuance of anticonvulsant therapy in patients with epileptic seizures. Epilepsia 5: 352–363
Juul-Jenson P 1968 Frequency of recurrence after discontinuance of anticonvulsant therapy in patients with epileptic seizures. Epilepsia 9: 11–16
Kellaway P 1979 An orderly approach to visual analysis: the parameters of the normal EEG in adults and children. In: Klass D W, Daly D D (eds) Current practice of clinical electroencephalography. Raven Press, New York, p 69–147
Kellaway P, Frost J D, Hrachovy R A 1978 Relationship between clinical state, ictal and interictal EEG discharges, and serum drug levels: partial seizures/phenobarbital. Annals of Neurology 4: 197
Kellaway P, Saltzberg B, Frost J D, Crawley J W 1979 Relationship between clinical state, ictal and interictal EEG discharges, and serum drug levels: Generalized epilepsy/ethosuximide. Neurology 29: 559
King D W, So E L, Marcus R, Gallagher B B 1986 Techniques and applications of sphenoidal recording. Journal of Clinical Neurophysiology 3: 51–65
Klass D W, Daly D D 1979 Appendix. In: Klass D W, Daly D D (eds) Current practice of clinical electroencephalography. Raven Press, New York, p 481–496
Klass D W, Westmoreland B F 1985 Nonepileptogenic epileptiform electroencephalographic activity. Annals of Neurology 18: 627–635
Kristensen O, Sindrup E H 1978 Sphenoidal electrodes. Their use in electroencephalographic investigation of complex partial epilepsy. Acta Neurologica Scandinavica 58: 157–166
Kubicki S T, Scheuler W, Brittenbecher H 1984 Short-term sleep in EEG recordings after partial sleep deprivation as a routine procedure in order to uncover epileptic phenomena: an evaluation of 719 EEG recordings. In: Degan R, Niedermeyer E (eds) Epilepsy, sleep and sleep deprivation. Elsevier, Amsterdam, p 249–271
Laplane R, Salbreaux R 1963 Convulsions hyperpyretiques. Revue Practique (Paris) 13: 753–761
Lennox M A 1949 Febrile convulsions in childhood: a clinical and electroencephalographic study. American Journal of Diseases of Children 78: 868–882
Lennox-Buchthal M A 1973 Febrile Convulsions: A reappraisal. Electroencephalography and Clinical Neurophysiology (Supplement 32)
Levy L L, Fenichel G M 1965 Diphenylhydantoin activated seizures. Neurology (Minneap) 15: 716–722
Maheshwari M C, Jeavons P M 1975 The effect of sodium valproate (Epilim) on the EEG. Electroencephalography and Clinical Neurophysiology 39: 429
Marcus R W, So E, King D W, Gallagher B B 1984 Comparison of sphenoidal, nasopharyngeal and surface electrodes in evaluating patients with partial complex seizures. Epilepsia 25: 652
Martin D, Hirt H R 1973 Clinical experience with clonazepam (Rivotril) in the treatment of epilepsies in infancy and childhood. Neuropädiatrie 4: 245–266
Martins da Silva A, Aarts J H P, Binnie C D et al 1984 The circadian distribution of interictal epileptiform activity. Electroencephalography and Clinical Neurophysiology 58: 1–13
Mattson R H 1980 Value of intensive monitoring. In: Wada J A, Penry J K (eds) Advances in epileptology (The Xth Epilepsy International Symposium). Raven Press, New York, p 43–51
Mattson R H, Pratt K L, Calverly J R 1965 Electroencephalograms of epileptics following sleep deprivation. Archives of Neurology 13: 310–315
Mattson R H, Cramer J A, Collins J F et al 1985 Comparison of carbamazepine, phenobarbital, phenytoin and primidone in partial and secondarily generalized tonic-clonic seizures. New England Journal of Medicine 313: 145–151
Metrakos K, Metrakos J D 1961 Genetics of convulsive disorders. II genetics and electroencephalographic studies in centrencephalic epilepsy. Neurology (Minneap) 11: 474–483
Meyer J S, Gotoh F 1960 Metabolic and electroencephalographic effects of hyperventilation. Archives of Neurology (Chicago) 5: 539–552
Miley M E, Forster F M 1977 Activation of partial complex seizures by hyperventilation. Archives of Neurology 34: 371–373
Millichap J G, Madsen J A, Aledort L M 1960 Studies in febrile seizures V. Clinical and electroencephalographic studies in unselected patients. Neurology (Minneap) 10: 643–653

Milligan N, Oxley M J, Richens A 1983 Acute effects of intravenous phenytoin on the frequency of interictal spikes in man. British Journal of Clinical Pharmacology 16: 285–289
Morgan M H, Scott D F 1970 EEG activation in epilepsies other than petit mal. Epilepsia 11: 255–261
Nanda R N, Johnson R H, Keogh H J, Lambie D G, Melville I D, Shakir R A 1977 Treatment of chronic epilepsy for 1 to 2 years with clonazepam. In: Penry J K (ed) Epilepsy The Eighth International Symposium. Raven Press, New York p 163–168
Newmark M E, Penry J K 1979 Photosensitivity and Epilepsy: A Review. Raven Press, New York
Niedermeyer E 1982 Sleep and EEG. In: Neidermeyer E, Lopes Da Silva F (eds) Electroencephalography: basic principles, clinical applications and related fields. Urban and Schwartzenberg, Baltimore, p 93–106
Overweg J, Rowan A J, Binnie C D, Oosting J, Nagelkerke N J D 1981 Prediction of seizure recurrence after withdrawal of antiepileptic drugs. In: Dam M, Gram L, Penry J K (eds) Advances in epileptology (Twelfth Epilepsy International Symposium). Raven Press, New York, p 503–508
Overweg J, Binnie C D, Oosting J, Rowan A J 1987 Clinical and EEG prediction of seizure recurrence following antiepileptic drug withdrawal. Epilepsy Research 1: 272–283
Oxley J, Roberts M 1985 Clinical evaluation of 4-channel ambulatory EEG monitoring in the management of patients with epilepsy. Journal of Neurology, Neurosurgery and Psychiatry 48: 930–932
Pampiglione G, Kerridge J 1956 EEG abnormalities from the temporal lobe studied with sphenoidal electrodes. Journal of Neurology, Neurosurgery and Psychiatry 19: 117–129
Pedley T A 1987 Epilepsy. In: Halliday A M, Butler S R, Paul R (eds) A textbook of clinical neurophysiology. Wiley, Chichester, p 231–267
Penry J K, Porter R J, Dreifuss F E 1972 Ethosuximide: relation of plasma levels to clinical control. In: Woodbury D M, Penry J K, Schmidt R O (eds) Antiepileptic drugs. Raven Press, New York, p 431–441
Penry J K, Porter R J, Dreifuss F E 1975 Simultaneous recording of absence seizures with videotape and electroencephalography. Brain 98: 427–440
Pinder R M, Brogden R N, Speight T M, Avery G S 1977 Sodium valproate: a review of its pharmacological properties and therapeutic efficacy in epilepsy. Drugs 13: 81–123
Porter R J 1985 Intensive monitoring: epileptic and non-epileptic seizures. In: Porter R J, Morselli P L (eds) The epilepsies. Butterworths International Medical Reviews, Stoneham
Porter R J, Penry J K 1983 Petit mal status. In: Delgado-Escueta A V, Wasterlain C G, Treiman D M, Porter R J (eds) Advances in neurology: status epilepticus — mechanisms of brain damage and treatment. Raven Press, New York, 34: 61–67
Porter R J, Penry J K, Lacy J R 1977 Diagnostic and therapeutic re-evaluation of patients with intractable epilepsy. Neurology 27: 1006–1011
Pratt K L, Mattson R H, Weikers N J, Williams R 1968 EEG activation of epileptics following sleep deprivation: a prospective study of 114 cases. Electroencephalography and Clinical Neurophysiology 24: 11–15
Proposal for Classification of Epilepsies and Epileptic Syndromes 1985 Epilepsia 26 (3): 268–278
Pryse-Phillips W E M, Jeavons P M 1970 Effect of carbamazepine (Tegretol) on the electroencephalograph and ward behavior of patients with chronic epilepsy. Epilepsia 11: 263–273
Ramsey R E 1982 Clinical usefulness of ambulatory EEG monitoring of the neurological patient. In: Stott F D, Wright S L, Raftery E B, Clement D L (eds) ISAM 1981 (Proceedings of The Fourth International Symposium on Ambulatory Monitoring.) Academic Press, London, p 234–243
Reilly E L, Peters J F 1973 Relationship of some varieties of electroencephalographic photosensitivity to clinical convulsive disorders. Neurology (Minneap) 23: 1050–1057
Rodin E A 1968 The prognosis of patients with epilepsy. Thomas, Springfield, Ill.
Rodin E A, John G 1980 Withdrawal of anticonvulsant medications in successfully treated patients with epilepsy. In: Wada J A, Penry J K (eds) Advances in epileptology (The Xth Epilepsy International Symposium). Raven Press, New York, p 183–186
Rose S W, Penry J K, Markush R E, Radloff L A, Putnam P L 1973 Prevalence of epilepsy in children. Epilepsia 14: 133–152
Roseman E 1961 Dilantin toxicity. A clinical and electroencephalographic study. Neurology (Minneap) 11: 912–921
Rovit R L, Gloor P, Rasmussen T 1961 Sphenoidal electrodes in the electrographic study of patients with temporal lobe epilepsy: an evaluation. Journal of Neurosurgery 18: 151–158
Rowan A J, Binnie C D, Warfield C A, Meinardi H, Meijer J W A 1979 The delayed effect of sodium valproate on the photoconvulsive response in man. Epilepsia 20: 61–68
Rowan A J, Binnie C D, Overweg J, DeVries J, Kamp A 1980a The value of prolonged EEG/video monitoring as a routine diagnostic procedure in epilepsy. In: Canger R, Angeleri F, Penry J K (eds) Advances in epileptology (XIth Epilepsy International Symposium). Raven Press, New York, p 139–142

Rowan A J, Overweg J, Sadikoglu S, Binnie C D, Nagelkerke N J D, Hünteler E 1980b Seizure prognosis in long-stay mentally subnormal epileptic patients: inter-rater EEG and clinical studies. Epilepsia 21: 219–226

Rowan A J, Veldhuizen R J, Nagelkerke N J D 1982 Comparative evaluation of sleep deprivation and sedated sleep EEGs as diagnostic aids in epilepsy. Electroencephalography and Clinical Neurophysiology 54: 357–364

Rowan A J, Meijer J W A, de Beer-Pawlikowski N et al 1983 Valproate-ethosuximide combination therapy for refractory absence seizures. Archives of Neurology 40: 797–802

Rowan A J, Siegel M, Rosenbaum D H 1987 Daytime intensive monitoring: comparison with prolonged intensive and ambulatory monitoring. Neurology 37: 481–484

Salinsky M, Kanter R, Dasheiff R M 1987 Effectiveness of multiple EEGs in supporting the diagnosis of epilepsy: an operational curve. Epilepsia 28: 331–334

Sato S, Dreifuss F E, Penry J K 1973 The effect of sleep on spike-wave discharges in absence seizures. Neurology (Minneap) 23: 1335–1345

Sato S, White B G, Penry J K, Dreifuss F E, Sackellares J C, Kupferberg H J 1982 Valproic acid versus ethosuximide in the treatment of absence seizures. Neurology (NY) 32: 157–163

Saunders M, Marshall C 1975 Isolated seizures: an EEG and clinical assessment. Epilepsia 16: 731–733

Saunders M G, Westmoreland B F 1979 The EEG in evaluation of disorders affecting the brain diffusely. In: Klass D W, Dale D D (eds) Current practice of clinical electroencephalography. Raven Press, New York, p 343–380

Scheffner D, Schiefer I 1972 The treatment of epileptic children with carbamazepine: follow-up studies of clinical course and EEG. Epilepsia 13: 819–828

Schmidt D 1985 Discontinuation of antiepileptic drugs. In: Porter R J, Morselli P L (eds) The epilepsies. Butterworths International Medical Reviews, Stoneham p 227–241

Schwab R S, Schwab M W, Withee D, Chock Y C 1954 Synchronized moving pictures of patient and EEG. Electroencephalography and Clinical Neurophysiology 6: 684–686

Scollo-Lavizzari G, Pralle W, De La Cruz N 1975 Activation effects of sleep deprivation and sleep in seizure patients: an electroencephalographic study. European Neurology 13: 1–5

Shinnar S, Vining E P G, Mellits E D et al 1985 Discontinuing antiepileptic medication in children with epilepsy after two years without seizures. New England Journal of Medicine 13: 976–980

Silverman D 1960 The anterior temporal electrode and the ten-twenty system. Electroencephalography and Clinical Neurophysiology 12: 735–737

Simon D, Penry J K 1975 Sodium di-n-propylacetate (DPA) in the treatment of epilepsy. A review. Epilepsia 16: 549–573

Spadetta V 1971 La privazione di sonno nella diagnosi elettroencefalografica di epilessia. Acta Neurologica (Napoli) 26: 7–13

Spenser S S 1980 Depth electroencephalography in selection of refractory epilepsy for surgery. Annals of Neurology 9: 207–214

Sperling M R, Engel J 1985 Electroencephalographic recording from the temporal lobes: a comparison of ear, anterior temporal, and nasopharyngeal electrodes. Annals of Neurology 17: 510–513

Stålberg E 1976 Experience with long-term telemetry in routine diagnostic work. In: Kellaway P, Petersen I (eds) Quantitative analytic studies in epilepsy. Raven Press, New York, p 269–278

Strobos R J, Kavallinis G P 1968 Changes in repeat electroencephalograms in epileptics. Neurology 18: 622–633

Takahashi T 1982 Activation methods. In: Niedermeyer E, Lopes DaSilva F (eds) Electroencephalography: basic principles, clinical applications and related fields. Urban and Schwartzenberg, Baltimore, p 179–196

Takahashi T, Niedermeyer E, Knott J R 1965 The EEG in older and younger adult groups with convulsive disorder. Epilepsia 6: 24–32

Theodore W H, Sato S, Porter R J 1984 Serial EEG in intractable epilepsy. Neurology (Cleveland) 34: 863–867

Thurston J H, Thurston D L, Hixon B B, Keller A J 1982 Prognosis in childhood epilepsy: 148 children 15 to 23 years after withdrawal of anticonvulsant therapy. New England Journal of Medicine 306: 831–836

Todt H 1984 The late prognosis of epilepsy in childhood: results of a prospective follow-up study. Epilepsia 25: 137–144

Treiman D M, Delgado-Escueta A V 1983 Complex partial status epilepticus. In: Delgado-Escueta A V, Wasterlain C G, Treiman D M, Porter R J (eds) Advances in neurology, status epilepticus mechanisms of brain damage and treatment. Raven Press, New York, 34: 69–82

Veldhuizen R, Binnie C D, Beintema D J 1983 The effect of sleep deprivation on the EEG in epilepsy. Electroencephalography and Clinical Neurophysiology 55: 505–512

Villarreal H J, Wilder B J, Willmore L J, Bauman A W, Hammond E J, Bruni J 1978 Effect of valproic acid on spike and wave discharges in patients with absence seizures. Neurology (Minneap) 28: 886–891
Westmoreland B F 1985 The electroencephalogram in patients with epilepsy. In: Aminoff M J (ed) Electrodiagnosis. Neurology Clinics 3: 599–613
Westmoreland B F, Klass D W 1981 A distinctive rhythmic EEG discharge of adults. Electroencephalography and Clinical Neurophysiology 51: 186–191
Wilkus R J, Green J R 1974 Electroencephalographic investigations during evaluation of the antiepileptic agent Sulthiame. Epilepsia 15: 13–25
Wilkus R J, Dodrill C B, Troupin A S 1978 Carbamazepine and the electroencephalogram of epileptics: A double blind study in comparison to phenytoin. Epilepsia 19: 283–291
Zivin L, Ajmone-Marsan C 1968 Incidence and prognostic significance of 'epileptiform' activity in the EEG of non-epileptic subjects. Brain 91: 751–778
Zwarts M J, Sie O 1985 A case report of phenytoin encephalopathy. Correlation between serum levels, seizure increase and EEG spike and wave activity. Clinical Neurology and Neurosurgery 87: 205–208

# 5. Teratogenicity of antiepileptic drugs

*M. S. Yerby*

## INTRODUCTION

Epilepsy is one of the most common neurological disorders with a prevalence of approximately 6/1000 (Hauser & Kurland 1975). Antiepileptic drugs (AED) permit a majority of persons with epilepsy to live with little interference from seizures. Changing public attitudes and the repeal of discriminatory legislation prohibiting marriage may encourage more women with epilepsy to bear children than in the past. Women with epilepsy now account for 1 of every 200 pregnancies (Svigos 1984). Despite many medical advances, women with epilepsy are at greater risk for complications of pregnancy and adverse pregnancy outcomes.

Low birth weight (< 2500 g) and prematurity occur more often in infants of epileptic mothers (IEM), ranging from 7–10% and 4–11% respectively (Svigos 1984 Levy & Yerby 1985, Bjerkdal & Bahna 1973, Nelson & Ellenberg 1982, Nakane et al 1980, Kallen 1986). Microcephaly has been demonstrated with increased frequency in IEM (Nelson & Ellenberg 1982, Neri et al 1983). Stillbirth rates are higher in IEM (1.3–14%) compared to controls (1.2–7.8%) (Nelson & Ellenberg 1982, Nakane et al 1980, Janz & Fuchs 1964, Nakane 1979). Other studies have also demonstrated increased rates of neonatal and perinatal death. Rates have ranged from 1.3–7.8% for IEM compared to 1.0–3.9% for controls (Bjerkedal & Bahna 1973, Nelson & Ellenberg 1982, Kallen 1986, Janz & Fuchs 1964, Knight & Rhind 1975, Higgins & Comerford 1974, Speidel & Meadow 1968).

Congenital malformations are the most widely reported as well as the most dramatic adverse outcome of pregnancy. Malformations are defined as a physical defect requiring medical or surgical intervention and causing major functional disturbance. Infants of epileptic mothers exposed to AED in utero are twice as likely to develop birth defects as infants not exposed to these drugs (Speidel & Meadow 1972, Fredrick 1983).

## HISTORICAL ASPECTS

The first report of a malformation attributed to AED described a child exposed to mephenytoin in utero with microcephaly, cleft palate, intestinal malrotation, a speech defect and an IQ of 60 (Muller-Kuppers 1963). The author first examined the child when he was 3 years 7 months of age and noted that the pregnancy was also complicated by vaginal bleeding.

A retrospective survey to evaluate the problem of AED-associated malformations was performed at the University of Heidelberg by Janz & Fuchs (1964). 426 pregnancies in 246 mothers with epilepsy were studied. The rates of miscarriages and stillbirths were increased for these patients, but the malformation rate was only 2.2%, not significantly different from that of the general population of West Germany. The authors concluded that AED were not associated with an increased risk of malformations.

Pantarotto (1965) described a neonate with aplasia of the bone marrow after phenytoin exposure in utero. Centa & Rasore-Quartino (1965) reported the first case of congenital heart disease with in-utero exposure to phenytoin and phenobarbital. Melchior et al (1967) described orofacial clefts with exposure to primidone or phenobarbital.

In a letter to Lancet, Meadow (1968) reported six cases of children with orofacial clefts, four of whom had additional abnormalities of the heart and dysmorphic facial features. All of these children had been exposed to AED in utero. He noted that similar abnormalities had been reported following the unsuccessful use of abortifactant folic acid antagonists. Since some AED act as folic acid antagonists, Meadow postulated that this might be the basis for AED teratogenicity.

In 1970, trimethadione was implicated as a teratogen in 8 of 14 pregnancies in which it was taken in the first trimester (German et al 1970). One mother had four malformed children while taking trimethadione. After discontinuing the drug, she had two normal children. This led the authors to survey retrospectively all of the deliveries of women with epilepsy in their institution. Over a 22 year period they found 278 such cases. Among these the congenital malformation rate was 5.8%, which was not considered a significant increase. German et al (1970) did find, however, that children exposed to trimethadione were at increased risk for birth defects with a 57% malformation rate.

Meadow collected 30 additional cases of IEM with congenital malformations and reported them in a retrospective survey by Spiedel & Meadow (1972) in which 427 pregnancies in 186 women with epilepsy were identified. For the first time a clear increase in the malformation rates of IEM was demonstrated.

The authors concluded that: (1) congenital malformations were twice as common in IEM exposed to AED; (2) no single abnormality was specific for AED exposure; and (3) a group of these children would have a characteristic pattern of anomalies which at its fullest expression consisted of trigonocephaly, microcephaly, hypertelorism, low set ears, short neck, transverse palmar creases, and minor skeletal abnormalities.

Unfortunately, subsequent studies have added little to this basic knowledge. Congenital malformations remain the most commonly reported adverse outcome in the pregnancies of epileptic mothers. Malformation rates in the general population range from 2–3% (Kalter & Warkany 1983, Kelly 1984a). Reports of malformation rates in various populations of IEM range from 1.25–11.5% (Nakane et al 1980, Meadow 1968, Philbert & Dam 1982). These combined estimates yield a risk of malformations in a pregnant women with epilepsy of 4–6%. Table 5.1 reviews the various studies which compare malformation rates in the offspring of epileptic and non-epileptic mothers.

## CURRENT CONCEPTS

The increased rate of malformations in offspring of epileptic mothers appears to be related in large part to AED exposure in utero. Evidence to support this association comes from four observations:

**Table 5.1** Malformation rates in the offspring of epileptic and control mothers

| | Control | | Epileptic mothers | |
|---|---|---|---|---|
| Authors | Malformation rate (%) | No. of pregnancies | Malformation rate (%) | No. of pregnancies |
| Sabin & Oxorn (1956) | | | 5.4 | 56 |
| Janz & Fuchs (1964) | | | 2.3 | 225 |
| German et al (1970) | | | 5.3 | 243 |
| Elshove & Van Eck (1971) | 1.9 | 12 051 | 15.0 | 65 |
| Speidel & Meadow (1972) | 1.6 | 483 | 5.2 | 427 |
| South (1972) | 2.4 | 7896 | 6.4 | 31 |
| Spellacy (1972) | | 50 | 5.8 | 51 |
| Bjerkedal & Bahna (1973) | 2.2 | 112 530 | 4.5 | 311 |
| Fedrick (1973) | 5.6 | 649 | 13.8 | 217 |
| Koppe et al (1973) | 2.9 | 12 455 | 6.6 | 197 |
| Kuenssberg & Knox (1973) | 3.0 | 14 668 | 10.0 | 48 |
| Lowe (1973) | 2.7 | 31 877 | 5.0 | 245 |
| Meyer (1973) | 2.7 | 110 | 18.6 | 593 |
| Millar & Nevin (1973) | 3.8 | 32 227 | 6.4 | 110 |
| Monson et al (1973) | 2.4 | 50 591 | 4.7 | 306 |
| Niswander & Wertelecki (1973) | 2.7 | 347 097 | 4.1 | 413 |
| Biale et al (1975) | | | 16.0 | 56 |
| Knight & Rhind (1975) | 3.65 | 69 000 | 4.3 | 140 |
| Starreveld & Zimmerman (1975) | | | 7.0 | 372 |
| Visser et al (1976) | 2.3 | 9869 | 3.7 | 54 |
| Weber et al (1977) | 2.2 | 5011 | 4.0 | 731 |
| Annegers et al (1978) | 3.5 | 748 | 8.1 | 259 |
| Seino & Miyokosh (1979) | | | 13.7 | 272 |
| Dieterich et al (1980) | | | | 37 |
| Majewshi et al (1980) | | | 16.0 | 111 |
| Nakawe et al (1980) | | | 11.5 | 700 |
| Hillesmaa et al (1981) | 2.0 | 5613 | 7.7 | 4795 |
| Beaussart et al (1986) | | | 7.8 | 295 |

1. Comparisons of the malformation rates in the offspring of treated mothers with epilepsy with those not exposed to AED treatment reveal consistently higher rates in the children of the treated group as illustrated in Table 5.2 (Nakane et al 1980, Speidel & Meadow 1972, Monson et al 1973, Annegers et al 1978, Lowe 1973, South 1972).

2. Mean plasma AED concentrations are higher in mothers with malformed infants than mothers with healthy children (Dansky et al 1980).

3. Infants of mothers taking multiple AED have higher malformation rates than those exposed to monotherapy (Nakane 1979, Lindout et al 1984).

4. Maternal seizures during pregnancy do not appear to contribute to the risk of congenital malformations (Fredrick 1983). In fact, there appears to be no association between seizures during pregnancy and the development of malformations, epilepsy or febrile convulsions in the offspring of women with epilepsy (Annegers et al 1978).

Virtually every type of congenital malformation has been reported in children of epileptic mothers, and every anticonvulsant medication has been implicated in their development. Cleft lip and/or palate and congenital heart disease account for a majority of all reported cases (Annegers et al 1978, Elshove & Van Eck 1971, Anderson 1976). Orofacial clefts are relatively common malformations in the general population occurring with a frequency of 1.5 per 1000 live births. Infants of epileptic mothers have

**Table 5.2** Malformation rates in the offspring of treated and non-treated epileptic mothers

| Authors | Malformation rate (%) Anticonvulsants | No anticonvulsants |
|---|---|---|
| Janz & Fuchs (1964) | 2.2 | 0 |
| Speidel & Meadow (1972) | 5.2 | 0 |
| South (1972) | 9.0 | 0 |
| Lowe (1973) | 6.7 | 2.7 |
| Monson (1973) | 5.3 | 2.9 |
| Annegers (1974) | 7.1 | 1.8 |
| Annegers (1978) | 10.7 | 2.4 |
| Nakane (1979) | 11.5 | 2.3 |

a rate of orofacial clefting of 13.8 per 1000, a nine fold increase in risk (Kelly 1984a). Early observations that persons with clefting of the lip or palate were twice as likely to have family members with epilepsy as controls suggested that orofacial clefts were associated with epilepsy (Friis et al 1986). Subsequent studies of the prevalence of facial clefts in the siblings and children of 2072 persons with epilepsy found observed/expected ratios increased only for maternal epilepsy. The risk was greater if AED were taken during pregnancy (4.7) than if no AED treatment was used (2.7). The authors concluded that there was no evidence that epilepsy itself contributed to the development of orofacial clefts (Friis et al 1986). Orofacial clefts account for 30% of the excess of congenital malformations in IEM.

Congenital heart defects are the second most frequently reported teratogenic abnormality associated with AED. Most studies do not give specific rates for congenital heart disease. Anderson collected data prospectively on maternal epilepsy and AED use in 3000 children with heart defects at the University of Minnesota. 18 IEM were identified, and 12 of these had ventricular septal defects. Although this was not a greater number of cases than one would expect given the prevalence of epilepsy in the general population, 9 of the 18 children had additional noncardiac defects and eight had orofacial clefts. The risk of a woman with epilepsy bearing a child with congenital heart disease was 0.6% (Anderson 1976).

No AED can be considered absolutely safe in pregnancy, but for the vast majority of drugs no specific pattern of major malformations has been identified. This lack of a particular or characteristic pattern of defects has been cited as evidence that AED are not teratogenic. When phenobarbital is giving during pregnancy for conditions other than epilepsy, no increase in malformation rates has been demonstrated (Shapiro et al 1976).

Some investigators have found increased malformation rates in the infants of epileptic fathers and suggest that epilepsy per se is associated with birth defects and not AED exposure (Dieterich et al 1980, Friis & Hauge 1985). Others have failed to demonstrate an increased malformation rate in IEM (Grosse et al 1972). These studies are for the most part retrospective, and thus case ascertainment is uncertain. The weight of the evidence tends to support some teratogenic effect of AED, for in addition to major malformations there are a variety of syndromes of anomalies associated with AED exposure.

## SYNDROMES OF ANOMALIES

In distinction to malformations which are deformaties of anatomy requiring medical or surgical intervention to maintain a functionally healthy person, anomalies are abnormalities of structure which, while varing from the norm, do not constitute a threat to health. Patterns of anomalies in infants of epileptic mothers (IEM) have been noted in respect to certain AED exposure. Three clinical syndromes have been reported in IEM: fetal trimethadione syndrome, fetal hydantoin syndrome, and fetal valproate syndrome. The clinical features of these syndromes are ouitlined in Table 5.3.

**Table 5.3** Syndromes of anomalies associated with anticonvulsants

| |
|---|
| *Fetal trimethadione syndrome* |
| Development delay |
| V-shaped eyebrows |
| Low set ears |
| IUGR |
| Cardiac anomalies |
| Speech difficulties |
| Epicanthal folds |
| Irregular teeth |
| Microcephaly |
| Inguinal hernia |
| Simian creases |
| *Fetal hydantoin syndrome* |
| Craniofacial anomalies |
| Broad nasal bridge |
| Short upturned nose |
| Low set ears |
| Prominent lips |
| Epicanthal folds |
| Hypertelorism |
| Wide mouth |
| Ptosis or strabismus |
| Distal digital hypoplasia |
| IUGR |
| Mental deficiency |
| *Fetal valproate syndrome* |
| Craniofacial anomalies |
| Epicanthal folds inferiorly |
| Small anteverted nose |
| Shallow philtrum |
| Flat nasal bridge |
| Long upper lip |
| Downturned mouth |
| Thin vermillion border |

## Fetal trimethadione syndrome

In 1970, German and colleagues described a case of a woman with epilepsy treated with trimethadione who had had four unsuccessful pregnancies. After trimethadione was discontinued, she went on to have two healthy children. Her physician then surveyed trimethadione exposed infants delivered at New York Hospital between 1946 and 1968. The records of 278 women with epilepsy were reviewed, and of these, 14 had taken trimethadione during pregnancy. Only 2 of these 14 children were normal. One had multiple hernias and diabetes; eight had developmental defects; three were spontaneously aborted; and only 3 of the 14 actually survived infancy.

The peculiar facial characteristics of these children were delineated by Zachai et al (1975), who noted that not only were these children short in stature and suffering from microcephaly, they had V-shaped eyebrows, epicanthal folds, low set ears, anteriorly folded helices, and irregular teeth. Other abnormalities were often frequent: inguinal hernias, hypospadias and simian creases. Feldman et al (1977) reviewed 53 pregnancies in which trimethadione was used. In 46 of these (87%), there was fetal loss or the development of a congenital malformation. Follow-up studies of the surviving children have reported significant rates of mental retardation (Goldman et al 1986).

**Fetal hydantoin syndrome**

Working at the Childrens Orthopedic Hospital in Seattle, Washington, Hanson & Smith (1975) reported five infants of epileptic mothers who had been exposed to hydantion in utero. These infants had multiple systemic abnormalities of the face, cranium and nails, distal digital hypoplasia, intrauterine growth retardation, and mental deficiencies. They noted that these infants resembled children with fetal alcohol syndrome, and described their cases as suffering from a fetal hydantoin syndrome. Only 1 of these 5 children was exposed to hydantoin monotherapy in utero. Of the others, three were also exposed to phenobarbital, one to mephobarbital, and the other to a combination of phenobarbital phensuximide and mephenytoin. Subsequent work by Hanson's group found that approximately 11% of infants exposed to hydantoin in utero demonstrated the complete syndrome, and an additional 30% would have some anomalous components (Hanson et al 1976). Many of the features of the hydantoin syndrome appear to be subjective, but some investigators believe that distal digital hypoplasia is a unique feature of the syndrome (Kelly 1984b). In fact 2 years before Hanson's and Smith's initial report, Loughman et al (1973) had described seven infants with variable degrees of hypoplasia and irregular ossification of the distal phalanges who had been exposed to hydantoin in utero. Researchers at the University of Virginia followed 98 women with epilepsy who took phenytoin during pregnancy and found that 30% of their offspring had distal digital hypoplasia with no other features of the fetal hydantoin syndrome (Kelly et al 1984b).

Long-term follow-up of children with the fetal hydantoin syndrome has been incomplete, and the long-term significance of these dysmorphic features is therefore unclear. Hanson (1986) feels that there are three components to the syndrome; (1) abnormal growth, (2) abnormal performance, and (3) dysmorphic cranial facial features. An unexpected sequela of the syndrome appears to be an increased risk of cancer. Four cases of neuroblastoma associated with the fetal hydantoin syndrome have been described since 1976, although all children were also exposed in utero to primidone or phenobarbital. There have also been reports of carcinoma, ganglioneuroblastoma, Wilms tumor, a melanotic neuroectodermal tumor, and a malignant mesenchymoma in children with fetal hydantoin syndrome (Ehrenband & Chaganti 1981).

A mouse model of phenytoin teratogensis was developed by Finnel (1981). Mice with spontaneous epilepsy who are treated with phenytoin during pregnancy bear pups with malformation rates that are directly related to the dose and concentration of phenytoin but not to the frequency of maternal seizures. Finnel explained differences in expression of the fetal hydantoin syndrome as being secondary to genotypic differences and susceptibility to a specific malformation. In three separate inbred strains of mice exposed to diphenylhydantoin in utero, all showed different frequencies of distributions of malformations, even though as a whole, malformations were increased in each group (Finnell & Chernoft 1984).

### Fetal valproate syndrome

Reports of dysmorphic children exposed to valproate in utero had previously been made by other investigators (Dalens et al 1980, Clay et al 1981), but it was DiLiberti et al (1984) who described a specific fetal valproate syndrome. They reported on seven infants exposed to valproic acid in utero who had facial abnormalities characterized by interior epicanthal folds, a flat nasal bridge, an upturned nose, a long upper lip, a thin vermilion border, a shallow philtrum, and downturned mouth. These children also had abnormalities of their distal digits, and they tended to have long thin overlapping fingers toes and hyper-convex nails. The prevalence of this syndrome has not yet been established. Jager-Roman et al (1986) described it in 5 of 14 children exposed to valproate monotherapy. In this same group, 43% of the children were distressed at labor, and 28% had low Apgar scores and other major malformations. In a review of 344 women who took valproate during the first trimester of pregnancy Jeavons (1984) described a 19.8% rate of abnormal deliveries.

The association of valproate with spina bifida is discussed further on.

### Benzodiazepine syndromes

Infants exposed to benzodiazepines in utero are at greater risk for intrauterine growth retardation, dysmorphic features and neurological dysfunction. Seven of 37 infants exposed to benzodiazepine drugs in utero were described as hypotonic and hyperexcitable, with dystonic postures and choreoathetotic movements (Laegreid et al 1987). Delayed hand-eye co-ordination, psychomotor slowing, and a learning disability were also noted. Four infants had major malformations and dysmorphic faces with wide set eyes, epicanthal folds, up turned noses, dysplastic oracles, high arched palates, webbed necks and wide spaced nipples (Laegreid et al 1987).

### Primidone embryopathy

Two groups of investigators have described children exposed to primidone in utero who have craniofacial abnormalities characterized by hirsute forehead, thick nasal root anteverted nostrils, long philtrum, straight thin upper lip and hypoplastic nails (Rudd & Freedom 1979, Gustavson & Chen 1985). These children were also likely to be small for their gestional age, have psychomotor retardation and heart defects.

### Current concepts of anomalies

In my view, clinical and laboratory evidence clearly support the association of certain anticonvulsants with teratogenic effects, especially facial and distal digital anomalies. However, the existence of specific syndromes remains controversial. Facial dysmorphism is difficult to quantify and clearly is not drug specific. Infants of epileptic mothers with similar dysmorphic features have been described in the pre-anticonvulsant era (Philbert & Dam 1982, Baptisti 1938). Follow-up of these infants into adult life has yet to be accomplished, and therefore the significance of these anomalies is unclear. The hypothesized association of dysmorphic features with mental retardation (Kelly et al 1984) has not been confirmed (Granstrom 1982, Hutch et al 1975). In the few cases which have been followed into early childhood, the dysmorphic features tend to disappear as the child grows older (Janz 1982).

The primary abnormalities in these syndromes involve the mid-face and distal digits. A retrospective study spanning 10 years of deliveries in Israel found hypertelorism to be the only anomaly seen more often in infants of epileptic mothers than in controls (Neri et al 1983). This was associated with all AED except primidone. It has been suggested that since a variety of similar anomalies of the mid-face and distal digits are seen in a small proportion of children exposed to anticonvulsants in utero, a better term for the entire group of abnormalities would be fetal anticonvulsant syndrome or AED embryopathy (Dietrich et al 1980, Vorhees 1986).

## MECHANISMS OF TERATOGENICITY

Over the last 10 years a body of evidence has accumulated supporting the hypotheses that:

1. An arene oxide metabolite of phenytoin is the ultimate teratogen.
2. A genetic defect in epoxide hydrolase (arene oxide detoxifying enzyme system) increases the risk of fetal toxicity.

### Epoxides

A large number of drugs and chemicals can be converted into epoxides, reactions which are catalyzed by the microsomal monoxygenase system (Jerina & Daly 1974, Sims & Grover 1974). Arene oxides are epoxides formed by aromatic compounds. Various epoxides are electrophilic and may elicit carcinogenic, mutagenic and other toxic effects by covalent binding with critical cell macromolecules (Nebert & Jensen 1979, Shum et al 1979). Epoxides are detoxified by two types of processes: (1) conversion to dihydrodiols catalyzed by the enzyme system epoxide hydrolase, and (2) conjugation with glutathione (spontaneously or mediated by glutathione transferase). In adult and fetal human liver, epoxide hydrolase activities have been found in the cytosol and in the microsomal subcellular fraction. Interestingly, epoxide hydrolase activity in fetal liver activity is much lower than that of adult liver (Pacifici et al 1983).

### Phenytoin teratogenicity

*Formation of an arene oxide by phenytoin*

Arene oxides are obligatory intermediates in the metabolism of aromatic compounds to trans-dihydrodiols. For over 15 years, it has been known that phenytoin forms a trans-dihydrodiol metabolite in several species (Chang et al 1970). This metabolite is also formed by neonates exposed to phenytoin in utero (Horning et al 1974). In vitro studies have shown that an oxidative (NADPH/02 dependent) metabolite of phenytoin binds irreversibly to rat liver microsomes (Martz et al 1977). This binding is increased by an inhibitor of epoxide hydrolase (trichloroponene oxide, TCPO) and decreased by glutathione (Martz et al 1977, Pantarotto et al 1982, Wells & Harbison 1985). Using a mouse hepatic microsomal system to produce phenytoin metabolites, and human lymphocytes to assess cell defense mechanisms against toxicity, Spielberg et al (1981) showed that cytotoxicity was enhanced by inhibitors of epoxide hydrolase.

*Phenytoin arene oxide as a teratogen*

In a study in mice, Martz et al (1977) showed that treatment with an inhibitor of epoxide hydrolase was associated with an increase in the rate of orofacial anomalies in fetal animals exposed to phenytoin. Furthermore, there was a correlation between the teratogenic effect and the amount of covalently bound material in fetal tissue.

*Phenytoin birth defects and lymphocyte cytotoxicity*

Recently, Strickler et al (1985) examined lymphocytes of 24 children exposed to phenytoin during gestation and lymphocytes from their families using the Spielberg test (Speilberg et al 1981) of cytotoxicity. Lymphocytes were incubated with phenytoin in a mouse microsomal system (with appropriate cofactors to generate oxidative metabolities) and a positive response was defined as increase in cell death over baseline. Cells from 14 children gave a positive response. Each positive child had a positive parent (as many mothers as fathers). A positive in vitro response was highly correlated with major birth defects. The authors concluded that 'a genetic defect in arene oxide detoxification seems to increase the risk of the baby having major birth defects' (Strickler et al 1985). However, no measurement of epoxide hydrolase activity was included in this study.

*Phenytoin birth defects and epoxide hydrolase activity*

In 1985, Buehler reported epoxide hydrolase activity in skin fibroblasts of a pair of dizygotic twins exposed to phenytoin in utero. The infant who had more features of the fetal hydantoin syndrome showed lower epoxide hydrolase activity. Although this finding supports the epoxide hydrolase hypothesis, it should be noted that a full report of the experimental details has not yet appeared.

*Intersubject variability in epoxide hydrolase activity*

Since 1977, several studies have examined the degree of intersubject variability in epoxide hydrolase activity measured in various organs obtained at autopsy or from biopsies (Kapitulnik et al 1977, Guengerich et al 1979, Glatt et al 1980, Thomas et al 1982, Lorenz et al 1984, Cresteil et al 1985). Generally, a large degree of variability was found. In the most recent study, Mertes et al (1985) measured microsomal and cytosolic epoxide hydrolase activity in liver biopsy samples from 166 subjects. Microsomal epoxiode hydrolase activity was found to vary by a factor of 53, while the cytosolic activity varied 539-fold.

The above findings provide strong support for the hypothesis that a relationship exists between phenytoin teratogenicity and defects in epoxide hydrolase activity.

**Valproic acid teratogenicity**

One of the factors necessary for classifying a substance as a teratogen is an increase in a specific adverse outcome associated with exposure. Phocomelia associated with exposure to thalidomide is one such example. Though orofacial clefts are the most commonly reported malformations associated with AED exposure, they are clearly not the majority of malformations, which have led some investigators to contend that true teratogenicity is not associated with AED.

The introduction of valproic acid (VPA) to the anticonvulsant armamentarium may modify our thinking in this regard. Dysmorphism has been associated with in utero exposure to VPA. The first such case was reported by Dalens et al (1980), who described an infant exposed to VPA in utero who was born with low birth weight, hypoplastic nose and fronto-orbital ridges, and levocardia. The baby died at 19 days of life. Subsequent reports of dysmorphism followed by Clay et al (1981) and a child with lumbosacral meningocele was described by Gomez (1981). Dickinson et al (1979) had previously demonstrated the ability of VPA to cross the placenta. As already noted, a fetal valproate syndrome has been described (DiLiberti et al 1984) and several additional cases reported (Jeavons 1984, Tein & MacGregor 1985).

A report in MMWR of October, 1982, made the first association of VPA with a specific malformation, neural tube defects. The Institut European de Genomutations in Lyon, France has developed a system of birth defect surveillance and between 1976 and 1982, registered 145 cases of spina bifida. They noted that of infants of epileptic mothers exposed to VPA, 34% had malformations, and 5 of 9 exposed to VPA monotherapy had spina bifida a rate 20 times that expected (MMWR 1982).

Robert et al (1984) sent questionnaires to 646 women with epilepsy, aged 15–45 years. Of 280 responses they collected 74 deliveries to which they added 74 additional cases collected from women delivering in Lyons, France. The malformation rate of the entire group was 13%, with a higher than expected rate of neural tube defects in children exposed to VPA.

Stanley & Chambers (1982) reported an infant exposed to VPA in utero with spina bifida whose two normal siblings were not exposed to the drug. Lindhout & Schmidt (1986) surveyed 18 epilepsy groups and collected 12 cases of infants and epileptic mothers with neural tube defects. A higher rate was seen in children exposed to VPA monotherapy (2.5%) than polytherapy (1.5%). The increased risk appears to be limited to spina bifida rather than other neural tube defects with an overall risk of an infant exposed to VPA in utero of 1.5%.

### *Possible mechanisms of valproate teratogenicity*

The actual mechanism of VPA teratogenicity is unknown. A combination of valpromide and carbamazepine results in an increase in carbamazepine 10–11 expoxide (Pacifici et al 1985). Epoxides have been implicated as teratogens, but carbamazepine's epoxide is quite stable and there appears to be a greater risk of spina bifida with VPA monotherapy than polytherapy.

VPA appears to be embryotoxic to cultured whole rat embryos, but none of the hydroxlyated metabolites have exhibited any significant embryotoxicity (Rettie et al 1986). This implies a direct teratogenic effect of the parent drug.

## CONCLUSIONS

Infants of epileptic mothers exposed to anticonvulsants in utero have a greater risk of developing congenital malformations than non-exposed infants or infants of mothers without epilepsy. The overall risk of a birth defect is between 4 and 6%. In addition, a subgroup of exposed children will have characteristic dysmorphic features of the mid-face and distal digits of uncertain long-term significance. The prevalence of this AED syndrome is unclear but with phenytoin exposure approaches 30% (Kelly et al 1984).

All commonly used AED cross the placenta and are present in the fetal circulation, and fetal and maternal free concentrations are equivalent (Yerby & Levy 1985). All commonly used AED have been associated with congenital malformations, and while many different types have been described, orofacial clefts are the most common accounting for approximately 30% of the total (Friis et al 1986). Specific major malformations associated with AED have been described only for VPA which causes a 1% risk of spina bifida in exposed infants. AED share many of the features of classic teratogens but generally do not produce a consistent pattern of major malformations. Hence, the factors contributing to birth defects in children exposed to these drugs must be, in part, multifactoral.

Generalized convulsions pose clear risks for maternal injury and miscarriage (Higgins & Comertord 1974, Stumpf & Frost 1978, Burnett 1946). For most women, anticonvulsant therapy needs to be continued during pregnancy. In our experience, risks of adverse outcome can be reduced by careful prenatal care, good seizure control, and maintenance of high serum folate levels.

Risks can also be reduced by good preconception counseling, the use of monotherapy where possible, and consistent administration of prenatal vitamins with folic acid. Women taking VPA should be informed of the additional risks of spina bifida. The unique nature of this defect permits detection in the prenatal period. A combination of real time ultrasonography and amniocentesis for an alpha fetal protein between 16 and 18 weeks gestation will detect over 90% of all cases of spina bifida. Despite the very real risks, over 90% of women with epilepsy taking AED will deliver children free of congenital malformations.

## ACKNOWLEDGEMENTS

I would like to thank the following persons for without their assistance this manuscript would not have been possible: Dr René Levy, Mr Patrick Friel, Ms Karen B. McCormick, RN, Ms Lois Mathews.

## REFERENCES

Anderson R C 1976 Cardiac defects in children of mothers receiving anticonvulsant therapy during pregnancy. Journal of Pediatrics 89(2): 318–319

Annegers J R, Elveback L R, Hauser W A, Kurland L T 1974 Do anticonvulsants have a teratogenic effect? Archives of Neurology 31: 364–373

Annegers, J F, Hauser W A, Elveback L R et al 1978 Congenital malformations and seizure disorders in the offspring of parents with epilepsy. International Journal of Epidemology 7: 241–247

Annegers J F, Hauser W A, Elveback L R, Anderson V E, Kurland L T 1978 Congenital malformations and seizure disorders in the offspring of parents with epilepsy. International Journal of Epidemology 7: 241–247

Anonymous 1982 Valproic acid and spinal bifida: a preliminary report. Morbiditidy and Mortality, Weekly Report 31: 565–566

Baptisti A 1938 Epilepsy and pregnancy. American Journal Obstetrics and Gynecology 35: 818–824

Beaussart-Defaye J, Bastin N, Demarcq C 1985 Epilepsies and reproduction. Grine Lille, France

Biale Y, Lewenthal H 1984 Effect of folic acid supplementation on congenital malformations due to anticonvulsant drugs. European Journal of Obstetrics, Gynecology, and Reproductive Biology 18: 211–216

Bjerkedal T, Bahna S L 1973 The course and outcome of pregnancy in women with epilepsy. Acta Obstetrica Et Gynecologica Scandanavica 52: 245–248
Buehler B A 1985 Epoxide hydrolase activity and the fetal hydantoin syndrome. Clinical Research 33: A129
Burnett C W F 1946 A survey of the relation between epilepsy and pregnancy. Journal of Obstetrics and Gynecology 53: 539–556
Centa E, Rasore-Quartino A 1965 La sindrome malformatina 'digitocardiaca' forme genetische e fenocopie. Probabile Azione Teratogena dei Farmaci Antiepilepttici Pathologica 57: 227–232
Chang T, Savory A, Glazko A J 1970 A new metabolite of 5,5 diphenylhydantoin. Biochemical Biochemical Research Communications 38: 444–449
Clay S A, McVie R, Chen H C 1981 Possible teratogenic effect of valproic acid. Journal of Pediatrics 98: 828
Cresteil T, Beaune P, Kremers P, Celier C, Guengerich F P, Leroux J P 1985 Immunoquantification of epoxide hydrolase and cytochrome P-450 isozymes in fetal and adult human liver microscomes. European Journal of Biochemistry 151: 345
Dalens B, Raynaud E J, Gaulme J 1980 Teratogenicity of valproic acid. Journal of Pediatrics 97: 332–333
Dansky L, Andermann E, Sherwin A L, Andermann F, Kinch R A 1980 Maternal epilepsy and congenital malformations: a prospective study with monitoring of plasma anticonvulsant levels during pregnancy. Neurology 3: 15
Dickinson R G, Harland R C, Lynn R K, Brewster-Smith W, Gerber N 1979 Transmission of valproic acid (Depakene) across the placenta: half-life of the drug in mother and baby. Journal of Pediatrics 94: 832–735
Dieterich E, Steveling A, Lukas A, Seyfeddinipur N, Spranger J 1980 Congenital anomalies in children of epileptic mothers and fathers. Neuropediatrics 11(3): 274–283
DiLiberti J H, Farndon P A, Dennis N R, Curry C J R 1984 The fetal valproate syndrome. American Journal of Medical Genetics 19: 473–481
Ehrenband L T, Chaganti R S K 1981 Cancer in the fetal hydantoin syndrome. Lancet 1: 97
Elshove J, Van Eck J H M 1971 Aangeboren misvorminge, met name gespleten lip met zonder gespleten verhemelte, bi j kinderen van moeders met epilepsie. Nederland T Geneesk 115(33): 1371–1375
Fedrick, J 1983 Epilepsy and pregnancy: a report from the Oxford record linkage study. British Medical Journal 2: 442–448
Feldman G L, Weaver D D, Lovrien E W 1977 The fetal trimethadione syndrome: report of an additional family and further delineation of this syndrome. American Journal of Diseases Child 131(13) 89–92
Finnell R H 1981 Phenytoin induced teratogenesis: a mouse model. Science 211: 483–484
Finnell R H, Chernoft G F 1984 Variable patterns of malformation in the mouse fetal hydantoin syndrome. American Journal Medical Genetics 19: 463–471
Friis M L, Hauge M 1985 Congenital heart defects in live born children of epileptic parents. Archives of Neurology 42: 374–376
Friis M L, Breng-Nielsen B, Sindrup E H, Lund M, Fogh-Andersen P, Hauge M 1981 Facial clefts among epileptic patients. Archives of Neurology 38: 227–229
Friis M L, Holm N V, Sindrup E H, Fogh-Andersen P, Hauge M 1986 Facial clefts in sibs and children of epileptic patients. Neurology 38: 346–350
German J, Kowal A, Ehlers K H 1970 Trimethadione and human teratogenesis. Teratology 3: 349–362
Glatt H R, Lorenz J, Fleischmann R et al 1980 Interindividual variations of epoxide hydrolase activity in human liver and lung biopsies, lymphocytes and fibroblast cultures. In: Conn M J, Conney A H, Estabrook R W, Gelboin H V, Gillette J R, O'Brien P J (eds) Microsomes, drug oxidations and chemical carcinogenesis. Academic Press, New York, p 551
Goldman A S, Zackai E H, Yaffe S J 1986 Environmentally induced birth defect risks. In: Sever J L, Brent R L (eds) Teratogen Update. Liss, New York, p 35–38
Gomez M R 1981 Possible teratogenicity of valproic acid. Journal of Pediatrics 9: 508
Granstrom M L 1982 Development of the children of epileptic mothers, preliminary results from the prospective Helsinki study. In: Janz D, Dam M, Richens A, Bossi L, Helge H, Schmidt D (eds) Epilepsy pregnancy and the child. Raven Press, New York, p 403–408
Grosse K P, Schwanitz G, Rott H D, Wissmuler H F 1972 Chromosomenuntersuchungen bei behandlung mit anticonvulsiva. Humangenetik 16: 209–216
Guengerich F P, Wang P, Mitchell M B, Mason P S 1979 Rat and human microsomal epoxide hydrolase. Journal Biological Chemistry 254: 122–488
Gustavson E E, Chen H 1985 Goldenhar syndrome, anterior encephalocele and aqueductal stenosis following fetal primidone exposure. Teratology 32: 13–17
Hanson J W 1986 Teratogen update: fetal hydantoin effects. Teratology 33: 349–353
Hanson J W, Smith D W 1975 The fetal hydantoin syndrome. Journal of Pediatrics 87: 285–290

Hanson J W, Myrianthopoulos N C, Sedgwich M A, Smith D W 1976 Risks to the offspring of woman treated with hydantoin anticonvulsants with emphasis on the fetal hydantoin syndrome. Journal of Pediatrics 89: 662–668

Hauser W A, Kurland L T 1975 Epidemiology of epilepsy in Rochester, Minnesota, 1935 through 1967. Epilepsia 16: 1–66

Hiilesmaa V K, Teramo K, Granstrom M L, Bardy A H 1981 Fetal head growth retardation associated with maternal antiepileptic drugs. Lancet 2: 165–167

Higgins T A, Comerford J B 1974 Epilepsy in pregnancy. Journal of Irish Medical Association 67: 317–329

Horning M G, Stratton C, Wilson A, Horning E C, Hill R M 1974 Detection of 5-(3,4-dihydroxy-1,5,cyclohexa-dien-1-yl)-5-phenylhydantoin as major metabolite of 5,5 diphenylhydantoin in the newborn human. Analytical Letters 4: 537–582

Hutch H C, Steinhouse H C, Helge H 1975 Mental development in children of epileptic parents. In: Hauser W A, Kurland L T (eds) Epidemiology of epilepsy in Rochester, Minnesota, 1935 through 1967. Epilepsia 16: 1–66

Jager-Roman E, Deichl A, Jakob S et al 1986 Fetal growth major malformations and minor anomalies in infants born to women receiving valproic acid. Journal of Pediatrics 108: 997–1004

Janz D 1982 Antiepileptic drugs and pregnancy: altered utilization patterns and teratogenesis. Epilepsia 23 (suppl 1): 853–863

Janz D, Fuchs U 1964 Are antiepileptic drugs harmful when given during pregnancy? German Medicine Monthly 9: 20–22

Jeavons P M 1984 Non dose related side effects of valproate. Epilepsia 25 (suppl 1): 550–55

Jerina D M, Daly J W 1974 Arene oxides: a new aspect of drug metabolism. Science 185: 573

Kallen B 1986 A register study of maternal epilepsy and delivery outcome with special reference to drug use. Acta Neurologica Scandinavica 73(3): 253–259

Kalter H, Warkany J 1983 Congenital malformations. New England Journal of Medicine 308: 491–497

Kapitulnik J, Levin W, Lu A Y H, et al 1977 Hydration of arene and alkene oxides by epoxide hydrolase in human liver microsomes. Clinical Pharmacology and Therapeutics 21: 158

Kelly T E 1984a Teratogenicity of anticonvulsant drugs 1: review of the literature. American Journal of Medical Genetics 19: 413–434

Kelly T E 1984b Teratogenicity of anticonvulsants III: radiographic hand analysis of children exposed in utero to diphenylhydantoin. American Journal of Medical Genetics 19: 445–450

Kelly T E, Edwards P, Rein M, Miller J Q, Dreifuss F E 1984 Teratogenicity of anticonvulsant drugs II: a prospective study. American Journal Medical Genetics 19: 435–443

Knight A H, Rhind E G 1975 Epilepsy and pregnancy: a study of 153 pregnancies in 59 patients. Epilepsia 16: 99–110

Koppe J G, Bosmon W, Oppers V M et al 1973 Epilepsie en aangeborn afwijkingen. Nederlands Tijdschrift voor Genesskunde 117: 220–224

Kuenssberg E V, Knox J D E 1973 Teratogenic effect of anticonvulsants. Lancet 1: 198

Laegreid L, Olegard R, Wahlstrom J, Conradi N 1987 Abnormalities in children exposed to benzodiazepines in utero. Lancet 1: 108–109

Levy R H, Yerby M S 1985 Effects of pregnancy on antiepileptic drug utilization. Epilepsia 26 (suppl 1): 525–557

Lindhout D, Schmidt D 1986 In utero exposure to valproate and neural tube defects. Lancet 1: 1392–1393

Lindhout D, Rene J E, Hoppener A, Meinardi H 1984 Teratogenicity of antiepileptic drug combinations with special emphasis on epoxidation (of carbamazepine). Epilepsia 25: 77–83

Lorenz J, Glatt H R, Fleischmann R, Ferlinz R, Oesch F 1984 Drug metabolism in man and its relationship to that in three rodent species: mono-oxygenase, epoxide hydrolase, and glutathione s-transferase activities in subcellular fractions of lung and liver. Biochemical Medicine 32: 43

Loughman P M, Gold H, Vance J C 1973 Phenytoin teratogenicity in man. Lancet 1: 70–72

Lowe C R 1973 Congenital malformations among infants born to epileptic women. Lancet 1: 9–10

Majewski F, Raft W, Fischer P, Huenges R, Petruch F 1980 Zur Teratogenitat von Antikonvulsiva. Deutsche Medizinische Wochenschrift 105: 719–723

Martz F, Failinger C, Blake D A 1977 Phenytoin teratogenesis: correlation between embryopathic effect and covalent binding of putative arene oxide metabolite to gestational tissue. Journal of Pharmacology Experimental Therapeutics 203: 231–239

Meadow S R 1968 Anticonvulsant drugs and congenital abnormalities. Lancet 2: 1296

Melchior I C, Svenswark O, Trolle D 1967 Placental transfer of phenobarbitone in epileptic women and elimination in newborns. Lancet 2: 860–861

Mertes I, Fleischmann R, Glatt H R, Oesch F 1985 Interindividual variations in the activities of cytosolic and microsomal epoxide hydrolase in human liver. Carcinogenesis 6: 219

Meyer J G 1973 The teratological effects of anticonvulsants and the effects of pregnancy and birth. European Neurology 10: 179–180

Millar J H D, Nevin N C 1973 Congenital malformations and anticonvulsant drugs. Lancet 2: 328
Monson R R, Rosenberg L, Hartz S C 1973 Diphenyhydantoin and selected congenital malformations. New England Journal of Medicine 289: 1049–1052
Mullers-Kuppers von M 1963 Embryopathy during pregnancy caused by taking anticonvulsants. Acta Paedopsychiatrica 30: 401–405
Nakane Y 1979 Congenital malformations among infants of epileptic mothers treated during prenancy. Folia Psychiatrica and Neurologica Japonica 33: 363–369
Nakane Y 1980 The teratological problem of antiepileptic drugs. Folia Psychiatrica et Neurologica Japonica 34: 277–287
Nakane Y, Oltuma T, Takahashi R et al 1980 Multi-institutional study on the teratogenicity and fetal toxicity of anticonvulsants: a report of a collaborative study group in Japan. Epilepsia 21: 663–680
Nebert D W, Jensen N M 1979 The Ah locus: genetic regulation of the metabolism of carcinogens, drugs, and other environmental chemicals by cytochrome P-450 mediated mono-oxygenases. CRC Critical Reviews in Biochemistry 6: 401–437
Nelson K B, Ellenberg J H 1982 Maternal seizure disorder outcomes of pregnancy and neurologic abnormalities in the children. Neurology 32: 1247–1254
Neri A, Heifetz L, Nitke S, et al 1983 Neonatal outcomes in infants of epileptic mothers. European Journal of Obstetrics Gynecology Reproductive Biology 16: 263–268
Niswander J D, Wertelecki W 1973 Congenital malformation among offspring of epileptic women. Lancet 1: 1062
Pacifici G M, Colizzi C, Giuliani L, Rane A 1983 Cytosolic epoxide hydrolase in fetal and adult human liver. Archives of Toxicology 54: 331
Pacifici G M, Tomson T, Beatilsson L, Rane A 1985 Valpromide/carbamazepine and the risk of teratogenicity. Lancet 1: 397–398
Pantarotto M F 1965 A case of bone marrow aplasia in a newborn attributable to anticonvulsant drugs used by the mother during pregnancy. Quad Clinical Obstetrics Gynecology 67: 343–38
Pantarotto C, Arboix M, Sezzano P, Abbruzzo R 1982 Studies on 5,5-diphenylhydantoin irreversible binding to rat liver microsomal proteins. Biochemical Pharmacology 31(8): 1501–1507
Philbert A, Dam M 1982 The epileptic mother and her child. Epilepsia 23: 85–99
Rettie A E, Rettenmeir A W, Beyer B K, Baille T A, Juchau M R 1986 Valproate hydroxylation by human fetal tissues and embryotoxicity of metabolites. Clinical Pharmacology Therapeutics 40: 172–177
Robert E, Lofkvist E, Maugiere F 1984 Valproate and spina bifida. Lancet 1: 1392
Rudd N L, Freedom R M 1979 A possible primidone embryopathy. Journal of Pediatrics 94: 835–837
Sabin M, Oxorn H 1956 Epilepsy and Pregnancy. Obstetrics and Gynecology 7(2): 175–179
Seino M, Miyakoshi M 1979 Teratogenic risks of antiepileptic drugs in respect to the type of epilepsy. Folia Psychiatrica et Neurologica Japonica 33(3): 379–385
Shapiro S, Slone D, Hartz S C et al 1976 Anticonvulsant and parental epilepsy in the development of birth defects. Lancet 1: 272–275
Shum S, Jensen N M, Nebert D W 1979 The Ah locus: in utero toxicity and teratogenesis associated with genetic differences in B(a)P metabolism. Teratology 20: 365–376
Sims P, Grover P L 1974 Epoxides in polycyclic aromatic hydrocarbon metabolism and carcinogenesis. Advances in Cancer Research 20: 165
South J 1972 Teratogenic effects of anticonvulsants. Lancet 2: 1154
Speidel B D, Meadow S R 1968 Anticonvulsant drugs and congenital anomalies. Lancet 2: 1296
Speidel B D, Meadow S R 1972 Maternal epilepsy and abnormalities of the fetus and newborn. Lancet 2: 839–843
Spellacy W N 1972 Maternal epilepsy and abnormalities of the fetus and newborn. Lancet
Spielberg, S P, Gordon G B, Blake D A, Mellits E D, Bross D S 1981 Anticonvulsant toxicity in vitro: possible role of arene oxides. Journal of Pharmacology and Experimental Therapeutics 217: 386–389
Stanley O H, Chambers T L 1982 Sodium valproate and neural tube defects. Lancet 2(8310): 1282–1283
Starreveld-Zimmerman A A E, Van Der Kolk W J, Meinardi H 1973 Are anticonvulsants teratogenic? Lancet 2: 48–49
Strickler S M, Dansky L V, Miller M A, Seni M H, Andermann E, Speiberg S P 1985 Genetic predisposition to phenytoininduced birth defects. Lancet 1: 746–749
Stumpf D A, Frost M 1978 Seizures, anticonvulsants, and pregnancy. American Journal of Diseases of Children. 132: 746–748
Svigos J M 1984 Epilepsy and Pregnancy. Australian and New Zealand Obstetrics and Gynaecology 24: 182–185
Tein I, MacGregor D L 1985 Possible valproate toxicity. Archives of neurology 42: 291–293
Thomas P E, Ryan D E, vonBahr C, Glaumann H, Levin W 1982 Human liver microsomal epoxide hydrolase: correlation of immunochemical quantitation with catalytic activity Molecular Pharmacology 22: 190

Visser G H, Huisjes H J, Elshove J 1976 Anticonvulsants and fetal malformations. Lancet 1: 970
Vorhees C V 1986 Developmental effects of anticonvulsants. Neurotoxicology 7(2): 235–244
Weber M, Schweitzer M, Mur J M, Andre M, Tridon P, Vett P 1977 Epilpsie medicaments antiepileptiques et grossesse. Archives Francaises de Pediatrie 34: 374–383
Wells P G, Harbison R D 1985 Significance of the phenytoin reactive arene oxide intermediate, its oxepin tantomer, and clinical factors modifying their roles in phenytoin-induced teratology. In: Hussell T M, Johnston M C, Dudley K H (eds) Phenytoin-induced teratology and gingival pathology. Raven Press, New York, pp 83–112
Yerby M S, Koepsell T, Daling J 1985 Pregnancy complications and outcomes in a cohort of women with epilepsy. Epilepsia 26: 631–635
Zachai E H, Mellman W J, Neideren B, Hanson J W 1975 The fetal trimethadione syndrome. Journal of Pediatrics 87(2): 280–284

# 6. Management of seizures during pregnancy

*I. E. Leppik*

Concerns about the medical-legal consequences of caring for women with epilepsy who are contemplating pregnancy have prompted a number of questions regarding proper treatment. As in most areas of medicine, answers from animal and clinical studies may be incomplete, inconclusive or contradictory. Specific issues of concern are the effect of pregnancy on seizure frequency, the effect of seizures on the fetus, the effect of antiepileptic drugs on the growth and development of the fetus, problems with labor and delivery, breast feeding, and the ability of the mother with seizures to care for a child. The most important aspect in managing a pregnant woman with epilepsy is maintenance of an open dialogue between the physician and the patient. Concerns must be discussed before pregnancy, and decisions regarding treatment should consider that conception may occur before the next patient-physician interaction. Questions raised by the woman should be answered with the best knowledge currently available with areas of uncertainty clearly delineated.

While some physicians believe that women with epilepsy are a very high risk group, the woman with epilepsy is at much less risk than women with other chronic disorders, for example, diabetes (Stanley et al 1985).

## SEIZURE FREQUENCY DURING PREGNANCY

The effect of pregnancy on the frequency of seizures has been studied for almost one century (Schmidt 1982). In one recent study of 84 pregnancies in 34 persons with 'idiopathic epilepsy,' seizures increased during 45% of pregnancies, decreased during 5%, and showed no change during 42% (Knight & Rhind 1975). Yet another study of 136 pregnancies in 122 women with various types of epilepsy, pregnancy did not affect seizure frequency in 50%, but seizures increased during 37% and decreased during 13% (Schmidt et al 1983). Thus, from 1/3 to 1/2 of women may have an increased number of seizures during pregnancy. The application of these findings derived from population studies, however, may be difficult for an individual patient. This is because variation of seizure frequency occurs from one patient to another and also during different pregnancies in the same patient.

Perhaps the most frightening and potentially serious exacerbation of seizures during pregnancy is the occurrence of status epilepticus. Fatal outcomes have been reported (Klein et al 1956). Recent experience has been more favorable if proper treatment is given (Ramsey et al 1978, Fougner et al 1985, Grunert & Field 1985).

The cause of increased seizures during pregnancy is not clearly understood. Pregnancy is associated with a number of physiological, endocrinological, and psychological changes, any or all of which might contribute to lowering the seizure threshold. Studies of seizure threshold and susceptibility to kindling in animal models have yielded contradictory results. Pregnant rats were found to be more susceptible to seizures produced by maximal electroshock or body-weight based doses of pentylenetetrazol than nonpregnant controls (Chou & Levy 1984). However, a study involving mice found just the opposite: pregnancy appeared to make mice less susceptible by increasing the seizure threshold (Nau et al 1985). Of two studies of the effect of pregnancy on kindling in the rat model, one found a mild facilitation of kindling during the second half of pregnancy (Ehlers et al 1980), while the other (Holmes & Weber 1985) found no effect.

During pregnancy there is often weight gain, some of which may be due to increased retention of water and sodium. This mechanism has been postulated to be responsible for an increase in seizure frequency (Suter & Klingman 1957). However, more recent studies in women with catamenial epilepsy have not shown a correlation between seizure frequency, body weight, and total body water (Backstrom 1976). Other metabolic factors such as decreases in serum electrolytes, calcium or magnesium have been considered as a cause for increased seizures.

Plasma progesterone and estradiol levels gradually increase during pregnancy, as does excretion of estriol, estrone, and estradiol. Chorionic gonadotropin peaks in the first trimester and then drops during the end of the pregnancy. A number of animal models of epilepsy have demonstrated that estrogen has the ability to increase susceptibility of animals to maximal electroshock seizures (Woolley & Timiras 1962). Furthermore, focal EEG spikes increase and clinical seizures are exacerbated by intravenous injection of estrogen (Logothetis et al 1959). However, progesterone may decrease seizure susceptibility in experimental animals and in patients (Landgren et al 1978). Intravenous infusion of progesterone to attain concentrations similar to those in the luteal phase were given to seven women with partial seizures. Four showed a significant decrease in interictal spike frequency (Backstrom et al 1984). No comprehensive studies correlating endocrinological changes during pregnancy with alteration in seizure frequency have been done. It is not clear, therefore, whether hormonal changes during pregnancy in patients with epilepsy affect seizure frequency.

Clinical factors which might be predictive of frequency during pregnancy have been studied. The best predictor appears to be seizure frequency prior to pregnancy (Knight & Rhind 1975). Almost all patients who had more than one seizure per month in this study had increased seizures during pregnancy, whereas individuals having less than one seizure every 9 months did not have an exacerbation.

Psychological stress factors, such as anxiety leading to lack of sleep, have been postulated to be important in lowering seizure threshold. Fear of antiepileptic drugs harming the fetus may also cause anxiety and lead to poor compliance in taking antiepileptic medication.

## ANTIEPILEPTIC DRUG CONCENTRATION DURING PREGNANCY

With the advent in the last decade of the ability to routinely measure antiepileptic drugs, alterations in the concentrations of medication appear to be evolving as a major cause of increased seizures during pregnancy. Change in antiepileptic drug concentrations can come about in two ways: altered pharmacokinetics or changes in a patient's compliance.

A number of studies have demonstrated decreased plasma levels of most antiepileptic drugs during pregnancy in compliant patients (Lander et al 1977, 1981). Many mechanisms may be operating to cause the decrease. These include alteration in hepatic clearance, change in bioavailability of a drug, alteration in the ratio of unmetabolized durgs eliminated through the kidney or in the gastrointestinal tract, alteration of protein binding, and metabolism by the fetus. The changes observed in humans have not been readily reproduced in experimental animals, and although the clinical phenomenon of increased antiepileptic drug clearance has been amply documented, the causative mechanisms remain unclear. Because clinical practice often dictates increased doses during pregnancy to maintain blood levels, one useful way in which to analyze the change of drug requirement is by evaluating the ratio obtained by dividing the daily dose by the concentration. This is often defined as apparent plasma clearance. However this ratio does not distinguish between decreased absorption, increased metabolism, or increased excretion. In addition, changes in this ratio could develop simply by changes in plasma protein binding.

A change by factor of two in the dose level ratio has been reported for phenytoin in carefully studied pregnancies (Dansky et al 1982, Bardy et al 1982). In a prospective study in Helsinki, plasma phenytoin levels in 111 pregnant women were monitored. Phenytoin clearance increased gradually within the first 32 weeks of pregnancy, reached twice preconception values during the last 8 weeks, and began to return to normal during the 12 week period after pregnancy (Bardy et al 1982). Thus, the most reasonable explanation of these observations would be a change in the hepatic capacity, most probably of the cytochrome P450 oxidative system. Because the kinetics of phenytoin are nonlinear, however, dose increases are not of the magnitude of the percent decrease in blood levels. In other words, a 50% reduction in blood level may need only a 20–30% increase in dose to restore the pre-pregnancy concentration.

In addition to increased clearance, other factors may lower phenytoin concentration. During pregnancy, the unbound (free) phenytoin fraction is higher than in the non-pregnant state (Chen et al 1982). The unbound fraction correlates well with the decrease in plasma albumin concentrations. Decreased bioavailability due to changes in diet, comedication or intestinal absorption may occur. In one patient, HPPH excretion was unchanged during and after pregnancy, and an increased fecal content of unmetabolized phenytoin was measured, documenting malabsorption during pregnancy (Ramsey et al 1978). In other studies, an increase in HPPH excretion during pregnancy was found, suggesting increased hepatic clearance (Kochenour et al 1980). Regardless of the precise mechanism, marked reduction in phenytoin levels during pregnancy, especially the third trimester, is a common phenomenon. Phenytoin concentrations should be monitored each trimester or more frequently, and dose changes made when necessary.

Most studies have shown a reduction in carbamazepine levels during pregnancy. This phenomenon, however, is not as striking as it is for phenytoin. In one study, the plasma drug clearance ratio in the third trimester compared to pre- or post-pregnancy state was 1.9 to 1 (Bardy et al 1982). A significant increase in the concentration of 10–11 carbamazepine epoxide has been observed, suggesting increased hepatic metabolism. Changes in the unbound carbamazepine fraction are usually too small to make a significant contribution to total concentrations.

Valproic acid has been less well studied than the other drugs, but decreased concentrations during pregnancy have been noted. In one study, the concentration of valproate by the third trimester decreased to less than half of the first trimester value (Nau et al 1982b). Stable-isotope labeled valproate was used in one patient to document increases in renal clearance, exhaled isotopic $CO_2$, and the fraction of the two ene metabolites (Nau et al 1982a). Paradoxically, the fraction of the dose excreted as valproate and measured metabolites decreased from 40 to 25% of the daily dose, suggesting that the increased clearance of valproate during the third trimester may have multiple mechanisms, some as yet unidentified. It has been suggested that some of valproic acid's metabolites may be more teratogenic than the parent compound (Nau et al 1981).

Decreased phenobarbital levels during pregnancy have been demonstrated. These may be less than for phenytoin or carbamazepine, but they can nevertheless be significant. Unlike phenytoin or carbamazepine, phenobarbital is partially eliminated by the kidney, and increased renal clearance is a factor during pregnancy.

Primidone is metabolized to phenobarbital and PEMA. Most studies, although small in number of patients observed, indicate that pregnancy does not significantly affect primidone concentrations. However, phenobarbital concentations in persons receiving only primidone decrease markedly (Battino et al 1984). The concentration of primidone-derived phenobarbital increases after delivery. These findings indicate that the conversion of primidone to phenobarbital is inhibited during pregnancy.

It is apparent that antiepileptic drug levels should be monitored during pregnancy. While there is some variation among studies, most indicate that a significant change occurs during the first trimester but the greatest change occurs in the third trimester. Within 2–3 months after delivery clearance values return to pre-pregnancy values.

It would seem logical that women concerned about the potential teratogenetic complications of medications, so widely publicized in recent years, would be likely to alter their drug dosage. Indeed, this has been born out in recent clinical studies. In a group of 125 Japanese women, 27% were considered to be poorly compliant and had a significant increase in seizure frequency during pregnancy. On the other hand, most of the women who were compliant showed no change in seizure frequency (Otani 1985). In a study of 136 women, noncompliance with medication was considered to be a major factor in aggravating seizure frequency (Schmidt et al 1983).

There is considerable disagreement as to what clinical course should be followed. Some experts suggest maintaining stable drug levels throughout pregnancy to prevent seizures from occurring. However, there are some women who do not have increased seizures even in the face of decreased antiepileptic drug levels. Furthermore, some evidence suggests that teratogenicity may be concentration related and that increasing dosage could theoretically enhance this side effect. Perhaps the most prudent course at this time would be to monitor antiepileptic drug levels and increase doses if there is any evidence of increasing seizures. Concentrations of antiepileptic drugs should be measured at least each trimester. Blood should be drawn at each breakthrough seizure to determine whether the threshold has changed (i.e. concentrations are as expected) or if there has been a change in clearance or compliance. Sometimes concentrations should be measured more often, such as every few weeks, and the variability between serial measurements may give an estimate of compliance (Leppik et al 1979).

Status epilepticus during pregnancy may occur in a woman with epilepsy whose seizures accelerate, or may represent a new onset of seizures in a woman with no prior history of epilepsy. Presently, intravenous loading with phenytoin may be the best treatment available. If given at a rate of no more than 50 mg per minute with simultaneous EKG monitor, a total dose of 20 mg per kg can be given safely (Leppik 1986). If this is not effective, intravenous phenobarbital in a dose of 10 or 20 mg/kg may be used. Diazepam has too short a central nervous system half-life to be effective for more than one convulsion. Because status epilepticus in a patient with no previous history of seizures has a high probability of being due to a brain lesion such as tumor, arteriovenous malformation, or other condition, evaluation should not be delayed until after delivery. Although little is yet published regarding this topic, seizures associated with eclampsia appear also to be better treated with phenytoin than with magnesium sulphate.

## EFFECT OF SEIZURES ON THE FETUS

While animal studies show dramatic effects of maternal generalized tonic-clonic seizures on the fetus, human evidence for similar adverse effects is based on a few case reports. Intracranial hemorrhage in utero following a maternal seizure has been described (Minkoff et al 1985). This involved a 28 year-old woman with a history of seizures since age 16 treated with phenytoin, 300 mg per day. During the 19th week of gestation she had a generalized seizure. A second seizure occurred in the 28th week of gestation after she missed several doses of medication. After the third seizure, between the 32nd and 33rd week of gestation, the patient felt decreased fetal movement. A sonogram revealed intracerebral hemorrhage with moderate hydrocephalus. There was no evidence of fetal cardiac activity or body motion. Eight days after the seizure labor was induced, and the patient delivered a still-born macerated male weighing 1815 g.

A dramatic report describes a 28-year-old woman who was being monitored during spontaneous labor at term. A spiral electrode had been attached to the fetal scalp to record heart rate. 43 minutes before delivery when the cervix was dilated to 6 cm, the patient unexpectedly had a generalized tonic-clonic seizure lasting 2–1/2 min. Immediately after the seizure, the patient became cyanotic and received 10 mg of diazepam intravenously. Fetal heart rate decelerated to less than 120 beats/min for over 13 min following the seizure. 29 min after the generalized seizure late deceleration brachycardia was still observed, and therefore, a cessarian was peroformed. Phenytoin concentration in maternal venous blood was only 0.9 μg/ml, suggesting noncompliance (Teramo et al 1979). Another birth monitored by Teramo developed a fetal heartbeat of less than 100. These observations indicate that a human fetus clearly can be asphyxiated, as judged by the fetal heart monitoring during and after generalized tonic-clonic seizures. The deceleration in heart rate can persist for some time and has the potential of significantly damaging the infant's development.

In a study of the population entered into the Collaborative Perinatal Project of the NIH, Nelson & Ellenberg (1982) found that 4.4 women per thousand of the approximately 45 000 women enrolled had one or more seizures during pregnancy. In addition, 4.5 per 100 had had one or more seizures 5 years prior to the study. The number of stillbirths, cerebral palsy, and mental retardation was significantly higher in the group of women defined as having a current seizure disorder. Head circumference of less than two standard deviations was significantly greater in women who had a seizure during pregnancy, as was the rate for mixed cerebral palsy and

mental retardation. Thus, it is evident from this study that, in addition to stillbirth, seizures occurring during pregnancy have a negative impact on fetal development (Table 6.1). Because of its retrospective design, this study could not detect differences
4

**Table 6.1** Outcomes of pregnancy in women who had seizures during pregnancy or within 5 years of pregnancy, 'current seizures' as compared to women who had never experienced a seizure. Modified from Table 4 of Nelson & Ellenberg (1982) by listing only significant differences between persons with seizures and controls

| | Current seizure disorders | | | |
|---|---|---|---|---|
| | In this pregnancy | Not in this pregnancy | Total | No seizures ever |
| *N* | 204 | 206 | 410 | 43 926 |
| Outcome (rate per 1000) | | | | |
| Stillbirth | 51.4[b] | 24.0 | 40.0[b] | 18.8 |
| Head size at 1 year | | | | |
| ≤2 SD | 55.9[a] | 46.0 | 50.5[b] | 22.9 |
| ≤3 SD | 18.6[a] | 17.2[a] | 17.8c | 3.6 |
| 7 year outcome | | | | |
| Mixed C.P. | 11.8[c] | 0.0 | 5.6[b] | 0.4 |
| Mental retardation | | | | |
| IQ < 70 | 80.5[b] | 51.0 | 65.2[b] | 34.0 |
| IQ < 50 | 47.0[c] | 12.7 | 29.3[b] | 4.3 |
| Any bad outcome | | | | |
| Without death | 178.6[c] | 120.8[a] | 151.7[c] | 72.7 |
| Including death | 262.8[c] | 181.3 | 226.4[c] | 129.1 |

[a] is $p < 0.05$; [b] is $p < 0.005$; [c] is $p < 0.001$ (Chi-squared).

in outcome to children of women who had been treated with antiepileptic medications compared to those who had not received medicines (Nelson & Ellenberg 1982).

While complex partial seizures would not be suspected of leading to direct damaging effects of the fetus, accidents or injuries sustained during seizures may have deleterious effects on the mother and thus indirectly on the fetus. One example would be that of a major burn suffered as a consequence of a complex partial seizure, necessitating prolonged treatment with a number of drugs and also subjecting the fetus to all the physiologic changes occurring with extensive third degree burns.

## FETAL MALFORMATIONS

This topic is developed in greater depth in Chapter 5. The risk of malformations in the offspring of women with epilepsy has been a topic of much debate. Some large population based studies have shown no risk (Stanley et al 1985), while others have shown a small but statistically significant risk (Table 6.2). Other studies have shown malformation rates as high as 18.9% that were possibly attributable to antiepileptic drugs (Darsky et al 1986).

The first systematic approach addressing the question of teratogenicity was a study in which a questionnaire was mailed to 246 mothers with epilepsy (Jane & Fuchs 1964). Information from 426 pregnancies was collected, but there were no controls, record reviews or examinations. Five malformations were noted in 262 pregnancies associated with antiepileptic drug use, and the authors concluded that the incidence of malformations was not higher in infants of women receiving antiepileptic drugs in the population at large (Janz & Fuchs 1964). In a case controlled study, Spidel

**Table 6.2** Rates of malformations in large population studies comparing offspring of women with epilepsy to women with diabetes (Stanley et al 1985) and to a control population matched for mother's age and place of birth of child (Bjerkedal 1982)

| | Mothers with: Diabetes | Epilepsy | All other mothers |
|---|---|---|---|
| *Australian study* | | | |
| Births | 225 | 244 | 62 265 |
| Number of malformed infants | 19 (8.4) | 9 (3.7) | 2099 (3.4%) |
| Relative risk | 2.5 | 1.1 | 1.0 |
| *Norwegian study* | | | |
| Births | | 3879 | 3879 |
| Number of malformed infants | | 170[a] (4.38%) | 136 (3.51%) |
| Relative risk | | 1.25 | 1.0 |

[a] $p = 0.023$.

& Meadows (1972) found that the incidence of congenital malformations was increased in the offspring of mothers with epilepsy, and concluded that some of the increase was apparently due to the medications. However, their study was relatively small, and questions regarding its design have been raised. 'A number of studies have been published but no single case control study has been sufficiently large enough to establish unequivocally that excess birth defects in infants with epileptic mothers is due to teratogenicity of antiepileptic drugs' (Kelly, 1984). Most studies do not clearly delineate the malformations or limit themselves to specific deformities, nor do they review a large enough population with controls. In a recent study of congenital heart defects of 2461 live born children of people with epilepsy, rates of malformation when the mother had epilepsy, the father had epilepsy and a control population was similar, and the authors conclude that antiepileptic treatment is not a major factor in etiology of congenital heart defects in the offspring of people with epilepsy (Friis & Hauge 1985). At this time, specific ranking of teratogenicity in humans is speculative with the exception of a few specific drugs. The American College of Obstetrics and Gynecology has recommended that only phenobarbital or no antiepileptic drugs be used during pregnancy. This represents an extreme position which does not consider the many and complex aspects of patient management including drug tolerance, potential damaging effects of phenobarbital on the fetus, and problems associated with switching patients from previously well-tolerated drugs to phenobarbital prior to pregnancy.

Most congenital malformations caused by drugs occur during the first trimester. Therefore, all patients of childbearing potential should be made aware of the possibility of teratogenicity of antiepileptic drugs at the time of first physician contact. The amount of detail discussed depends on the individual woman's plans for the future. Rational decisions should be made before pregnancy. The need for antiepileptic drug therapy should be constantly reassessed in women of childbearing potential.

Of all the available agents, trimethadione is the most teratogenic and it should be avoided in any women of childbearing potential. In one study of multiple births to one women, all four births which occurred while the patient was being treated with trimethadione resulted in malformations, but there were no ill effects in two children born while the patient was being treated with other drugs (German et al 1970). Women of childbearing potential should not be exposed to trimethadione.

The teratogenic potential of phenytoin has been the subject of numerous reports. Animal studies indicate that it has a dose-related propensity for causing cleft lip, cleft palate, and cardiac defects (Finnel 1981). Results from human studies are not as clear. The major suspected malformations associated with phenytoin are cleft lip, cleft palate, and cardiac lesions. Less common are bifid ureter and other organ malformations. The types of malformations and the relative frequency associated with phenytoin do not differ from those occurring spontaneously, and thus the effect of phenytoin may be to simply increased the rate of spontaneously occurring defects. In one study, the rate of malformations to mothers receiving phenytoin alone was 27.3% (Dansky et al 1986), but other studies have reported much lower rates (Granstrom & Hulesmaa 1982).

A syndrome specific to phenytoin has been called the fetal hydantoin syndrome (Hanson et al 1976). Its features are similar to the fetal alcohol syndrome and consist of major and numerous 'minor' congenital anomalies. The major features are microcephaly, growth retardation and impaired intellectual functioning. Minor anomalies include strabismus, ptosis, ocular hypertelorism, broad and/or distal phalanges with or without nail hypoplasia, hyperextensible joints, hypotonia, pilonidal sinus, inguinal hernia, umbilical hernia, abnormal dermatoglyphic patterns, and minor club deformities of the feet. These may lead to a characteristic facial appearance. However, these features have also been observed with maternal use of other antiepileptic drugs and the term 'fetal antiepileptic drug syndrome' may be more appropriate.

Recently, significant neural tube defects associated with valproic acid have been reported. Data from a registry of spina bifida and anencephaly revealed that treatment with valproate was present in a much higher frequency than expected in children with these defects (Robert & Giubaud 1982). In one study of 12 children born to 11 epileptic mothers, two children were born with microencephaly (Robert et al 1983). Thus, unlike the other commonly used antiepileptic drugs, valproate may have a specific teratogenic effect. The risk appears to be 1 to 2 per 100 births, but genetic factors may also play a role.

Animal models indicate that cleft lip and palate are not significantly increased by carbamazepine. Too few reports in humans are available to make definitive statements. Many of the features seen in the 'fetal hydantoin' syndrome may be seen with barbiturates (Sepi 1976). Primidone appears to be more teratogenic than phenobarbital by itself (Myhre & Williams 1981). Statements to the effect that barbiturates are less teratogenic than other antiepileptic drugs, with the exception of Tridione, cannot be substantiated by literature currently available.

Use of multiple drugs in the treatment of epilepsy is common, and most studies show that the risk of malformations increases with the number of drugs used (Nakane et al 1980). Interestingly, the incidence of malformation was the highest (12.7%) in medicated patients who had seizures during pregnancy (Nakane et al 1980). Thus, the highest risk of fetal injury occurs in women whose seizures are incompletely controlled even with mutliple drug use.

There appears to be a possible association between maternal folic acid efficiency and spontaneous abortion, placental abruption and fetal malformations. A retrospective study examining the effect of folic acid supplementation on congenital malformations due to antiepileptic drugs reported that 66 children born to 24 women who received antiepileptic drugs without folic acid had a 15% rate of malformation (Biale

& Lewenthal 1984). These consisted of congenital heart disase, cleft lip and palate, neural tube defects and skeletal abnormalities. A prospective study by the same investigators found that 33 infants born to 22 epileptic women were without congenital malformations and of normal body weight. From these dramatic results, the authors recommended folic acid supplementation during pregnancy (Biale & Lewenthal 1984). However, the results may be biased because there was no control group and retrospective data were compared with prospective outcomes. Nevertheless, a study by Dansky et al (1987) support these results, although not as dramatically. Use of folic acid supplement during pregnancy is currently recommended.

A confounding variable is the genetic influence on malformations. One study indicated that children born to fathers with epilepsy had a higher rate of malformations than controls, but other studies have not confirmed these findings (Annegers et al 1976). It appears, then, that although some studies have reported exceedingly high rates of malformations in women with epilepsy, the weight of evidence, especially from larger well controlled studies, is that offspring of women with epilepsy either have no increased risk or only a small risk of deformities. While some of the increased risk is attributable to antiepileptic drugs, it is likely that there is a complex interaction of genetic factors and environmental factors (drugs, vitamin deficiences, etc.) working in concert to affect the few individuals involved.

## LABOR AND DELIVERY

A frequent problem encountered during labor and delivery is increased tendency for bleeding in the neonate. This can be overcome by the use of vitamin K. The mechanism for this deficit is thought to be induction of hepatic enzymes by antiepileptic drugs. In general, infant mortality is slightly higher in children born to epileptic mothers than in controls. Vitamin D levels may often be below normal. Interestingly, neonatal jaundice occurs very seldom in children exposed to antiepileptic drugs in utero, possibly because of fetal liver enzyme induction. Bone mineralization does not appeart to be different in children born to mothers receiving antiepileptic drugs (Christiansen et al 1981).

Complications of labor and delivery such as pre-eclampsia, abruptio placenta, polyhydramnios, assisted delivery, cesarean section, prematurity, and intrauterine growth retardation may be increased to a small degree in women with epilepsy (Kallen 1986).

## INFANT CARE

Breastfeeding has been an issue of great concern. Most all antiepileptic drugs are transferred in breast milk. The milk to serum concentration for phenytoin is 18%, for phenobarbital 36%, primidone 70%, carbamazepine 40%, and for valproic acid only 4 to 5% (Kaneko et al 1982). The problem of breastfeeding is compounded by the fact that half-lives for drugs may be increased in the neonatal period. However, feeding difficulties and decreased weight gain been definitely correlated only with maternal ingestion of phenobarbital and primidone. On the other hand, abrupt withdrawal of antiepileptic drugs has been thought to be a factor in neonatal convulsions on isolated occasions. The frequency of this is not well established, although in one study it was observed in 4 of 42 infants.

Most mothers with epilepsy are able to care for their infants, especially if seizures are partial elementary. Most problems with child care can usually be attributed to factors other than maternal epilepsy. Precautions such as having another person available during bathing of the infant, however, should be taken.

## TREATMENT OF THE WOMAN WITH EPILEPSY DURING CHILDBEARING YEARS

Although the woman with epilepsy faces greater risks than a person with no chronic illnesses or deleterious life style, these risks are not great enough, with a few exceptions, to preclude pregnancy. The woman and her husband or other companion have the responsibility of deciding to bear children. The physician's role is limited to providing information regarding risks of childbearing and offering medical care which will reduce the risks as much as possible. Often overlooked in this regard are risk factors other than epilepsy which may be of much greater consequence than seizures or antiepileptic drugs. These include, to list only a few, advancing maternal age, heavy smoking, substance abuse, prescription drugs, inadequate prenatal care, and genetic factors.

The most critical step in properly caring for a woman of childbearing age is accurate diagnosis. A substantial number of persons diagnosed as having intractable epilepsy have nonepileptic events (pseudoseizures), and possibly can escape the risks posed by antiepileptic medication and convulsions. Some women whose seizures have been well controlled may have their antiepileptic medication discontinued. Attempts to withdraw drugs should be made well in advance of contemplated pregnancy. If medication cannot be discontinued, attempts should be made to reduce drugs to a minimum number and dosage. At this time, it is not clear if significant differences in risk of teratogenicity exist among carbamazepine, phenytoin, and phenobarbital. Many physicians prefer use of carbamazepine in women of childbearing potential because of its preceived lower risk during pregnancy, although sound clinical studies have not yet conclusively demonstrated this. In general, if an antiepileptic drug has been effective prior to pregnancy and its use has been carefully reviewed, there is no need to change to another before or during pregnancy. Women of childbearing age who wish to avoid pregnancy should be counseled about the interactions between oral contraceptives and antiepileptic drugs. In general, use of oral contraceptives does not exacerbate seizures, but antiepileptic drugs may diminish the effectiveness of oral contraceptives.

Correct classification of seizure types is essential to proper drug treatment. Partial seizures (simple or complex, with or without secondary generalization) are the most common type of seizures in this age group. Carbamazepine, phenobarbital, phenytoin and primidone are the most widely used drugs for these seizures, and no study has demonstrated these drugs to differ in terms of their ability to control seizures. Phenobarbital and primidone appear to have more side effects than the others. Treatment with carbamazepine or phenytoin appears to be the most reasonable course of action when it has been concluded that a woman would be at risk for having seizures. For women with idiopathic generalized tonic-clonic seizures in whom valproate has been successful in controlling seizures, changing antiepileptic drugs prior to or during pregnancy may cause more problems than the small risk of neural tube defects. Other drugs appear to have malformation rates similar to those seen with valproate, although the types of malformations are different. Furthermore, other drugs may not control generalized tonic-clonic seizures as well in some women. Women on valproate should be warned of the potential for neural tube defects and be followed by a specialist able to monitor for these anomalous developments. Seizures occurring during pregnancy appear to be more dangerous to the fetus than risks posed by antiepileptic drug therapy.

Antiepileptic drug concentrations should be measured every trimester or more frequently if a change in seizures occurs. Doses should be increased if necessary and decreased after pregnancy to maintain stable antiepileptic drug concentrations.

Quality pre-natal care must be provided. Folic acid supplementation of 1–5 mg may lower the incidence of malformations (Dansky et al 1987). Vitamin K supplementation is necessary to reduce bleeding problems during labor and delivery.

With optimal care, both the patient and physician can expect a favorable outcome of pregnancy in the vast majority of instances, and epilepsy should not preclude a woman from childbearing and child rearing.

## ACKNOWLEDGEMENTS

This work was supported in part by NINCDS contract #P50 NS1-16308.

## REFERENCES


Annegers J F, Hauser W A, Elveback L R, Anderson V E, Kurland L T 1976 Seizure disorders in offspring of parents with a history of seizures — a maternal-paternal difference? Epilepsia 17: 1–9

Backstrom T 1976 Epileptic seizures in women related to plasma estrogen and progesterone during the menstrual cycle. Acta Neurologica Scandinavica 54: 321–347

Backstrom T, Zetterlund B, Blom S, Romano M 1984 Effects of intravenous progesterone infusions on the epileptic discharge frequency in women with partial epilepsy. Acta Neurologica Scandinavica 69(4): 240–248

Bardy A H, Teramo K, Hiilesmaa V K 1982 Apparent plasma clearances of phenytoin, phenobarbitone, primidone and carbamazepine during pregnancy: results of the prospective Helsinki study. In: Janz D, Bossi L, Dam M, Helge H, Richens A, Schmidt D (eds) Epilepsy, pregnancy and the child. Raven Press, New York, p 141–145

Battino D, Binelli S, Bossi L, Como M L, Croci D, Cusi C, Avanzini G 1984 Changes in primidone/phenobarbitone ratio during pregnancy and the puerperium. Clinical Pharmacokinetics 9: 252–260

Biale Y, Lewenthal H 1984 Effect of folic acid supplementation on congenital malformations due to anticonvulsive drugs. European Journal of Obstetrics, Gynecology and Reproductive Biology 18: 211–216

Bjerkedal T 1982 Outcome of pregnancy in women with epilepsy, Norway 1967 to 1978: Congenital malformations. In: Janz D, Bossi L, Dam M, Helge H, Richens A, Schmidt D (eds) Epilepsy, pregnancy, and the child. Raven Press, New York, p 289–295

Chen S S, Perucca E, Lee J N, Richens 1982 A serum protein binding and free concentration of phenytoin and phenobarbitone in pregnancy. British Journal of Pharmacology 13: 547–54

Chou R C, Levy G 1984 Kinetics of drug action in disease states III: Effect of pregnancy on the relationship between phenytoin concentration and antiseizure activity in rats. Journal of Pharmaceutical Sciences 73(10): 1348–1351

Christiansen C, Brandt N J, Ebbesen F, Sardemann H, Trolle D 1981 Bone mineral content during pregnancy in epileptics on anticonvulsant drugs and in their newborns. Acta Obstetricia Et Gynecologica Scandinavica (Sweden) 60(5): 501–503

Dansky L, Andermann E, Andermann F, Sherwin A L, Kinch R A 1982 Maternal epilepsy and congenital malformations: correlation with maternal plasma anticonvulsant levels during pregnancy. In: Janz D, Bossi L, Dam M, Helge H, Richens A, Schmidt D (eds) Epilepsy, pregnancy, and the child. Raven Press, New York, p 251–258

Dansky L, Andermann E, Sherwin A L, Andermann F 1982 Plasma levels of phenytoin during pregnancy and the puerperium. In: Janz D, Bossi L, Dam M, Helge H, Richens A, Schmidt D (eds) Epilepsy, pregnancy and the child. Raven Press, New York, p 155–162

Dansky L, Andermann E, Roseblatt D, Sherwin A L, Andermann F 1987 Anticonvulsants, folate levels, and pregnancy outcome: A prospective study. Annals of Neurology 21: 176–182
Ehlers C L, Clifton D K, Sawyer C H 1980 Amygdala kindling during pregnancy in the rat. Physiological Behavior 25: 599–601
Finnel R H 1981 Phenytoin induced teratogenesis: a mouse model. Science 211: 483–84.
Fougner A C, Wilson S J, Seltzer V L 1985 Status epilepticus in pregnancy. A case report. Journal of Reproductive Medicine 30(12): 948–950
Friis M L, Hauge M 1985 Congenital heart defects in live-born children of epileptic patients. Archives of Neurology 42: 374–376
German J, Kowal A, Ellers K H 1970 Trimethadione and human teratogenesis. Teratology 3: 349–362
Granstrom M L, Hulesmaa V K 1982 Malformations and minor anomalies in the children of epileptic mothers: Preliminary results of prospective helsinki study. In: Janz D, Bossi L, Dam M, Helge H, Richens A, Schmidt D (eds) Epilepsy, pregnancy and the child. Raven Press, New York, p 303–307
Grunert G M, Field D R 1985 Refractory status epilepticus in pregnancy. A case report. Journal of Reproductive Medicine 30(1): 69–73
Hanson J W, Myrianthopoulos N C, Sedgwick-Harvey M A, Smith D W 1976 Risks of the offspring of women treated with hydantoin anticonvulsants with emphasis on the fetal hydantoin syndrome. Journal of Pediatrics 89: 662–668
Holmes G L, Weber D A 1985 Effect of pregnancy on development of seizures. Epilepsia 26: 299–302
Janz D, Fuchs 1964 Are antiepileptic drugs harmful when given during pregnancy. German Medical Monthly 9: 20–22
Janz D, Dam M, Richens A, Bossi L, Helge H, Schmidt D (eds) 1982 Epilepsy, pregnancy, and the child. Raven Press, New York
Kallen B 1986 A register study of maternal epilepsy and delivery outcome with special reference to drug use. Act Neurologica Scandinavica 73: 253–259
Kaneko S, Suzuki K, Sato T, Ogawa Y, Nomura Y 1982 The problems of antiepileptic medication in the neonatal period: Is breast feeding advisable? In: Janz D, Bossi L, Dam M, Helge H, Richens A, Schmidt D (eds) Epilepsy, pregnancy and the child. Raven Press, New York, p 343–348
Kelly T 1984 Teratogenicity of anticonvulsant drugs I: Review of the literature. American Journal of Medical Genetics 19: 413–434
Klein M D, Goodfriend M J, Shey I A 1956 Status epilepticus and pregnancy. American Journal of Obstetrics and Gynecology 72: 188–190
Knight A H, Rhind E G 1975 Epilepsy and pregnancy: a study of 153 pregnancies in 59 patients. Epilepsia 16: 99–110
Kochenour, N K, Emery M G, Sawchuck R J 1980 Phenytoin metabolism in pregnancy. Obstetrics and Gynecology 56(5): 577–582
Lander C M, Edwrds V E, Eadie M J, Tyrer J H 1977 Plasma anticonvulsant concentrations during pregnancy. Neurology 27: 128–131
Lander C M, Livingstone I, Tyrer J H, Eadie M J 1981 The clearance of anticonvulsant drugs in pregnancy. Clinical and Experimental Neurology 17: 71–78
Landgren S, Backstrom T, Kalistratov G 1978 The effect of progesterone on the spontaneous interictal spike evoked by topical application of penicillin to the cat's cerebral cortex. Acta Physiologica Scandinavica 102: 81A–83A
Leppik I E 1986 Status epilepticus. Neurologic Clinics 4(3): 633–643
Leppik I E, Cloyd J C, Sawchuk R J, Pepin S M 1979 Compliance and variability of plasma phenytoin levels in epileptic patients. Therapeutic Drug Monitoring 1: 475–483
Logothetis J, Harner R, Morrell F, Torres F 1959 The role of estrogens in catamenial exacerbation of epilepsy. Neurology 9: 352–360
Minkoff H, Schaffer R M, Delke I, Grunebaum A N 1985 Diagnosis of intracranial hemorrhage in utero after a maternal seizure. Obstetrics & Gynecology 22S–24S
Myhre S A, Williams R 1981 Teratogenic effects associated with maternal primidone therapy. Journal of Pediatrics 99(1): 160–162
Nakane Y, Okuma T, Takahaski R et al 1980 Multi-institutional study on the teratogenicity and fetal toxicity of antiepileptic drugs: a report of a collaborative study group in Japan. Epilepsia 21(6): 663–680
Nau H, Rating D, Koch S, Hauser I, Helge H 1981 Valproic acid and its metabolites: placental transfer, neonatal pharmacokinetics, transfer via mother's milk, and clinical status in neonates of epileptic mothers. Journal of Pharmacology and Experimental Therapeutics 219(3): 768–777
Nau H, Wittfoht W, Rating D, Jakobs C, Schafer H, Helge H 1982a Pharmacokinetics of valproic acid and its metabolites in a pregnant patient: stable isotope methodology. In: Janz D, Bossi L, Dam M, Helge H, Richens A, Schmidt D (eds) Epilepsy, pregnancy and the child. Raven Press, New York, p 131–139

Nau H, Schmidt D, Beck-Mannagetta G, Rating D, Koch S, Helge H 1982b Pharmacokinetics of primidone and metabolites during human pregnancy. In: Janz D, Bossi L, Dam M, Helge H, Richens A, Schmidt D (eds) Epilepsy, pregnancy, and the child. Raven Press, New York, p 121–129

Nau H, Kuhnz W, Loscher W 1985 Effects of pregnancy on seizure threshold and the disposition and efficacy of antiepileptic drugs in the mouse. Life Science 36(7): 663–669

Nelson K B, Ellenberg J H 1982 Maternal seizure disorder, outcome of pregnancy, and neurologic abnormalities in children. Neurology 32(11): 1247–1254

Otani K 1985 Risk factors for the increased seizure frequency during pregnancy and puerperium. Folia Psychiatrica Neurologica Japonica 39(1): 33–41

Philbert A, Dam M (1982) The epileptic mother and her child. Epilepsia 23(1): 85–99

Ramsey R E, Strauss R G, Wilder B J, Willmore J 1978 Status epilepticus in pregnancy: effect of phenytoin malabsorption on seizure control. Neurology 28: 85–89

Robert E, Giubaud P 1982 Maternal valproic acid and congenital neural tube defects. Lancet 2: 937

Robert E, Robert J M, Lapras C 1983 L'acide valproique est-il teratogene? Revue Neurologique 139: 445–447

Robertson I G 1986 Epilepsy in pregnancy. Clinics in Obstetrics and Gynecology 13: 365–384

Schmidt D 1982 The effect of pregnancy on the natural history of epilepsy: Review of the literature. In: Janz D, Bossi L, Dam M, Helge H, Richens A, Schmidt D (eds) Epilepsy, pregnancy and the child. Raven Press, New York, p 3–14

Schmidt D, Canger R, Avanzini G et al 1983 Change of seizure frequency in pregnant epileptic women. Journal of Neurology, Neurosurgery and Psychiatry 46(8): 751–755

Seip M 1976 Growth retardation dysmorphic facies and minor malformations following massive exposure to phenobarbital in utero. Acta Paediatrica Scandinavica 65: 617–621

Spidel B D, Meadows S R 1972 Maternal epilepsy and abnormalities of the fetus and newborn. Lancet 2: 839–843

Stanley F J, Priscott P K, Johnston R, Brooks B, Bower C 1985 Congenital malformations in infants of mothers with diabetes and epilepsy in Western Australia, 1980–1982. The Medical Journal of Australia 143: 440–442

Stevenson M M, Gilbert E F 1970 Anticonvulsants and hemorrhagic diseases of the newborn infant. Journal of Pediatrics 77: 516

Suter C, Klingman W O 1957 Seizure states and prgnancy. Neurology 7: 105–118

Teramo K, Hiilesmaa V, Bardy A, Saarikoski S 1979 Fetal heart rate during a maternal grand mal epileptic seizure. Journal of Perinatal Medicine 7: 3–6

Woolley D E, Timiras P S 1962 Estrous and circadian periodicity and electroshock convulsions in rats. American Journal of Physiology 202: 379–382

# 7. Epilepsy and parasitosis of the central nervous system

*P. R. M. Bittencourt C. M. Gracia P. Lorenzana*

## INTRODUCTION

The relationship of parasitosis to epilepsy is more important than is indicated by current research publications. The greater mobility of people everywhere has increased awareness of parasitic diseases in developed countries and also increased world wide the number of areas with parasite reservoirs. Central nervous system (CNS) involvement in parasitic diseases as a whole is infrequent but its relevance in clinical practice is increasing. The relationship of epilepsy to parasitic disorders has rarely been studied systematically. A computer search of the papers published between 1966 and 1987 (Medline) produced little original material relating epilepsy directly to parasitosis of the CNS.

**Table 7.1** Countries or regions with high prevalence of seven major parasitoses of the CNS. Data adapted from text

| | Americas | Europe | Africa | Asia | Oceania |
|---|---|---|---|---|---|
| Schistosomiasis | Latin (Mexico to Brazil) | — | North, central | Southeast | — |
| Hydatid disease | Uruguay, Chile, Argentina | Southern | North, south | Middle East, Southeast | Australia, New Zealand |
| Cysticercosis | Latin | Southwest | Central, south | Southeast | Some islands |
| African trypanosomiasis | — | — | Sub-Saharan | — | — |
| American trypanosomiasis | Latin (Panamá to Brazil) | — | — | — | — |
| Malaria | Latin (tropical) | East mediterranean | Central, south | Southeast | Many islands |
| Toxoplasmosis in AIDS | USA, Brazil | Western | Central | — | — |

Intracranial involvement is more frequent in malaria, cysticercosis and toxoplasmosis than in disease caused by other protozoan agents, such as round worms, tape worms or fluke (Bia & Barry 1986). Toxoplasmosis has recently assumed special status because of its frequency as an opportunistic infection in Acquired Immuno-Deficiency Syndrome (AIDS, Navia et al 1986a, b).

Seizures may complicate parasitosis acutely or later as sequelae to chronic infection and brain scarring. The severity and characteristics of the seizure disorder may vary with disease stage and with the individual seizure threshold. In acute schistosomiasis, in 'encephalitic' cysticercosis and in acute cerebral malaria, seizures are a more severe clinical problem than in other stages of these disorders. It is unclear how frequently epilepsy may be a chronic sequelae to malaria, schistosomiasis or trypanosomiasis.

In contrast epilepsy is well recognized as a consequence of cysticercosis, toxoplasmosis and hydatid disease.

**Table 7.2** Some characteristics of neurological involvement and of epilepsy in seven major parasitosis of the CNS. Data adapted from text

| | Cerebral involvement | Neurological presentation | Frequency of epilepsy | Nature of epilepsy |
|---|---|---|---|---|
| Schistosomiasis | Frequent in acute forms<br>1/4 chronic severe forms | Acute meningo-encephalopathy<br>Chronic granulomas | 2–4% with cerebral ova | Partial ± GTC |
| Hydatid disease | 3% of all cases | Focal signs (90%)<br>Raised ICP (90%) | 30% before surgery<br>10% after surgery | Partial ± GTC<br>Frequent status |
| Cysticercosis | 90% of all cases | Raised ICP (60%)<br>Mental changes (15%) | 60% | Partial ± GTC<br>Frequent status |
| African trypanosomiasis | All cases at late stage | Chronic meningo-encephalopathy | Common | Partial ± GTC |
| American trypanosomiasis | Frequent in acute form<br>Rare in chronic form | Acute meningo-encephalopathy<br>Cerebral embolism | Rare | Partial ± GTC |
| Malaria | 10% of *P. falciparum* malaria | Acute encephalopathy | 28% of cerebral malaria | GTC<br>Febrile convulsions* |
| Toxoplasmosis in AIDS | 13% of AIDS in USA | Somnolence<br>Confusion<br>Focal deficits | 25% of cases | Partial ± GTC |

GTC, generalized tonic-clonic seizures; ICP, intracranial pressure; *, in uncomplicated malaria.

Cerebral involvement in parasitosis with associated inflammation, vasculitis or mass effect results in 'symptomatic localization-related epilepsies' (Commission on Classification and Terminology of the ILAE 1985), with partial seizures with or without secondary generalization. This is clinically evident with hydatid disease and cysticercosis. In cerebral malaria, seizures are more often generalized from the outset. Systemic, non-cerebral malaria is very commonly associated with febrile convulsions in African children.

## SCHISTOSOMIASIS

### Epidemiology and microbiology

Some 300 000 000 people carry *Schistosoma mansoni* in Africa and Latin America while similar numbers carry *S. heamatobium* in Africa or *S. japonicum* in southeast Asia (Pawlowski 1981). Schistosomes are digenetic trematodes which multiply in the intermediate snail host before infecting vertebrates. Cercarie released from the snail penetrate the vertebrate host through the skin, subcutaneous tissue, venous blood vessels and peripheral lymphatics (Neves & Souza 1983). They reach the portal system or liver where they mature and mate. They then migrate to the mesenteric or vesical veins where egg production begins. Adult parasites are 6–28 mm long, produce up to 3000 eggs daily, and survive for 5–10 years (Neves & Souza 1983).

**Pathophysiology and clinical course**

Acute schistosomiasis or Katayama syndrome occurs in a small proportion of patients usually due to *S. japonicum*. It is possibly an immune-complex mediated disorder secondary to antigenic schistosomal stimuli (Dennert 1981). Malaise, myalgia, fever, abdominal pain and diarrhoea occur, and there is occasionally an encephalopathy with mental changes leading to stupor, visual impairment, papilledema, focal cerebral involvement, and partial and generalized seizures. A myelopathy may also be part of the picture. Some degree of intracranial hypertension develops (Dennert 1981, Neves & Souza 1983, Scrimgeour & Gadjusek 1985). Clinical manifestations subside, and neurological signs and symptoms are said to resolve completely (Scrimgeour & Gadjusek 1985). Local reaction may lead to disappearance of the parasites, and to calcifications or fibrotic scarring in the liver, spleen, intestines, genito-urinary tract, lungs and, more rarely, brain (Neves & Souza 1983).

Schistosomal eggs may travel retrogradely in deep iliac veins, vena cava, meningeal veins and vertebral venous plexus. Development of cor pulmonale is probably antecedent to cerebral schistosomiasis as this would allow eggs to pass to the arterial circulation through pulmonary shunts or lesions and embolize to the brain (Scrimgeour & Gadjusek 1985). The frequency with which ova reach the brain varies from 0–56% of cases studied, independent of the urinary or hepatosplenic forms (Scrimgeour & Gadjusek 1985). Cerebral deposition of ova was found in 26% of 46 patients with hepatosplenic schistosomiasis who also had cor pulmonale (Pitella & Lana-Peixoto 1981). Although ova have been reported in the leptomeninges, choroid plexus, brainstem, cerebellum, hippocampus, temporal and occipital lobes and basal ganglia, clinically significant granulomas rarely develop in the CNS. Scrimgeour & Gadjusek (1985) found only three cases of mass lesions due to granulomata of the cerebrum or cerebellum, and three other cases of intracranial haemorrhage. A number of patients who died of unrelated causes had silent cerebral granulomas or parasites.

Levy et al (1975) described eight patients with cerebral schistosomiasis, six of whom had epilepsy during an acute meningo-encephalitic phase of the disease. In other studies, between 2.4 and 3.8% of 68 patients with confirmed cerebral ova deposition had epilepsy (Alves 1958, Monteiro de Barros et al 1956; Pitella & Lana-Peixoto 1981, Queiroz 1974). The prevalence of epilepsy in urban Latin America is approximately 1% (Bittencourt 1988). It is unclear whether this relatively minor increase in prevalence is related to schistosomal involvement of the brain or to other non-specific factors likely to occur in this population.

**Diagnosis**

Parasites can be demonstrated in feces or by rectal biopsy. Peripheral blood examination may show eosinophilia, and a CSF pleocytosis, occasionally with eosinophils may occur (Neves & Souza 1983, Scrimgeour & Gadjusek 1985). Cerebrospinal fluid (CSF) protein may be slightly increased, but is probably markedly elevated only with obstruction to CSF flow by granulomata. Radioimmuno- and enzyme-linked immunosorbent assays applied to serum or CSF may indicate previous exposure to schistosomes (Scrimgeour & Gadjusek 1985) in 83% of minor and in 98% of severe infections (Pelley et al 1977). Demonstration of ova by biopsy is the final proof of CNS involvement, although therapeutic tests with schistosomicidal drugs may be advocated in specific cases.

**Management and prognosis**

Therapy of cerebral schistosomiasis involves steroids and etiological therapy in the Katayama syndrome and in schistosomal encephalopathy. Of schistosomicidal agents available, praziquantel is preferable to oxamniquine and metrifonate because it kills parasites and decreases immunological reactions (Scrimgeour & Gadjusek 1985). Regimens for neurological involvement have not been fully investigated in view of the rarity of the condition, but those proposed for cysticercosis may be adequate. Prognosis is generally good, depending on disease stage at the time of treatment. Late epilepsy may complicate schistosomiasis in a substantial number of the half billion carriers in the planet, but this has not been determined.

## ECHINOCOCCOSIS (HYDATID DISEASE)

**Epidemiology and microbiology**

Man, sheep, cows or pigs are intermediate hosts in which the larval form of a small taenia, echinococcus granulosus, grows into the hydatid cysts which may reach 20 cm in diameter and be localized in the liver (60%), lungs (20%), and more rarely in the brain (3%) or other internal organs. In dogs, the hydatid cyst evolves to the final tape-worm. Humans are infected by fecal material. Hydatid disease is endemic in sheep-growing areas of southern Europe, North Africa, South Africa, Middle East, Australia and New Zealand. The highest rates of infection are found in Uruguay, Chile and Argentina (Shantz 1984).

**Pathophysiology and clinical course**

In humans, the hexacanth embryo perforates the intestinal mucosa to reach liver, vena cava and lungs, from where it may embolize to the brain. Symptoms are due mostly to compression by the slowly growing cysts. The lack of a systemic syndrome indicating an acute early phase is possibly related to the minimal if any immune reaction to the intact cyst. Minor leaks in cyst wall may cause asthma or skin rashes; cyst rupture with spilling of liquid and scolices may lead to pain, anxiety, headache, dyspnoea, nausea, anaphylactic shock, seizures, coma and rapid death.

Saus et al (1973) reported 90 cases of cerebral hydatidosis operated upon or autopsied in Montevideo between 1932–1973. The commonest clinical presentations were focal signs (95%), intracranial hypertension (92%), and seizures (31%). Cysts were prerolandic (69%), post-rolandic (29%) or located in the posterior fossa (2%). They were single in 43 cases, and multilocculated in four. These findings are comparable to those of Arseni & Marinescu (1974) in Bulgaria. Arseni & Marinescu (1974) found that approximately 1/3 of patients had clinical seizures. Saus et al (1973) found that 1/3 had seizures and another 1/3 had EEG 'spike-activity' and included the latter as 'clinical evidence of epilepsy'.

Clinical studies of etiology of epilepsy in Uruguay have not shown hydatidosis (De Pasquet et al 1972) or a prevalence of 1% (De Pasquet et al 1976).

Rarer presentations of hydatidosis are spinal cord compression and hypothalamic dysfunction (Pamir et al 1984, Tiberin et al 1984).

Arseni & Marinescu (1974) reported 62 children and adults seen between 1938–1979, 59 of whom were operated upon. Twenty-two developed epilepsy before surgery. Seizures were simple partial with or without secondary generalization in all but one case. Complex partial seizures were not reported. Signs of focal cerebral involvement or raised intracranial pressure were found at the onset of epilepsy in all patients.

Four patients had seizures only after operation. Of the 22 patients operated on after seizures began, seven had further seizures immediately, six between 3 and 12 months, and three others more than 1 year after surgery. Tonic-clonic status epilepticus was infrequent, but partial status or 'bursts' of partial seizures of various kinds were common before and after surgery. Focal motor deficits following a seizure were common including in the only patient who presented with a generalized tonic-clonic seizure. Ten patients had EEGs which demonstrated slowing of varying severity and localization, and two had paroxysmal discharges. Saus et al (1973) found EEG 'evidence of epilepsy' in 3 of 19 cases examined before surgery, and in all 13 examined after surgery.

The literature from 1929 to 1967 reviewed by Arseni & Marinescu (1974) indicated epilepsy was present in 3–40% of cerebral hydatidosis cases. Arseni & Marinescu (1978) concluded that seizures, focal neurological deficits, and increased intracranial pressure were a direct result of hydatid cyst size and location with resulting parenchymal compression and ischemia rather than edema or other manifestation of the host's immune response.

**Diagnosis**

Epidemiological, clinical and radiological information provides clear clues to diagnosis. Serological tests are of limited value, being negative in up to 50% of confirmed cases (Bia & Barry 1986). Computerized tomography (CT) is now basic to diagnosis and staging of the disease. In most cases, hydatids can be differentiated from cysticercosis by the absence of associated parenchymal edema or bizarre patterns of hydrocephalus. CSF studies are also helpful.

**Management and prognosis**

In systemic hydatidosis, 20–60% of non-operated cases die within 3 years. Early or late postsurgical mortality ranges from 4–20% (Shantz 1984). Leaking of cyst contents leads to the reappearance of many cysts approximately 1 year later, and mortality increases with the number of operations (Fabiani et al 1980).

The role of surgery in hydatid disease of the brain is likely to be much greater than in cysticercosis, since cysts are larger and usually single. Furthermore, the consequences of cyst rupture are circumvented by steroid or diuretic therapy in cysticercosis; the benefit of these treatments are as yet unknown in hydatidosis.

Medical therapy of hydatid disease includes mebendazole, fluoromebendazole and praziquantel. The former two have been used more extensively, in regimens of 10–40 mg/kg/day for 30 days. The effect of any medical treatment on CNS hydatids is unclear, however. Praziquantel was used successfully in 101 cases of abdominal hydatidosis (Ping Li et al 1985). A 10 day course of 25–30 mg/kg/day led to 'mortality of protoscolices' in more than 90% of hydatid cysts recovered from 39 patients who were operated upon immediately after therapy.

At the moment, surgery is indicated for excision of large hydatid cysts, but medical therapy should be recommended in specific patients with smaller cysts and as adjunctive treatment to surgical procedures.

Arseni & Marinescu (1974) used phenobarbitone and phenytoin to treat seizures but did not evaluate results. Apparently 16 of 22 patients went on having seizures and a few had status epilepticus after surgery despite antiepileptic drugs. All seizure relapses between 3 and 12 months after surgery heralded recurrence of hydatids.

## CYSTICERCOSIS

### Epidemiology and microbiology

Ingestion of *Cysticercus cellulosae*, the larval form of *Taenia solium*, leads to taeniasis when the larva grows to the full taenia in the intestines or to cysticercosis when it crosses to the blood stream and reaches body tissues (Campos & Perpétuo 1983). Reports of neurocysticercosis in utero, in the first days post-partum, and in non-pork-eaters indicate infection by means other than ingestion of pork or fecal-oral transmission (Bittencourt et al 1986a). Even though contaminated vegetables, air and transplacental mechanisms may play a role, pigs provide the reservoir for transmission. The disease is common in Latin America, Central and Southern Africa and Eastern Asia. It is less frequent in south and west Europe, but it is becoming more frequent in North America and Europe.

In the 19th century, 2% of human autopsies carried out in Berlin showed cysticerci (Blacklock & McArthur 1934). Recent autopsy rates have been 2% in Mexico, 0.4% in other Latin American countries, and 0.45% in Zimbabwe. In a village in Bali, 3% of the 199 inhabitants had subcutaneous cysticercus nodules, and at another village 8% of the population had epilepsy possibly related to neurocysticercosis (Gelfand 1948, Rabiella-Cervantes et al 1982, Simanjuntak et al 1977, Woodhouse et al 1982).

### Pathophysiology and clinical course

Once in the systemic circulation, the hexacanth embryo reaches tissues by passive venous and lymphatic transport with subsequent passage through the lungs and systemic embolization. It then develops into *Cysticercus cellulosae* when it has the scolex (live larva) or *Cysticercus racemosae* when it does not (Zavala 1983). The parasite evolves through the vesicular, colloidal, granular-nodular and calcified stages over a period of 2–5 years. There may be varying degrees of immune reaction to the cyst locally, with granulomatous changes and vasculitis (Escobar 1983).

The larvae show great preference for muscle, brain, choroid plexi, and CSF cavities, possibly due to the extensive blood supply (Zavala 1983). Much more rarely cysts develop in other organs (Escobar 1983). They are common in the ventricles and subarachnoid spaces. Contrary to traditional knowledge (Escobar 1983), chronic meningeal forms are rare and the proportion of extraparenchymal neurocysticercosis is less than previously thought (Table 3, Bittencourt et al 1985, Botero & Castaño 1982, Grisolia & Wiederholt 1982, Lombardo et al 1983).

An acute 'encephalitic' form of cysticercosis occurs predominantly in children and adolescents. Its rapid clinical course to death or resolution, and the observation that CT shows multiple areas of edema with ring-enhancement (Fig. 7.1), appear to indicate that initial invasion of the CNS by a cysticercus takes place with an immune-mediated parenchymal reaction. Support of this assumption is given by the subsequent evolution of surviving cases to a final stage of multiple calcifications (Fig. 7.1). Mazer et al (1983) and Minguetti & Ferreira (1983) reported that about 20% of their cases belonged

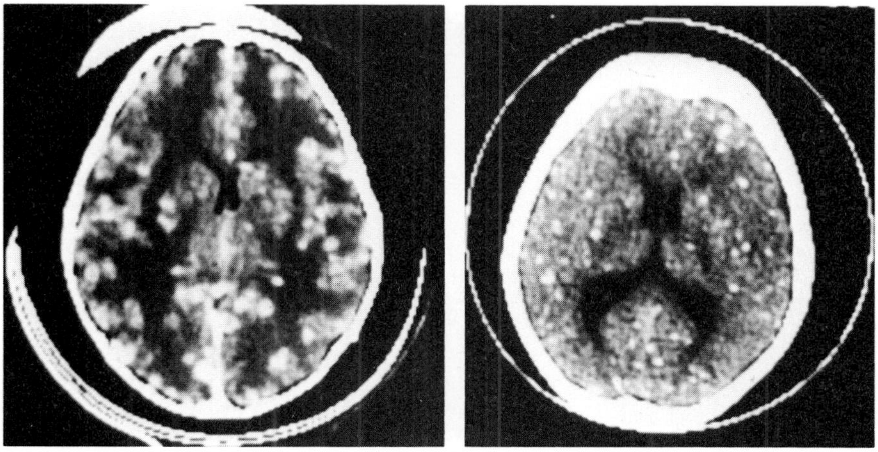

**Fig. 7.1** CT scans of a 5-year-old girl with acute 'encephalitic' cysticercosis, at clinical presentation after administration of intravenous contrast (left) and 3 years later (right). During this period she underwent extensive steroid treatment and had a lumbar-peritoneal shunt inserted for intracranial hypertension and received antiepileptic drugs. The severe edema with contrast-enhanced ring or dot-shaped areas gave place to multiple cerebral calcifications. (Courtesy of Dr S. Mazer, Hospital Nossa Senhora das Graças, Curitiba, Brazil.)

to this acute 'encephalitic' group, while Rodriguez-Carbajal et al (1983) gave a figure of 65%. These studies were based on radiological-surgical samples. Clinically-based studies indicate a prevalence of acute 'encephalitis' in approximately 10% (Costa et al personal communication).

The interval between initial infection and clinical disease may vary from weeks to many years. Focal signs of parenchymal brain involvement, of hydrocephalus of various types, of compression by large cysts, and of meningeal irritation due to spilling of cyst material may present in various combinations (Bittencourt et al 1986a).

Neurocysticercosis has been compared with multiple sclerosis with regard to its clinical course marked by relapses and remissions related to local parenchymal or CSF immune reactions to cyst components (Livramento et al 1985). Fluctuating clinical, CSF and CT evidence of neurocysticercosis may be related to the presence of cysts at various stages of development in many patients (Fig. 7.2, Bittencourt et al 1986a,b) with varying degrees of local and meningeal inflammatory reaction and structural compression (Fig. 7.3).

The frequency of the various clinical presentations has varied depending upon whether the series has been based on radiological, pathological or neurosurgical data (Bia & Barry 1986, Escobar 1983, Minguetti & Ferreira 1983). Analysis of clinically-based material shows that the commonest presentations are epilepsy and intracranial hypertension, with or without meningeal signs, followed by psychiatric syndromes (Table 7.3 and 7.4). Canelas (1963), found intracranial hypertension alone in 36% and in association with epilepsy in 25% of cases.

A host of rarer clinical forms have been described including spinal cord compression and stroke-like syndromes (Botero & Castaño 1982, Grisolia & Wiederholt 1982, Loo & Braude 1982, Manreza 1982, Takayanagui & Jardim 1983). Some patients present with an isolated generalized tonic-clonic seizure, and subsequent investigation discloses an isolated ring-enhancing area surrounding a probable cyst, with white-

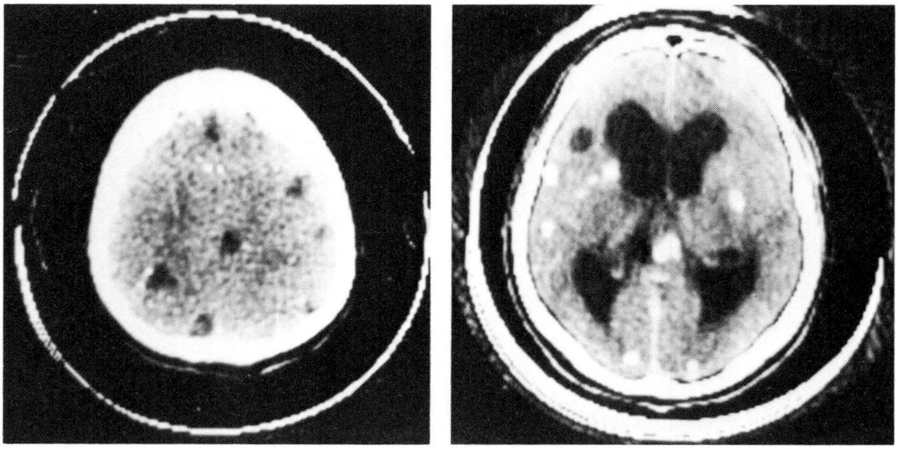

**Fig 7.2** CT scans of a patient with active neurocysticercosis with partially calcified cysts, cysts in the parenchyma and in the subarachnoid spaces (left) and of another with asymetrical hydrocephalus, intraparenchymal cysts and calcifications (right). (Courtesy of Dr S. Mazer, Hospital Nossa Senhora das Graças, Curitiba, Brazil.)

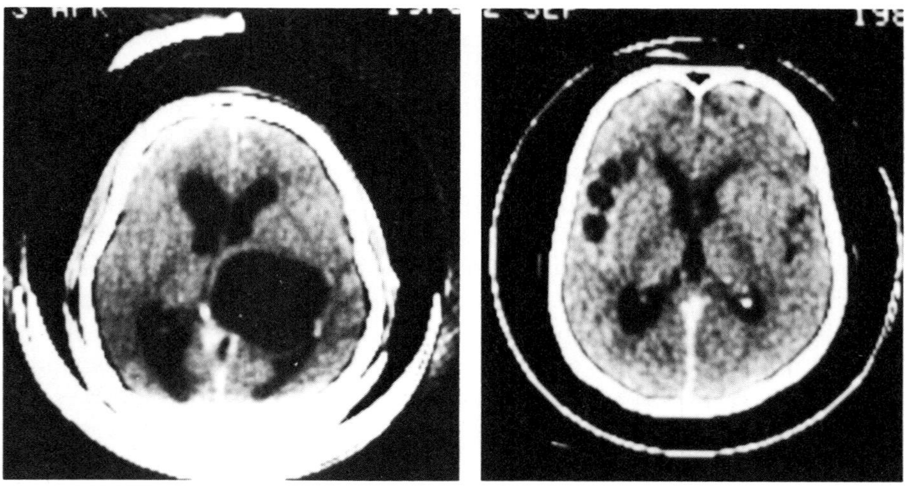

**Fig 7.3** CT scans before (left) and after (right) administration of intravenous contrast in patients with a large intra-ventricular cyst with obstructive hydrocephalus (left) and with cysts in the Sylvian fissure (right). (Courtesy of Dr S. Mazer, Hospital Nossa Senhora das Graças, Curitiba, Brazil.)

matter edema (Fig. 7.4) In endemic areas this is most likely cysticercosis, but in other areas this diagnosis can only be confirmed when the lesion shows progressive calcification (Mazer, personal communication).

Arseni & Cristescu (1972) reported their retrospective limited observations on 104 patients aged 4–63 years with epilepsy and neurocysticercosis, seen at a neurosurgical unit in Bucharest between 1935–1970. At least 83% had partial seizures with or without secondary generalization, while five patients had grand-mal seizures and 10 had 'loss of consciousness'. Partial seizures were unilateral motor (12 patients), unilateral sensory (17), unilateral sensory-motor (7) and complex partial (approximately 20). The

**Table 7.3** Symptoms presented by 42 patients classified according to whether they had the mixed, intraparenchymal or extraparenchymal forms of active neurocysticercosis. (Costa et al personal communication)

| Symptoms | Mixed | | Intraparenchymal | | Extraparenchymal | |
|---|---|---|---|---|---|---|
| | n | % | n | % | n | % |
| Headache | 10 | 53 | 5 | 42 | 10 | 83 |
| Epilepsy | 12 | 74 | 11 | 92 | 1 | 9 |
| Nausea ± vomiting | 4 | 21 | 2 | 17 | 8 | 73 |
| Psychiatric features | 3 | 16 | 3 | 25 | 1 | 9 |
| Double vision | 3 | 16 | 0 | 0 | 0 | 0 |
| Decreased visual acuity | 1 | 5 | 0 | 0 | 1 | 9 |
| Dizziness and ataxia | 1 | 5 | 1 | 8 | 2 | 18 |
| Dysarthria | 1 | 5 | 0 | 0 | 0 | 0 |
| Total | 19 | | 12 | | 11 | |

**Table 7.4** Signs observed on physical examination on admission of 42 patients with mixed, intraparenchymal or extraparenchymal types of neurocysticercosis. (Costa et al personal communication)

| Signs | Mixed | | Intraparenchymal | | Extraparenchymal | |
|---|---|---|---|---|---|---|
| | n | % | n | % | n | % |
| Nuchal rigidity | 3 | 16 | 0 | 0 | 2 | 18 |
| Bilateral papilledema | 4 | 21 | 2 | 17 | 2 | 18 |
| Hyper-reflexia | 3 | 16 | 0 | 0 | 1 | 9 |
| Ataxia | 3 | 16 | 1 | 8 | 0 | 0 |
| 6th nerve paresis | 3 | 16 | 0 | 0 | 0 | 0 |
| Nystagmus | 1 | 5 | 1 | 8 | 0 | 0 |
| Total | 19 | | 12 | | 11 | |

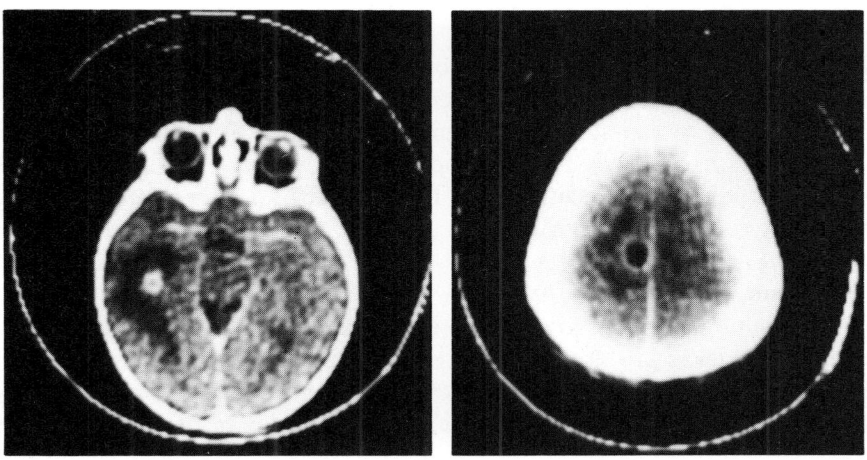

**Fig. 7.4** CT scans after administration of intravenous contrast in patients who presented with isolated generalized tonic-clonic seizures showing ring-enchancement and surrounding white-matter edema.

authors emphasize the polymorphism of the seizures in 20 patients who had 'Jacksonian' seizures alternating between right and left sides or even more complex patterns related to multiple cortical cysts (Arseni & Cristescu 1972).

Gracia et al (personal communication) studied 24 epileptic patients drawn from a group of 42 patients with neurocysticercosis, admitted consecutively to a neurological unit (Curitiba Prospective Study). Patients had had epilepsy for 48 ± 68 months (mean ± standard deviation) and symptoms of cysticercosis for 34 ± 77 months. Seizures were simple partial (2 cases) complex partial (1), simple (14) or complex (3) partial with secondary generalization or generalized tonic-clonic (4).

Marques-Assis & Ortiz (1972) compared 131 patients with cysticercosis-related epilepsy aged 2–68 years to 1217 patients from their epilepsy clinic. The higher frequency of tonic-clonic seizures in both these groups is in disagreement with data from Bucharest and from the Curitiba Prospective Study (Arseni & Cristescu 1972, Gracia et al personal communication), as well with other prospective studies of epilepsy (Bittencourt 1988).

Partial or tonic-clonic status epilepticus were reported in 7 of 104 patients with epilepsy and cysticercosis by Arseni & Cristescu (1972), and in 6 of the 24 patients of Gracia et al (personal communication). The latter found that seizure disorders were more severe before than after admission to a neurological unit for treatment of neurocysticercosis (Table 7.5).

**Table 7.5** Seizure status of patients with neurocysticerosis before and after admission to a neurological unit. During admission 1 patient had 10 partial seizures and another had 3 partial seizures with secondary generalization. Status epilepticus after discharge was related to interruption of therapy. (Gracia et al personal communication)

| | Before admission | After discharge |
|---|---|---|
| ⩾ 1 seizure monthly | 19 | 8 |
| ⩽ 1 seizure monthly | 5 | 5 |
| Seizure free | 0 | 11 |
| Status epilepticus | 4 | 2 |

Ahuja & Mohanta (1982) found neurocysticercosis to be the etiology in 5.1% of 253 patients aged 25 years or more consecutively evaluated for recent-onset epilepsy in New Delhi. A similar study by Bittencourt (in press) in Curitiba, Brasil, found evidence of cysticercosis in 4% of 107 patients above 16 years of age. Both were prospective studies of consecutive cases in a neurological rather than neurosurgical environment, carried out after the advent of CT.

## Classification

The concepts of disease activity, fluctuating course, and overlapping symptoms and signs have been taken into account in the classification of neurocysticercosis presented in Figure 7.5 modified from Bittencourt et al (1986a). As argued by Campos & Perpétuo (1983), previous syndromic, pathological and radiological classifications create unnecessary complexity and are by definition incomplete. Disease activity is defined as CT or CSF evidence of immune reaction to the cysts or demonstration of the cysts themselves. In extraparenchymal neurocysticercosis, CT shows no involvement

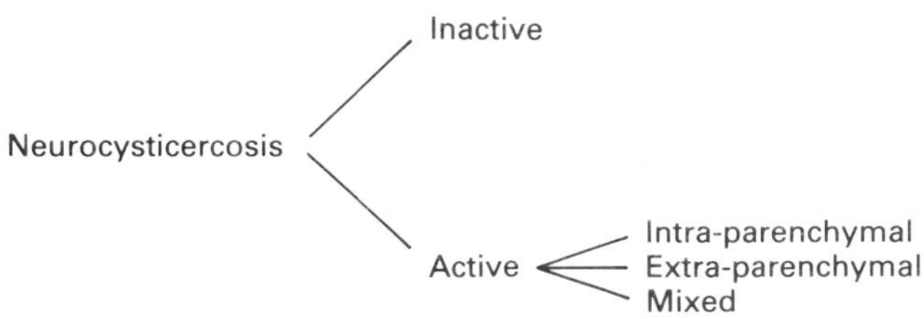


**Fig. 7.5** Classification of neurocysticercosis.

**Table 7.6** Findings on CT scan of 42 patients with mixed, intraparenchymal and extraparenchymal forms of neurocysticercosis admitted consecutively to a neurological unit

| CT scan | Mixed | Intraparenchymal | Extraparenchymal |
|---|---|---|---|
| Normal | — | — | 6 |
| IP cysts | 4 | 5 | — |
| IP cysts + other findings | 14 | 7 | — |
| Calcifications | 9 | 5 | 2 |
| Hydrocephalus | 7 | 1 | 3 |
| Ventricular asymmetry | 4 | 2 | 1 |
| Generalized edema | 2 | 1 | 0 |
| Total | 19 | 12 | 11 |

IP, intraparenchymal.

**Table 7.7** Findings on examination of cerebral spinal fluid (CSF) of 42 patients with mixed, intraparenchymal and extraparenchymal forms of cysticercosis admitted consecutively to a neurological unit. (Costa et al personal communication)

| CSF | Mixed | Intraparenchymal | Extraparenchymal |
|---|---|---|---|
| Cells (n) | 36 ± 71 | 1 ± 1 | 72 ± 90 |
| Mononuclear (%) | 94 ± 13 | 75 ± 45 | 88 ± 21 |
| Eosinophils (%) | 2 ± 8 | 0 | 11 ± 21 |
| Polymorphs (+) | 3 ± 12 | 0 | 0.3 ± 0.6 |
| Protein (mg%) | 65 ± 69 | 36 ± 19 | 53 ± 44 |
| Glucose (mg/dl) | 69 ± 23 | 67 ± 12 | 59 ± 14 |
| Complement fixation test (% positive) | 47 | 0 | 36 |
| Total | 19 | 12 | 11 |

of the cerebral parenchyma (Table 7.6) while in the parenchymal type CSF studies are normal (Table 7.7). In the mixed form, both CSF and brain parenchyma are involved.

The acute 'encephalitic' form of cysticercosis may be intraparenchymal or mixed (intra and extraparenchymal) depending on CSF findings. The previously commonly seen basal meningitic and racemose forms (Escobar 1983) can be classified similarly. The current classification is also based on the fact that drugs most likely achieve different concentrations in the cerebral parenchyma and CSF.

Many reports published before the era of CT do not make clear which cases are of active or inactive disease. In some reports after CT became available inactive cases are a large proportion (Minguetti & Ferreira 1983). The data of Costa et al (personal

**Table 7.8** Age, sex, length of history and number of 42 patients classified according to whether they had mixed, intraparenchymal or extraparenchymal forms of active neurocysticercosis. (From Costa et al personal communication)

| | Mixed | Intraparenchymal | Extraparenchymal |
|---|---|---|---|
| Age { m ± s.d. months | 35 ± 14 | 24 ± 14 | 30 ± 14 |
| Age { range (years) | 2–62 | 6–51 | 5–54 |
| Male sex | 12 | 5 | 7 |
| Female sex | 7 | 7 | 4 |
| Length of history (m ± s.d., months) | 54 ± 88 | 21 ± 55 | 20 ± 50 |
| Number | 19 | 12 | 11 |

communication, Tables 7.3, 7.4, 7.6–7.8) show clear distinction between the forms of active disease. Intraparenchymal cysticercosis is present in a younger age group and more frequent in women. Epilepsy is very rare in extraparenchymal neurocysticercosis, while headache, nausea and vomiting are more common than in intraparenchymal or mixed forms. In the same study, three patients with the mixed form had epilepsy and intracranial hypertension, and two had epilepsy and a psychiatric syndrome. In the intraparenchymal form, two patients had epilepsy and intracranial hypertension, one had psychiatric symptoms and intracranial hypertension, and two had epilepsy and psychiatric symptoms. In the extraparenchymal form, only one patient had epileptic seizures which were superimposed on signs and symptoms of intracranial hypertension and meningeal irritation.

## Diagnosis

### *Serum, blood and CSF*

The peripheral blood may show an elevated eosinophil count without evidence of inflammation. Complement fixation, immunofluorescence, protein electrophoresis and hemogglutination tests either yield low sensitivity (Table 7.7) or are non-specific (Ramirez 1986). Diwan et al (1982) described an enzyme-linked immunosorbent assay (ELISA) for detection of antibody to cysticerci of taenia solium based on a pork muscle antigen control. This detected serum antibodies in 79% of Mexican patients with confirmed disease, in 61% of patients with presumed disease from Irian Jaya, and in no healthy Americans and residents of Papua New Guinea. An IgM ELISA technique used by Costa et al (1985) was positive in 46.2% of CSF samples from confirmed cases, and its specificity was confirmed by samples becoming negative after 2-mercaptoethanol treatment. This raises the possibility that this test may be useful for defining disease activity.

CSF studies help exclude other etiologies and demonstrate disease activity when CT is normal or shows only calcifications (Table 7.7, Bittencourt et al 1986a,b). CSF sugar is decreased in 20% of the cases and total protein is slightly increased with elevated gammaglobulins in 88%. The typical cellular reaction is made up of mononuclear cells, polymorphs and eosinophils (Fishman 1980). Eosinophils are highly suggestive of cysticercosis in endemic areas, being found in 20–77% of cases (Fishman 1980). This classical CSF picture denotes disease activity with spilling of cyst contents in the CSF (Lange 1940, Spina França Netto 1961, Livramento et al 1985).

*Imaging techniques*

Parenchymal calcifications, found in up to 70% of patients in radiological series (Mazer et al 1983), are usually multiple, each between 1–7 mm in diameter. Cysts average 10 mm in diameter and may have a peripheral calcification, denoting cyst degeneration. Intraventricular and subarachnoid cysts have the same density as CSF, but when large enough they cause deformation of surrounding structures. Intrathecal contrast is useful in demonstrating non-parenchymal cysts. Hydrocephalus, found in 7–44% of patients in radiological series (Mazer et al 1983, Minguetti & Ferreira 1983) is more frequently obstructive and asymmetrical due to varying degrees of foramina and aqueduct stenosis secondary to cyst impaction and inflammation (Escobar 1983, Mazer et al 1983, Figs. 7.2 and 7.3).

The 'acute encephalitic form' consists of multiple areas of edema of the white matter, with small ring-shaped or nodullary areas of contrast absorption in their midst. Edema may also surround cysts of various sizes in the parenchyma and may vary in severity (Mazer et al 1983, Figs 7.1, 7.3, 7.4).

In clinically-based studies of active neurocysticercosis, CT has more commonly shown mixed findings with cysts, with or without surrounding contrast enhancement, calcifications and hydrocephalus (Bittencourt et al 1985, 1986a, López-Hernandez & Garaizar 1982). Magnetic resonance Imaging (MRI) allows visualization of intraventricular (Figs 7.6, 7.7) and subarachnoid cysts as well as precise definition of the various forms of hydrocephalus (Radvany personal communication). It may be that MRI will be especially useful in follow-up of ventriculo-peritoneal shunting in view of the notorious tendency of ventricular shunts to malfunction due to cyst impaction or their location within closed cavities in the ventricles (Fig. 7.7, Radvany personal communication). Initial evaluation of MRI shows that small parenchymal and intraorbital cysts are precisely visualized (Fig. 7.8) and occasionally even the live scolex can be seen (Fig. 7.9).

## Management

Therapy of neurocysticercosis is both symptomatic and specific. Intracranial hypertension is a lethal complication and needs to be treated rapidly. Furosemide, mannitol and glycerol are usually sufficient to control raised intracranial pressure (Bittencourt et al 1986b). Dexamethazone is very efficient in controlling edema if present on CT (Minguetti & Ferreira 1983). In the presence of hydrocephalus ventriculo-peritoneal shunting may be a necessary adjunct to medical therapy of raised intracranial pressure. Other medications used frequently consist of analgesics, antacids and H-3 receptor blockers for frequent iatrogenic gastritis and duodenitis. Drugs with sedative side effects should be avoided as they may obscure the clinical manifestations of the underlying disorder.

Gracia et al (personal communication) found that patients had more seizures before being admitted for symptomatic and etiological therapy than after discharge. Seizures during admission occurred in two cases and were manageable. Status epilepticus had occurred in four cases before admission. Treatment of cysticercosis and changes in antiepileptic drug regimens may have influenced this improvement. Table 7.9 shows

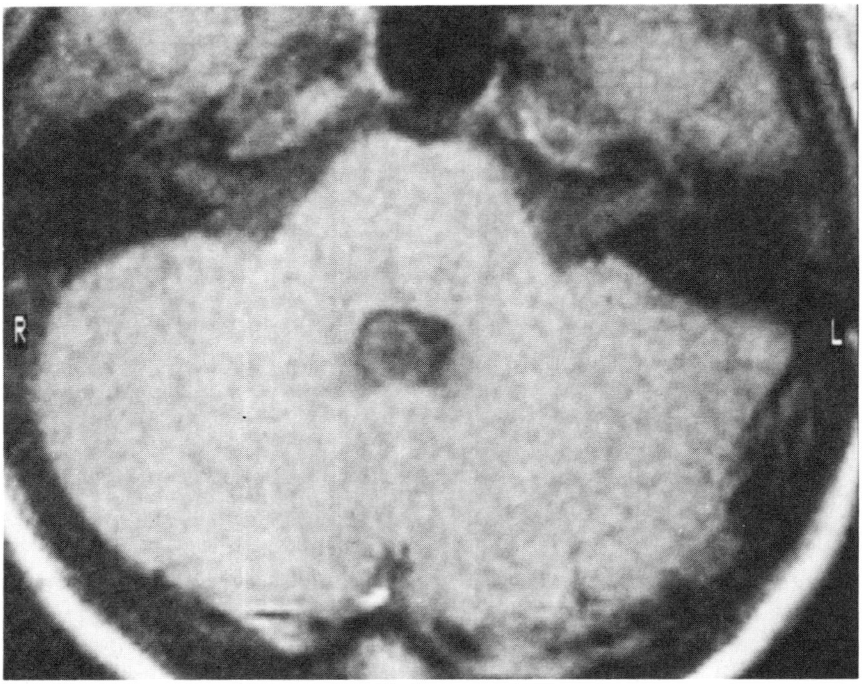


**Fig. 7.6** Fourth-ventricular intact cyst shown by MRI in a 4-year-old girl with seizures, raised intracranial pressure and a right frontal calcification on CT. (Courtesy of Dr J. Radvany, Hospital Israelita Albert Einstein, São Paulo, Brazil.)

that patients were changed to regimens which emphasize use of carbamazepine and phenytoin rather than phenobarbitone.

Surgical excision of cysts, which was previously recommended (Facure et al 1978, Mazer et al 1983) should be deferred until pharmacological therapy has been tried. Surgery, in any event, is of limited use when multiple cysts are present.

Sotelo et al (1984) showed unequivocally that praziquantel is effective in decreasing cyst size and number in the cerebral parenchyma, as had been tentatively indicated by a large number of prior publications with respect to all forms of active neurocysticercosis (Groll 1981). The usual regime consists of 50 mg/kg/day given orally 4 times daily for periods of 15 or 21 days (Sotelo et al 1984, Spina França et al 1982). Sotelo et al (1984) did not use steroids and patients were thus exposed to the acute relapses which may occur during treatment associated with cyst destruction. Episodes of meningeal reaction and increased intracranial pressure have led to occasional deaths during therapy (de Guetalde et al 1983, Groll 1981, Sotelo et al 1984), but are not unexpected from the immune response to cyst eradication. Judicious use of steroids, diuretics and ventriculo-peritoneal shunting can minimize complications during treatment as shown in the Curitiba Prospective Study of 42 patients who received more than 55 courses of praziquantel in doses of 50–100 mg/kg/day (Bittencourt et al, personal communication).

A novel therapeutic regimen with higher praziquantel dose, 100 mg/kg/day for 10 days, has been administered to 20 patients in the Curitiba Prospective Study (Gracial

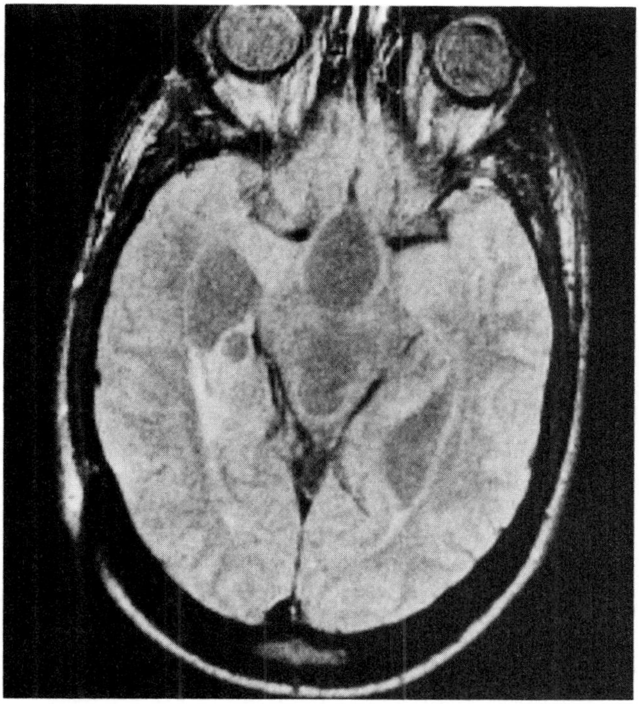

**Fig. 7.7** New onset of diplopia in a 26-year-old patient with known neurocysticercosis and shunted hydrocephalus prompted MRI which showed cyst obstructing the anterior portion of left temporal horn, large third ventrical and normal right temporal horn, indicating the inflammatory nature of the hydrocephalus. (Courtesy of Dr J. Radvany, Hospital Israelita Albert Einstein, São Paulo, Brazil.)

et al, personal communication) with no complications indicating that this regimen is as effective as others previously used and reduces the cost of hospitalization.

Management of acute 'encephalitis' due to neurocysticercosis is the same as for the other forms of disease.

Albendazol, a new broad-spectrum anti-helmintic, should become available for treatment of cysticercosis in the near future (Penne et al 1982).

**Prognosis**

Prolonged remission rather than cure should be the objective of therapy in view of the fluctuating course of the disease. The usual praziquantel regimens generally produce a remission rate of about 2/3 when patients are followed for 1 to 2 years (Groll 1981, Sotelo et al 1984, Spina França et al 1982). In the Curitiba Prospective Study (Bittencourt et al, personal communication) repeated treatment with praziquantel in doses of 50, later 75 and finally 100 mg/kg/day for periods of 10 to 15 days gave improved results over previously used regimens. Of 26 treated patients, 88% were clinically in remission or much improved and leading normal lives 19 months later; one patient died of late shunt complications. This outcome may be compared to the findings of Torrealba et al (1984). Thirty-two patients were followed for 40 months

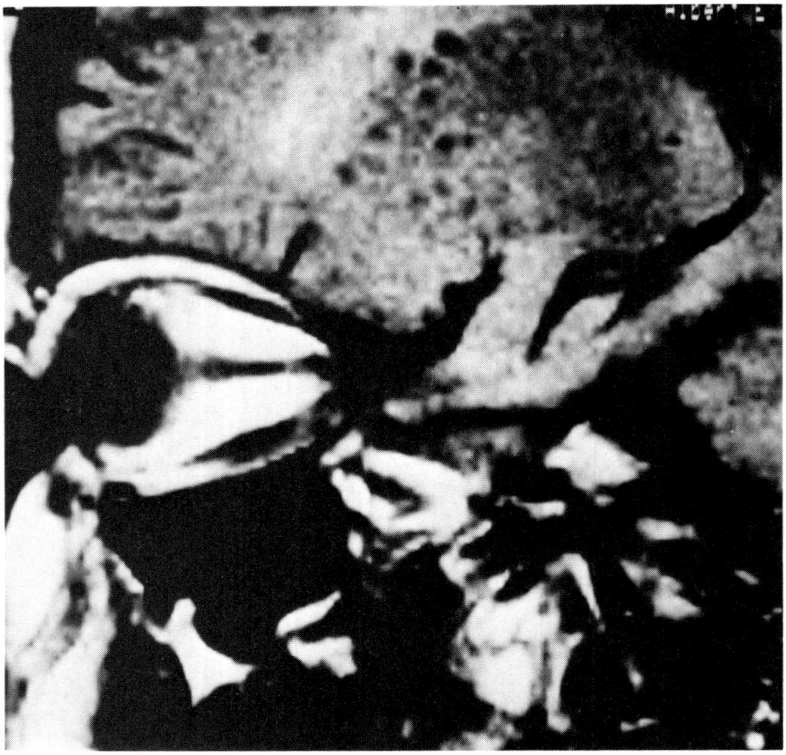

**Fig. 7.8** MRI scan showing multiple small cysts not seen on CT in a patient with clinical and CSF evidence of extra-parenchymal neurocysticercosis. An intra-orbital cyst is visible. (Courtesy of Dr J. Radvany, Hospital Israelita Albert Einstein, São Paulo, Brazil.)

during which time they received only anticonvulsants and steroids, underwent 11 craniotomies for cyst resection, 18 shunting procedures and one external-internal carotid bypass surgery. At the end of follow-up 38% were dead, 9% severely disabled and 53% were well.

## AFRICAN TRYPANOSOMIASIS

### Epidemiology and microbiology

Humans develop sleeping sickness upon transmission of *Trypanosoma brucei* by tse-tse flies in a sub-Saharan area extending from the western to the eastern coasts and south to Zambia and Zimbabwe (Lumsden 1981). About 40 000 000 people are at risk of infection (Dumas et al 1985).

There are three subspecies of *T. brucei*: *brucei, rhodesian* and *gambiense*. The brucei strain does not infect man. In rhodesian disease, patients either die or respond quickly to treatment. Infection is found mainly in fish and men who hunt. Gambiense disease has a more protracted course which allows human-fly-human transmission and equally affects men, women and children (Ferreira & Rocha 1982, Lumbsden 1981). An unknown number of infected persons do not develop clinical disease. The case-fatality

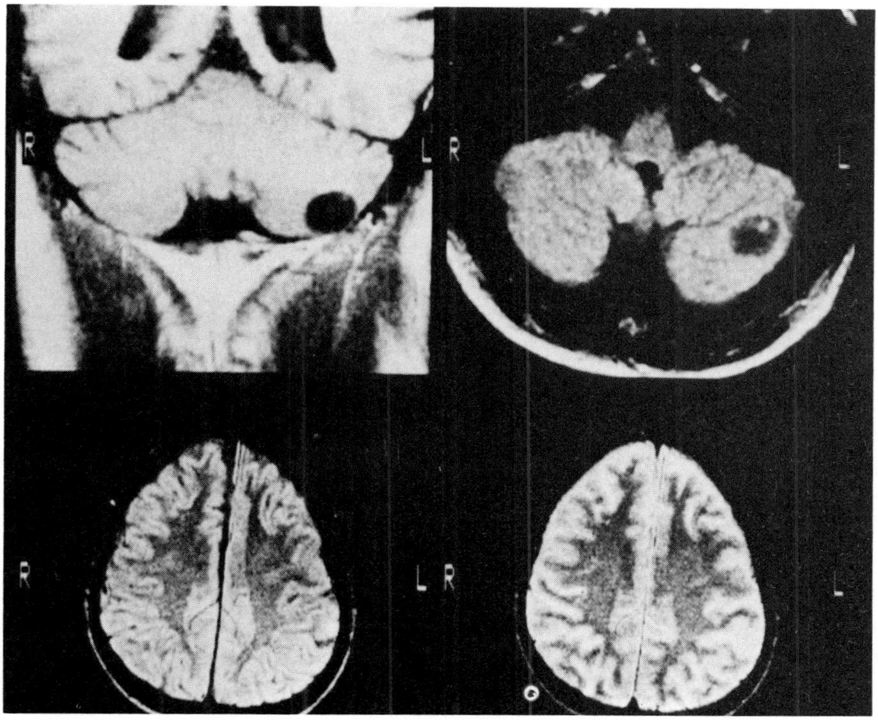


**Fig. 7.9** MRI scan of a 38-year-old man with neurocysticercosis. The T1-weighted images show the cerebellar cyst (above left), the cyst and the live scolex (above right) and hemispheric lesions at different stages of development (below). (Courtesy of Dr J. Radvany, Hospital Israelita Albert Einstein, São Paulo, Brazil.)

**Table 7.9** Number of patients on carbamazepine (CBZ), phenytoin (DPH), phenobarbitone (PHB), on two concomitant drugs (CBZ, DPH or PHB) and on no drugs before, during and after admission to a neurological unit for therapy of neurocysticercosis associated with epilepsy. One patient was left on no medication due to infrequent seizures. (From Gracia et al personal communication.)

| | Before admission | During admission | After admission |
|---|---|---|---|
| CBZ | 3 | 6 | 9 |
| DPH | 2 | 6 | 6 |
| PHB | 12 | 4 | 1 |
| 2 drugs | 5 | 7 | 7 |
| No drugs | 2 | 1 | 1 |

rate in rhodesian and gambiense disease approximates 90% making sleeping sickness one of the most lethal infections.

### Pathophysiology and clinical course

Upon entering the vertebrate host, *T. brucei* changes its outer glycoprotein layer every few days, leading to successive antigenic stimuli and production of large amounts of IgM. There is accompanying reticuloendothelial hyperplasia, atrophic changes in the lymph nodes and spleen, and immune suppression (Lumsden 1981, Neves 1983). High IgM levels, raised erythrocyte sedimentation rate and immune-complex mediated disease probably underlie the pathological characteristics of the disease including anemia, thrombocytopenia, glomerulonephritis, myocarditis with valvulitis and pericarditis, and a late-evolving diffuse meningoencephalitis with edema and arachnoiditis (Ferreira & Rocha 1982, Lumsden 1981, Neves 1983). The typical CNS lesion is intense perivascular cuffing with lymphoid cells.

The trypanosome chancre, a local reaction, is followed by the acute stage, in which trypomastigotes multiply and invade body fluids. The parasitemia produces waves of fever, weakness, anemia, and cardiac signs and symptoms (Lumsden 1981). Lymphadenopathy, localized edema, skin rashes, intravascular coagulation, and thrombocytopenia may occur during this acute stage which evolves into a variable period of latent disease. In the third stage, there is progressive neurological involvement with mood changes, pyramidal, extrapyramidal and cranial nerve signs, tremor, progressive rigidity, choreoathetoid movements, muscle fasciculations and prominent cerebellar ataxia (Ferreira & Rocha 1982). Most texts on African trypanosomiasis mention the occurrence of generalized and partial seizures during the neurological stage of both gambian and rhodesian varieties (Neves 1983, Ferreira & Rocha 1983).

In a congenital case reported by Lingam et al (1985), the mother had acquired trypanosomes by transfusion 4 years before she gave birth to a child who at 18 months developed progressive somnolence and retarded milestones, generalized tonic-clonic seizures, and a picture compatible with meningoencephalitis. Treatment was started 10 months after initial presentation, and brain damage had already occurred. The CT showed atrophy and areas of low attenuation. The disease process was arrested by treatment with suramin and melarprosol, but the child remained retarded and continued having complex partial seizures despite carbamazepine treatment. This case has raised the possibility that many cases of so-called 'viral encephalitis' or 'febrile encephalopathies of unknown etiology' which commonly underlie mental retardation and seizure disorders in Africa (Edgell & Stanfield 1972) may be due to treatable infections.

### Diagnosis

Epidemiological and clinical clues are basic to the diagnosis. In the acute disease, parasites can be demonstrated in body fluids or tissues. Complement fixation and immunofluorescent techniques are complicated by the antigenic variation of the organism (Lumsden 1972). An ELISA technique has been positive in 70% of serum samples of confirmed cases. When high IgM levels were also considered, diagnostic sensitivity increased to 78% (Barret-Connor 1981, Whittle et al 1977). The lymphocytic pleocytosis and high CSF IgM concentration are further evidence of active disease.

**Management and prognosis**

The untreated disease leads to death in less than 18 months in the rhodesian form and in less than 3 years in the gambian form, usually of intercurrent bacterial infection (Barrett-Connor 1981, Lumsden 1981). Death typically ensues 6 months after neurological involvement in the former and 12 months after in the latter.

Prognosis in gambian disease may be radically altered by early treatment with suramin sodium alone if neurological involvement has not occurred or with suramin followed by melarprosol in patients with evidence of central disease. Both suramin and melarprosol should be used in rhodesian disease after 4 weeks of the initial contact, with or without neurological involvement (Medical Letter 1986). Only melarprosol crosses the blood-brain barrier efficiently (Dumas et al 1985). Malnutrition and intercurrent infections are frequently present, and suramin and melarprosol are rather toxic. The former may cause shock, rashes and renal damage, while the latter carries all the problems associated with arsenic poisoning (Barrett-Connor 1981) including severe encephalopathy in 5% of treated cases (Dumas et al 1985). A number of other trypanosomicidal agents were reviewed by Dumas et al (1985). Concomitant use of steroids is recommended in advanced cases where survival may be prolonged enough for specific therapy to have its effect, and in the prophylaxis of side effects.

## AMERICAN TRYPANOSOMIASIS

**Epidemiology and microbiology**

There are some 7 000 000 patients with Chagas' diseases in Latin America between Panama and central Argentina, half of them in Brasil. Transmission of *Trypanosoma cruzi* depends on the presence of insects of the triatominae subfamily in wooden shacks in rural areas. Transmission by blood transfusion has become a hazard in the continent. Trypomastigotes deposited in the feces of the insects when they suck blood nocturnally enter the skin and transform into amastigotes (Dias et al 1983).

**Pathophysiology and clinical course**

If dissemination takes place, *T. cruzi* multiplies rapidly within cell cytoplasm especially in muscle and nerves of the intestines and heart. In the acute phase, direct cell damage takes place. Of five patients who died in this phase who were studied pathologically by Queiros (1978a), one had had clear clinical findings of meningoencephalitis. All five patients had pathological evidence of cerebral involvement, with meningeal inflammation (2), cerebral edema and congestion (4), varying degrees of inflammation and glial nodules in the cerebral and cerebellar parenchymal (5), focal neuronal lesions (2) and amastigote trypanosomes in the glial cells (3). This early inflammatory phase appears to be related to the release of trypomastigotes and toxins from ruptured cells.

In the chronic phase, few organisms remain (Dias et al 1983), and there is progressive destruction of nerve cells in autonomic ganglia, in the esophagus and intestines, as well as in muscle cells of various organs. Ruptured or intact pseudo-cysts (cells populated by trypanosomes) may become granulomatous.

Clinically, the disease starts with a Chagoma, the local reaction to the innoculation, followed by an acute stage with malaise, fever, headache, generalized or localized edema, skin rashes, lymphadenopathy, liver and spleen enlargement, myocarditis, and meningoencephalitis. Signs vary in severity from subclinical (the majority of cases) to life-threatening (a small minority), and may lead to severe neurological impairment including frequent epileptic seizures (Dias et al 1983). Queiros (1973) described a trypanosomal mass occupying both occipital lobes and extending to the parietal lobe in a patient who apparently succumbed to the acute phase of Chagas' disease. He had partial motor seizures at the onset of his neurological syndrome characterized by dysphasia and motor incoordination.

The disease process then abates and an unknown number of patients pass on to the chronic stage with slowly progressive morphological and functional disturbances of hollow organs, especially the heart, esophagus and colon. The latter may become very large and impacted with food or feces, when they are termed megaesophagus and megacolon. Cardiomegaly, often extreme, is accompanied by severe conduction disturbances, Adams–Stokes syndrome, cerebral and peripheral embolization, and heart failure. The chronic phase may take 10–20 years after innoculation to become evident (Dias et al 1983). Involvement of other organs in the chronic phase is uncommon. Direct involvement of the CNS is very rare. Of 114 cases studied pathologically 70% had normal brains, 15.7% had cerebral atrophy (similar frequency to that of a control group), and 26.3% had cerebral infarcts from cardiogenic thrombo-embolism (Queiros 1978b). Jardim & Takayanagui (1981) compared epileptic patients with (44) and without (approximately 90) Chagas' disease. They found those with Chagas' disease had more frequent onset of epilepsy after 25 years of age and more partial seizures with elementary symptomatology, as well as EEGs with more localized slowing. Their report is incomplete, and at least five of the Chagas' patients had had cerebral infarcts secondary to cardiogenic embolism. Faria et al (1976b) looked at 438 epileptic and 441 paired-control orthopedic patients in São Paulo, Brasil, and found that 6.8% of the former and 4% of the latter, as well as 7.48% of those with partial epilepsy and 3.6% of their paired controls were serologically positive for Chagas' disease (not statistically significant). Faria et al (1976a) found that of 19 epileptic patients seropositive for Chagas' disease, seven had normal ECGs as did 13 of 18 seronegative epileptics and 13 of 16 controls ($p < 0.05$). Only by considering together the ECG abnormality, dysphasia and dyspnoea were they able to find a statistical difference indicating a relationship of Chagas' and epilepsy. As dysphasia and dyspnoea may occur in many other disorders not controlled for in this retrospective study of a small group of patients, there is no definite proof of an epileptic syndrome secondary to trypanosomal involvement of the brain except in very rare instances (Queiros 1978b). The EEG studies of Girardelli (1969a,b) are similarly difficult to interpret due to methodological factors.

We conclude that epilepsy in Chagas' disease is most often secondary to cerebral embolization of cardiac blood clots, and that direct involvement of the brain by trypanosomes is very rare.

### Diagnosis

The most widely-used serological test is a complement-fixation technique, practically as specific and sensitive as hemogglutination and fluorescent antibody tests for detection of past infection (Cerisola et al 1969). The fluorescent antibody test became positive immediately after acute infection was diagnosed in 80% of patients, 1 month later in 90% and 2 months later in 100%. The two other techniques are slower (Cerisola et al 1969). In the acute infection, trypomastigotes may be demonstrated by microscopy in peripheral blood and CSF (Memoranda 1984). Staging of disease is clinically determined and by demonstration of hollow organ involvement using radiological or other methods.

**Management and prognosis**

Nifurtimox and benzonidazol are trypanosomicidal in therapeutic doses and appear to suppress clinical and serological disease in the acute phase when *T. cruzi* is in the blood stream. In the chronic phase preliminary results are not encouraging, and serological positivity persists (Dias et al 1983). In view of the natural history of the disorder, treatment with nifurtimox, 8–20 mg/kg/daily for 120 days may be advocated in acute as well as in chronic stages (Medical Letter 1986). Symptomatic care involves management of megaesophagus, megacolon, heart failure, and cardiac arrythmias. Many patients need to be anticoagulated chronically, but compliance is poor as a rule. Epileptic seizures may warrant therapy with carbamazepine or phenytoin. Although there are no clear data, the prognosis for seizure control is presumably as good as in other infarct-related seizure disorders, even though the prognosis of Chagas' disease itself is poor, evolving to refractory cardiac failure.

## MALARIA

**Epidemiology and microbiology**

Malaria is endemic in tropical America, Africa, Asia and in subtropical areas of the East Mediterranean. One quarter of humanity is exposed to the disease which is held responsible for the death of at least 10% of African children under 3 years of age. In South America, the highest prevalence is found in El Salvador, Haiti, Colombia and Brasil (Espinal & Toro 1986, WHO 1986). Despite the efforts of the WHO, 3 000 000 cases were identified in 1972, and 8.5 million in 1976 (Espinal & Toro 1986). An increase in morbidity in endemic zones of the Americas from 56 in 1960 to 352 per $10^5$ inhabitants in 1984 is thought to be related to increased mobility of populations and to failure of health programs (Gabaldon 1968, Oficina Sanitaria Panamericana 1986). Human malaria is caused by four species of the genus plasmodium: *P. vivax, P. falciparum, P. malarie* and *P. ovale. P. vivax* is the most widely distributed in endemic and nonendemic regions (Gilles 1981). In some regions of Africa malaria is the commonest cause of fever associated with febrile convulsions. This is the commonest pediatric emergency in the Ilesha area of western Nigeria (McGucken 1975).

*P. falciparum* malaria represents between 40 and 90% of the total number of cases in some areas (Espinal & Lopez 1987a, White et al 1983b).

Cerebral malaria is the commonest clinical presentation and cause of death in severe malaria. Its frequency in disease caused by *P. falciparum* varies from 1.6–12.5% (Betancur et al 1974, Daroff et al 1967, Uribe et al 1969, Warrell et al 1982). Morbidity is high and mortality ranges from 0–50%, with a mean of approximately 37% (Toro & Vergara 1978). In adults, cerebral disease predominates in previously unexposed males, frequently after prophylactic medication has been interrupted. Pregnant women are at high risk even when native to endemic areas, with severe clinical pictures especially common in first pregnancies (Toro et al 1983a, WHO 1986). Carriers in endemic zones have few clinical symptoms except pregnant women, immunosuppressed patients and splenectomized individuals (Gilles 1981).

**Clinical course**

Many combinations of symptoms and signs have been described in cerebral malaria. Daroff et al (1967) found that disturbance of consciousness was the commonest neurological presentation followed in frequency by an acute organic mental syndrome with confusion and disorientation, movement disorders, and acute personality changes. Focal neurological signs were rare and transient. Cerebral malaria, caused by *P. falciparum* malaria, may develop suddenly from a rather uneventful clinical picture. Characteristically, there is somnolence, hyperthermia, tachycardia and rapid progression to stupor and coma with nucchal rigidity. Seizures are common (Toro et al 1983a). Other cases may present with acute personality changes with delirium or paranoid psychosis (Daroff et al 1967, Toro et al 1983a). Sometimes malarial encephalopathy is a final complication of severe *P. falciparum* malaria associated with renal failure, hemoglobinuria, hepatitis and adult respiratory distress syndrome (Toro et al 1983a).

A diagnosis of cerebral malaria depends on unarousable coma, exclusion of other encephalopathies, and confirmation of *P. falciparum* infection (WHO 1986). In a patient with confirmed parastaemia, unexplained confusion may signal imminent cerebral complications. Retinal hemorrhages are found in 15% of cases and may presage the development of cerebral signs and symptoms (Looareesuwan et al 1983).

Hypoglycemia in patients with severe *P. falciparum* malaria and in pregnant women with malignant or benign disease may be related to quinine treatment (Looareesuwan et al 1985, Migasena 1983). Quinine is a potent stimulant of insulin secretion, and its serum levels correlate with the degree of hypoglycaemia in normal controls and in patients with cerebral malaria (White et al 1983a). As the clinical picture is similar to that of patients without hypoglycemia, blood sugar estimations should be carried out frequently in cerebral malaria (Migasena 1983). Pregnant women are at a special risk of developing hypoglycemia (Looareesuwan et al 1985).

Fluid and electrolyte imbalances are common in severe *P. falciparum* malaria. Patients are often hypovolemic due to high fever, sweating, vomiting and diarrhoea. Mild hyponatremia is common but severe hyponatremia with hypoosmolarity is rare (WHO 1986).

Renal failure due to *P. falciparum* malaria is often transient. In most patients, renal function will improve with treatment using antimalarial drugs and fluid replacement, but acute tubular necrosis may develop (Phillips & Warrell 1986, White 1986). Severe malaria with pigmented urine has been called 'blackwater fever' and is due to intravascular hemolysis and hemoglobinuria. It is more frequent in patients with glucose 6-phosphate dehydrogenase deficiency (Phillips & Warrell 1986).

Impaired liver function is common in malaria, but hepatocyte destruction and frank liver failure are rare (Phillips & Warrell 1986, White 1986). Hepatomegaly and jaundice may be associated with anemia and renal failure resulting in a high mortality (White 1986).

The prevalence of seizures in patients with *P. falciparum* malaria ranges from 11–49% in the different series published, with a mean of 22.3% (Table 7.10). Reports indicate seizures to be generalized tonic-clonic. There is no evidence of a partial component except in the context of a syndrome of late complications in survivors of cerebral malaria mentioned briefly in the German literature (Lyon 1966, Rothenberg

**Table 7.10** Source, date of publication, number of patients and prevalence of seizures in studies of *P. falciparum* malaria

| Source | No of patients | Prevalence |
|---|---|---|
| Daroff et al (1967) | 19 | 11% |
| Hendrickse et al (1971)[a] | 500 | 45% |
| Betancur et al (1974) | 30 | 23% |
| Toro et al (1976) | 19 | 21% |
| Warrell et al (1982) | 100 | 41% |
| White et al (1983) | 153 | 49% |
| Total | 921 | 22% (mean) |

[a] Quoted in WHO (1986) from pediatric population.

& Schubert 1983). Even African publications do not offer more information on this subject (Osuntokum 1983).

There is a special link between malaria and seizures, especially febrile convulsions, a combination which may lead to some 5% of pediatric emergency consultations in endemic areas (Espinal & Toro 1986, Toro et al 1983a). Seizures are generalized without focal features. They may be followed by coma, and if the latter persists for more than 6 hours, cerebral involvement should be diagnosed (WHO 1986). An idea of the impact of malaria on the etiological spectrum of epilepsy in Africa is given by the report of a pioneer pediatric neurology clinic in Kampala (Edgell & Stanfield 1972). The commonest problems were mental retardation and epilepsy. Of 138 children evaluated at the clinic 86 (63%) had had normal birth and post-natal onset of neurological insult, frequently with seizures. In 38 cases, the onset of neurological disability was sudden, and in 27 a febrile illness with seizures preceded the more severe neurological picture. Edgell & Stanfield (1972) consider cerebral malaria, bacterial meningitis or febrile encephalopathy of unknown etiology the commonest underlying causes of seizures with fever.

Senga et al (1985) found that 9.6% of all children aged 1 month–6 years, admitted to Brazzaville General Hospital (Congo) between 1981–1983, presented with seizures. Of the 525 children evaluated 84% had tonic-clonic, 13% had tonic and 3.5% had atonic seizures. Lateralized or focal seizures were found in only 3.4%. Status epilepticus occurred in 13.6% of the cases, and 67% of these were related to benign malaria. Febrile seizures occurred in 73.5% of all cases, and 81% of them were related to malaria, almost always benign (89%). Most cerebral malaria patients were aged 1–3 years and presented with status epilepticus. Cerebral involvement was diagnosed in 10% of all malaria patients (Senga et al 1985). These numbers may speak by themselves: approximately 60% of all seizure disorders between 1 month and 6 years of age in a large general hospital were related to benign or malignant forms of malaria, and seizures were the reason for admission in 10% of all children in that age group.

**Pathophysiology**

Brain edema secondary to increased permeability of the blood-brain barrier and subsequent compression of small vessels have been considered key elements in malaria encephalopathy (Jerusalem et al 1984). Other investigators have argued that data obtained from primate experiments using severe *P. knowlesi* infections do not resemble human disease (White 1986). Phillips & Warrell (1986) reported that the majority of their human cases had normal CSF pressure and that pressures were lower in fatal cases.

Toro et al (1976) demonstrated pathologically that there is a disseminated vasculomyelinopathy secondary to a vasculopathy caused by a hyperergic reaction of the CNS to antigens of *P. falciparum*. Alteration of the endothelium is followed by brain edema, perivascular infiltrates, hemorrhages and perivascular demyelination (Fig. 7.10).

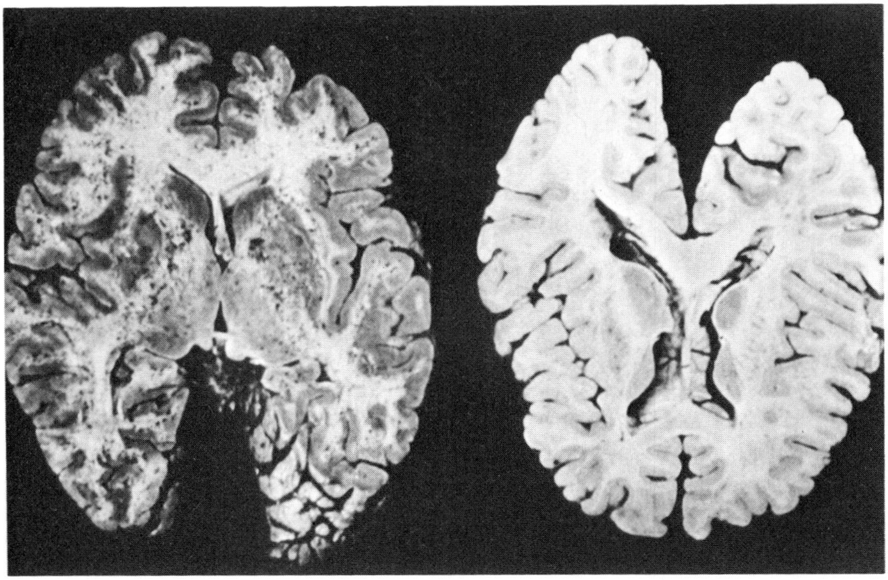

**Fig. 7.10** Cerebral malaria: diffuse petechial haemorrhages in the white matter (left) in sharp contrast with a normal brain (right). (Courtesy of Professer Gabriel Toro, Universidad Nacional de Colombia, Bogotá.)

The thrombocytopenia noted to occur in malaria (Neva et al 1970) has been attributed to disseminated intravascular coagulation, but examination of experimental animal and human brains has not shown the widespread fibrin deposition or microvascular thrombosis characteristic of this condition. Furthermore, coagulation studies in *P. falciparum* malaria have failed to show unequivocal evidence of intravascular coagulation (Neva et al 1970, Phillips & Warrell 1986, White 1986, WHO 1986). Permanent neurological sequelae are rare in patients surviving cerebral malaria (Espinal & Toro 1986, Toro et al 1983a, Phillips & Warrell 1986) which make it 'difficult to reconcile a theory of widespread cerebrovascular thrombosis as the cause of malaria with the dramatic recovery which occurs in survivors' (Phillips & Warrell 1986).

Sequestration of erythrocytes containing mature forms of the parasite in deep vascular territories of the brain, explains why encephalopathy is such a prominent feature of severe malaria (Winslow et al 1971). Selective adhesion of red cells containing mature forms of the parasite accounts for the pathological observation of sequestration (White 1986). Electron microscopy of parasitized red blood cells shows protrusions or 'knobs' which contain specific parasite antigens and bind to protein receptors in the vascular endothelium. This suggests that strain specific antibodies might be used to reverse cytoadherence in a clinically useful manner (Phillips & Warrell 1986).

The vigorous general immune response observed about a week after parasites are detected in the peripheral blood (Neva et al 1970) may be delayed until after parasite multiplication to lethal numbers in *P. falciparum* disease. The virulence of *P. falciparum* is also related to hepatic schizonts releasing approximately 30 000 merozoites, twice the number released in more benign malarias. Furthermore, the hepatic phase of development is shorter, and *P. falciparum* invades erythrocytes of all ages which offer greater growth potential. *P. vivax* and *P. ovale* prefer young cells (White 1986).

**Diagnosis**

Proof of malarial infection is provided by finding parasites in routine blood films by examination with an oil immersion lens. Broad-spectrum antibiotics and insufficient doses of antimalarial drugs may eliminate parasites from the peripheral blood but do not cure the infection (Gilles 1981). The degree of parasitemia correlates with the severity of infection and is a useful measure of the response to treatment. When rapid examination of blood films is impossible, or parasites are not found but there is clinical evidence of malaria, treatment should be started. Delay in diagnosis is usually related to low diagnostic threshold of suspicion when history of travel to endemic zones is not obtained. Gram-negative septicemia has been associated with severe malaria (Phillips & Warrell 1986, White 1986). Other infections such as viral or bacterial meningoencephalitis must be excluded (Toro & Vergara 1978).

**Prognosis**

Reports of mortality in cerebral malaria have varied from almost none to over 50%, with a mean of 34% (Toro et al 1983a). Prognostic factors include the patient's immune status related to previous exposure to plasmodia and to the presence of factors producing immunodepression, pregnancy, the velocity of onset of the neurological picture, degree of parasitemia, and delay in initiating appropriate medical therapy. It has been calculated that 50% of pregnant women who become unarousable eventually do not survive; there is a corresponding high fetal mortality.

The density of parasitemia correlates with clinical severity (Hall 1976, Neva et al 1970). Parasitemias of up to 25 000 per $mm^3$ resulted in a mortality of 0.2%. Parasite counts of 100 000 to 500 000 per $mm^3$ were associated with mortality rates up to 15%. Counts above $10^6/mm^3$ correlated with a mortality of greater than 70% (Neva et al 1970).

**Management**

The treatment of uncomplicated malaria has been reviewed elsewhere (Bruce-Chwatt 1981, Espinal 1982, Medical Letter 1986). Patients suffering from cerebral malaria are as a rule critically ill, and most deaths occur in the first 48 hours following admission to hospital (Warrell et al 1982). Such patients should be cared for in intensive care units where rapid decision making may improve prognosis (Neva et al 1970, WHO 1986).

Resistance of *P. falciparum* to chloroquine is a growing problem (Peters 1982). It has been documented in Asia since 1980, and recent reports indicate resistance in Asia, Latin America and Africa (Table 7.11) (Bruce-Chwatt 1981, Botero & Restrepo 1984a, CDC 1985, Éspinal et al 1985, Peters 1982, Restrepo et al 1980).

Parasiticidal concentrations of effective antimalarial drugs should be achieved

**Table 7.11** Countries in which Chloroquine-resistant *Plasmodium falciparum* have been reported. (Adapted from Centers for Disease Control 1985.)

| Africa | Asia and Oceania | South America |
|---|---|---|
| Angola | Burma | Bolivia |
| Burundi | China (southern parts) | Brazil |
| Central African Republic | Indonesia | Colombia |
| Cameroun | Kampuchea | Ecuador |
| Gabon | Laos | French Guiana |
| Kenya | Malaysia | Guyana |
| Madagascar | Philippines | Panama |
| Malawi | Thailand | Peru |
| Mozambique | Vietnam | Surinam |
| Namibia | Papua New Guinea | Venezuela |
| Rwanda | Solomon Islands | |
| Sudan | Vanuatu | |
| Tanzania | Bangladesh | |
| Uganda | India | |
| Zaire | Pakistan | |
| Zambia | | |

quickly. Quinine is rapidly acting and the only available parenteral treatment for severe chloroquine-resistant falciparum malaria (Hall 1976, White et al 1983a). The drug should not be given by intramuscular or subcutaneous injection because of tissue necrosis (Toro et al 1983a). An initial loading dose of quinine reduces parasitemia more rapidly (White et al 1983a, Espinal & Toro 1986). Quinine dihydrochloride (or gluconate) should be diluted in saline or dextrose solutions and infused intravenously over 4 hours. The loading-dose is 20 mg/kg and the 8-hourly maintenance dose is 10 mg/kg. As soon as possible, oral dosing should substitute the parenteral route, until the 7-day course is completed. The daily dose is 20–25 mg/kg and should not exceed 1800 mg (Espinal & Toro 1986, Medical Letter 1986, Toro et al 1983a, White et al 1983a).

When chloroquine is indicated, the loading-dose is 10–15 mg/kg infused over 4 hours, followed by two 6-hourly and four 12-hourly doses of 5 mg/kg (chloroquine phosphate, base). Total dose is 25–50 mg/kg base. The conversion of base to salt is made on 3:5 ratio (Espinal & Toro 1986, Medical Letter 1986, WHO 1986).

Concomitant administration of pyrimethamine, sulfadizine, tetracycline, doxycycline, clyndamicin, minocycline or sulphadoxine lower the rate of recurrence (Medical Letter 1986, WHO 1986).

Antimalarial drugs as a whole are safe, and side effects are infrequent (Gilles 1981). Cinchonism is a symptom complex noted during treatment with quinine and characterised by headache, nausea, tinnitus, vertigo and blurred vision. It is usually transient and does not warrant withholding therapy (Espinal & Toro 1986). High concentrations of quinine in the blood stream (above 250 μg/ml) may lead to hypotension, myocardial conduction deficits, deafness, blindness and depression of consciousness. These complications are best avoided by slow continuous intravenous infusion especially when the volume of distribution is decreased by fever, sweating, vomiting and diarrhoea (White et al 1983a). Oral administration may lead to abdominal discomfort, vomiting, headache, diarrhoea, blurred vision and pruritus (Bruce-Chwatt 1981, Gilles 1981). Dyskinesias and hearing loss are rare (WHO 1986). Sudden collapse and death after intramuscular injection in children is thought to be related to irregular sudden absorption from the chloroquine injection site (Bruce-Chwatt 1981, WHO 1986). As parenteral use is necessary only in severe malaria, intravenous infusion in saline or dextrose is preferable to intramuscular injection.

Chloroquine-induced retinopathy, ototoxicity and myopathy have been reported with chronic exposure to weekly doses of 600–900 mg taken for 1 year.

Although seizures occur frequently in malaria and are typically of a generalized tonic-clonic nature, specific therapeutic regimens have not been proposed. Status epilepticus may occur and appropriate treatment should be available (Delgado-Escueta et al 1982, Simon 1985). For emergency situations carbamazepine given by nasogastric tube is useful if gastric stasis is not suspected. In critically ill adults 600 mg given in this manner will produce effective serum concentration in 2–4 hours (Leite et al in press).

Hyperthermia leads to seizures and mental changes and should be treated promptly. Hypoglycemia is so frequent, easy to treat and at the same time difficult to recognize clinically in severely ill patients that it should be suspected as contributing to any neurological deterioration. Regular determinations of blood glucose are indicated (WHO 1986).

Dexamethasone and other steroids were in the past strongly recommended for cerebral malaria (Neva et al 1970, Toro & Vergara 1978). It is now recognized that there is no definite pathophysiological basis for their utilization, and indeed prognosis was worse in the steroid-treated group of a double-blind controlled trial (Espinal & Toro 1986, Warrell et al 1982). Heparin is contraindicated (WHO 1986).

## TOXOPLASMOSIS

### Epidemiology and microbiology

*Toxoplasma gondii* is an intracellular parasite of domestic and wild animals distributed world-wide (Table 7.12, Krich & Remington 1978). Humans are infected by ingestion of undercooked meat contaminated with cysts or by food contaminated with oocysts

**Table 7.12** Prevalence of antitoxoplasma antibodies (1 : 16, dye test) in children and adults. (Taken from: a, Apt 1984; b, Desmonts & Courvreur 1974c; Julião et al 1983.)

| Country or city of origin | % positive, age 6 months–10 years | % positive, age 30–40 years |
|---|---|---|
| Austria (a) | 7 | 62 |
| El Salvador(a) | 40 | 93 |
| Finland (a) | 8 | 45 |
| England and Wales (a) | 8 | 25 |
| Paris (b) | 33 | 87 |
| Trinidad (a) | 29 | 45 |
| Colombia (c) | 32 | 54 |
| Arizona (Navajo Indians, USA (a)) | 0 | 5 |
| New Orleans, USA (a) | 21 | 42 |
| Pittsburg, USA (a) | 8 | 45 |
| Portland, Oregon, USA (a) | 7 | 26 |
| South California, USA (a) | 10 | 27 |

from cat feces. Transplacental transmission, blood transfusion and organ transplantation are other documented routes of infection (Frenkel 1971, Saravia 1986, Toro et al 1983b).

**Congenital toxoplasmosis**

Approximately one third of fetuses become infected during acute infection of seronegative pregnant women, but only 10% develop severe clinical disease. The remainder have either mild disease or infection is subclinical at birth (Desmonts & Couvreur 1974). Severity of involvement depends on the time of intrauterine infection. Disease is more severe if acquired in the first two trimesters. Subclinical cases should be followed and probably treated since ocular lesions may not become clinically apparent until months or even years after birth (Desmonts & Couvreur 1974, Saravia 1986). In severe congenital toxoplasmosis, chorioretinitis is found in 75–86% of cases (Toro et al 1983b, Saravia 1986), hydrocephalus with aqueduct stenosis and cerebral calcifications in 60%, and mental retardation with seizures and cerebral palsy or blindness in 80–90% (Stern et al 1969). Some 40–60% of these patients have seizures (Feldman 1958). It has been calculated that 2–3% of all mental deficiencies are related to congenital rubella or toxoplasmosis (Stern et al 1969).

The prevalence of congenital toxoplasmosis aetiologically related to specific seizure syndromes is not clear. Dennis (1978) found no cases of toxoplasmosis in 50 babies with neonatal convulsions. Only one case was found by Riikonen & Donner (1979) and Riikonen (1978) in 312 cases of infantile spasms in Finland. Aicardi & Chevrie (1978) reviewed the literature on infantile spasms and concluded that toxoplasmosis was a possible etiology in a small but indeterminate number of patients. Grossi-Bianchi & Pistone (1968) described a case of 'hypsarrythmic syndrome' reversible with treatment of congenital toxoplasmosis. Gastaut & Gastaut (1976) did not find toxoplasmosis in 500 patients with epilepsy examined by CT, including six with West's syndrome and 42 with Lennox–Gastaut syndrome. Chevrie & Aicardi (1972) found one case of congenital toxoplasmosis in 80 cases of the Lennox–Gastaut syndrome.

In children born with subclinical toxoplasmosis neurological complications are as frequent as in those with overt disease, but they are less severe. Epilepsy occurred in 4 of 25 such cases (Wilson et al 1980).

**Acquired toxoplasmosis**

In the otherwise healthy host acquired toxoplasmosis is asymptomatic or a mild febrile illness resembling mononucleosis with malaise and lymphadenopathy (Krich & Remington 1978), peripheral atypical lymphocytosis and spontaneous resolution within a few months (Frenkel 1971, Frenkel 1978). Rarely encephalitis, myocarditis or pneumonitis may occur (Krich & Remington 1978, Toro et al 1983b). Chorioretinitis may be an isolated manifestation of acquired infection, or occur as a late sequela of congenital infection.

Ruskin & Remington (1976) reported 81 cases of acquired toxoplasmosis in patients with decreased immunity. More than 50% had diffuse encephalopathy, meningoencephalitis or cerebral mass lesions. CNS toxoplasmosis is common in patients with AIDS. Cytomegalovirus (CMV), herpes, *Cryptococus neoformans*, atypical mycobacteria or other infections may occur concomitantly (Luft et al 1984). The multiplicity of infections and the high prevalence of retrovirus related AIDS-dementia complex often makes it difficult to identify signs and symptoms related to each pathological process, but seizures occurred at presentation in 4 of 24 patients with toxoplasmosis (Navia et al 1986a, b).

**Diagnosis**

Diagnosis may be confirmed by serological tests, isolation of the parasite, or biopsy. Progressive rise of antibody titers over a 2-week interval indicates acute infection. IgM antibodies appear in the first week of infection and usually peak within a month, returning to negative after 3 months. Negative tests rule out recent but not longer-standing infection. IgM antibodies may be detected by the indirect fluorescent antibody test or by the dye test, by indirect hemagglutination and complement fixation tests. Titers of 1:1000 or higher are considered positive but occur in many asymptomatic patients. Documentation of a rise in titer is more diagnostic (Krich & Remington, 1978). In immunocompromised hosts, antibody titers fail to rise (Levy et al 1985, Ruskin & Remington 1976, Snider et al 1983) and biopsy may be the only means of confirming the diagnosis (Bia & Barry 1986, Snider et al 1983). In selected patients, a 2-week trial of antibiotics may be an alternative to immediate cerebral biopsy (Navia et al 1986b). The CSF may show moderate elevation of protein, mononuclear pleocytosis and normal or slightly reduced sugar, or it may be normal CT scan shows single or multiple lesions, mainly of subcortical structures with enhancing margins in 50% of cases (Bia & Barry 1986, Horowitz et al 1983, Snider et al 1983, Navia et al 1986a, b). MRI may be more sensitive, but also less specific in AIDS patients.

**Management and prognosis**

Treatment of CNS toxoplasmosis using pyrimethamine and sulphadizine aims at stopping proliferation until natural immunity develops (Frenkel 1971). In the immune-compromised host, continued administration may be required even weeks after the lesions have resolved on CT. Relapse has been observed in 30% of cases (Bia & Barry 1986). Of 22 AIDS patients treated by Navia et al (1986b), 18 responded well to anti-toxoplasma therapy, but 14 died within 1 year from intercurrent medical problems including status epilepticus. Of the other four patients, three were on long-term maintenance therapy. Treatment may result in improvement in 80% of immune-compromised hosts (Ruskin & Remington 1976). Pregnant women are treated with spiramycin or clindamycin due to the teratogenic effects of pyrimethamine (Frenkel 1978, Toro et al 1983b). Treatment of toxoplasmosis acquired at any time during pregnancy decreases the chance of congenital infection (Krich & Remington 1978).

Drug regimens include pyrimethamine 75 mg daily in the first 3 days followed by 25 mg daily in adults and sulphadiazine 2000 mg daily throughout the period. In children the daily dose of pyrimethamine is 2 mg/kg in the first 3 days followed by 1 mg/kg, while the dose of sulphadiazine is 100 mg/kg. Folinic acid and yeast are given to counteract bone marrow suppression due to pyrimethamine.

Preventive measures are directed towards pregnant women, children and immuno-compromised patients. Cat transmission of the disease may be much improved by elimination of wild cats and by feeding well cooked meat to domestic cats (Frenkel 1971). Pregnant women should avoid cat contact, and manipulation of raw meat should be followed by hand washing. Seropositive individuals should not donate blood or organs for transplant (Saravia 1986).

## OTHER PARASITOSES OF THE CNS

Primary amebic encephalitis (PAM) is a rapidly fatal disease caused by several amebo-flagellates, *Naegleria fowleri* being the most common in the more than 60 published cases (Bia & Barry 1986, Botero & Restrepo 1984b, Duma et al 1971, Duque 1978). These free-living amebas are found in the soil, in decaying vegetable material and in lakes or pools (Duma et al 1971, Duque 1978). Clinically, sudden severe frontal headache is followed by fever, anorexia, nausea and vomiting in previously healthy children or young adults with a recent history of swimming in pools or lakes. Meningeal signs develop very rapidly and seizures, coma and death may take place within 72 hours (Bia & Barry 1986). CSF shows pleocytosis of up to 20 000 per $mm^3$, and trophozoites may be seen in wet-mount preparations. One case of chronic meningoencephalitis due to hartmannella has been published (Cleland et al 1982). Epidemiological and CSF data are critical clues to diagnosis as the disease is otherwise undistinguishable from acute pyogenic or other forms of meningoencephalitis (Toro et al 1983c). The free-living amebas penetrate the nasal mucosa, cribriform plate, olfactory bulb and nerves to more posterior regions of the brain, leading to hemorrhagic and purulent basal meningitis with swollen cerebral hemispheres and superficial hemorrhagic necrosis. Amebas may be seen microscopically around small blood vessels or adjacent to necrotic areas (Bia & Barry 1986, Duma et al 1971). Treatment is unsatisfactory, and the majority of published cases come from autopsy material. Intravenous (1 mg/kg/day) and intrathecal (0.1 mg/kg in alternate days) amphotericin B is the standard treatment. Tetracycline, rifampicin and miconazole are known to act synergistically (Bia & Barry 1986, Botero & Restrepo 1984b). The source of infection should be reported to authorities. Host/parasite relationships are not fully understood, but clearly a large number of individuals are exposed whereas only a few develop the disease.

Entamoeba histolytica infection of the CNS is rare (Perez-Tamayo & Brandt 1971). Parasites reach the CNS from the intestine probably by hematogenous dissemination through the lung, followed by embolization to the brain, even in the absence of demonstrable pulmonary lesions (Duque 1978). Lombardo and associates (1964) found 96 published cases with parasite confirmation in 27. They published 17 further cases, 11 of which were confirmed. Cerebral lesions may be single or multiple, varying from a few millimeters to 5 cm in diameter, and from small areas of softening with petechial hemorrhages to large areas of necrosis or true abscesses. Meningeal involvement is indistinguishable from other types of acute purulent meningitis. Most cerebral abscesses are associated with hepatic or lung abscesses (Perez-Tamayo & Brandt 1971). Patients are severely ill with fever, weight loss and malaise. There may or not be a history of intestinal disorder. The diagnosis should be suspected in patients with focal neurological signs, including seizures, occurring on the background of a hepatic or lung abscess (Zuluaga et al 1984). Serum antibodies against *E. histolytica* are useful (Toro et al 1983c). Prognosis is bleak. Only three cases of survival have been published (Duque 1978, Toro et al 1983c). Metronidazole and chloroquine are effective in cerebral lesions (Bia & Barry 1986, Toro et al 1983c).

Cerebral involvement is rare in other parasitic diseases. In cerebral angiostrongyloidiasis the picture is of a meningoencephalitis occasionally with cranial nerve involvement (Rosen 1981). Cerebral paragonimiasis is a rare complication of the lung-fluke infection in the Far East, Africa and South America. It may present with subacute onset of meningitis, space-occupying lesions, dementia and seizures; recovery is prompt with early treatment using bithionol. Trichinosis and toxocariasis are also uncommon causes of cerebral disease which could lead to seizures (Bell et al 1982).

In conclusion we present a therapeutic summary of the seven major parasitoses (Table 7.13).

**Table 7.13** Summary of main therapeutic guidelines and prognosis in seven major parasitic diseases of the CNS. Adapted from text

| | Specific therapy | Supportive therapy | Prognosis with therapy |
|---|---|---|---|
| Schistosomiasis | Praziquantel<br>Oxamniquine<br>Metrifonate | Steroids<br>Surgery (spinal) | Arrests progress |
| Hydatid disease | Mebendazole<br>Fluoromebendazole<br>Praziquantel (?) | Surgical excision of cyst | Frequent cyst recurrence |
| Cysticercosis | Praziquantel (multiple regimens) | Steroids<br>Diuretics<br>V-P shunting | 80% remission in 2 years |
| African trypanosomiasis | Suramin sodium and melarprosol | Steroids | Arrests progress |
| American trypanosomiasis | Nifurtimox<br>Benzonidazol | Diuretics and anticoagulants in chronic phase | Good in acute phase |
| Cerebral Malaria | Quinine<br>Chloroquine<br>Antibiotics | Intensive care unit<br>Hypoglycemia | 34% mortality |
| Toxoplasmosis in AIDS | Pyrimethamine +<br>Sulphadiazine | Concurrent infections | Good with maintenance therapy |

V-P, ventriculo-peritoneal.

## ACKNOWLEDGEMENTS

Collecting material and preparing the manuscript was possible only with the assistance and sometimes active contribution of Ms M. Barbara, Ms J. Meister and Dr S. Mazer (Hospital Nossa Senhora das Graças, Curitiba, Brazil), Dr J. Radvany (Hospital Israelita Albert Einstein, São Paulo, Brazil), Dr N. de Franco Júnior (Ciba-Geigy, Brazil), Dr R. Martins (Merck, Brazil), Ms Christine Bylik (Children's Hospital Research Foundation, Cincinnati, USA), Ms M. Lorenzana, Dr C. A. Espinal, Dr I. Vergara, Dr J. Saravia and Professor G. Toro (Universidad Nacional de Colombia, Bogotá).

## REFERENCES

Ahuja G K, Mohanta A 1982 Late onset epilepsy: a prospective study. Acta Neurologica Scandinavica 66: 216–226

Aicardi J, Chevrie J J 1978 Les spasmes infantiles. Archives Françaises de Pediatrie 35: 1015–1023

Alves W 1958 The distribution of schistosoma eggs in human tissues. Bulletin of the World Health Organization 18: 1092–1097

Apt W 1984 Epidemiologia de la toxoplasmosis. In: Guhl F, Marinkelle C J, Rodriguez N (eds) Simpósio Interamericano de Toxoplasmosis. Editora Guadalupe. Bogotá, p 37–46

Arseni C, Cristescu A 1972 Epilepsy due to cerebral cysticercosis. Epilepsia 13: 253–258

Arseni C, Marinescu V 1974 Epilepsy in cerebral hydatidosis. Epilepsia 15: 45–54

Barrett-Connor E 1981 African sleeping sickness. In: Braude A I, Davis C E, Fierer J (eds) Medical microbiology and infectious diseases. Saunders, Philadelphia, p 1287–1292
Bell W E, Chun R W M, Jabbour J T, Meloff K L 1982 Infections of the brain and spinal cord. In: Swaiman K F, Wright F S (eds) The practice of pediatric neurology, vol 2. Mosby, St Louis, p 9–80
Betancur S, Ricaurte M E, Ramírez R 1974 Malaria cerebral. Antioquia Médica 24: 27–34
Bia J F, Barry M 1986 Parasitic infections of the central nervous system. In: Boos J, Thornton G (eds) Infectious diseases of the central nervous system. Neurologic Clinics 4: 171–207
Bittencourt P R M Epilepsy in developing countries: Latin America. In: Laidlaw J, Richens A, Oxley J (eds) Textbook of epilepsy, 3rd edn, Churchill Livingstone, Edinburgh 1988
Bittencourt P R M, Oliveira T V, Mazer S 1985 Praziquantel for neurocysticercosis. Journal of Neurology 232 (S): 217
Bittencourt P R M, Gorz A M, Oliveira T V, Mazer S 1986a Neurocisticercosis: conceptos básicos de clínica, diagnóstico y tratamiento. Parte I Acta Neurologica (Colombia) 2: 11–15
Bittencourt P R M, Gorz A M, Oliveira T V, Mazer S 1986b Neurocisticercosis: conceptos básicos de clínica, diagnóstico y tratamiento. Parte II Acta Neurologica (Colombia) 2: 11–14
Blacklock D B, McArthur W P 1934 Cysticercosis as seen in the British Army, with special reference to the production of epilepsy. Transactions of the Royal Society of Tropical Medicine and Hygiene 27: 343–363
Botero D, Castaño S 1982 Treatment of cysticercosis with praziquantel in Colombia. American Journal of Tropical Medicine and Hygiene 31: 810–821
Botero D, Restrepo M 1984a Malária. In: Botero D, Restrepo M (eds) Parasitosis humanas. Ediciones Corporación para Investigaciones Biológicas. Medellín, p 199–236
Botero D, Restrepo M 1984b Meningoencefalitis amebiana primária. In: Botero D, Restrepo M (eds) Parasitosis humanas. Ediciones Corporación para Investigaciones Biológicas. Medellín, p 50–52
Bruce-Chwatt L J 1981 Chemotherapy of malaria. 2nd edn. World Health Organization, Geneva, p 120–140
Campos G B, Perpétuo F O L 1983 Neurocisticercosis. In: Neves J (ed) Diagnóstico e tratamento das doenças infectuosas e parasitárias 2nd edn. Guanabara-Koogan, Rio de Janeiro, p 959–965
Canelas M H 1963 Neurocysticercosis its incidence, diagnosis and clinical forms. In: Van Bogaert L, Pareyrakfer J, Poch J F (eds) Tropical neurology. Buenos Aires, Tropical Neurology Libreros Editores
Centers for Disease Control 1985 Revised recommendations for preventing malaria in travelers to areas with chloroquine-resistance. Plasmodium falciparum MMWR 34: 185–190
Cerisola J A, Alvarez M, Lugones H, Rebosolán J 1969 Sensibilidad de las reacciones serológicas para el diagnóstico de la enfermedad de Chagas. Boletin Chileno de Parasitologia 24: 2–8
Chevrie J J, Aicardi J 1972 Childhood epileptic encephalopathy with the slow spike-wave. A statistical study of 80 cases. Epilepsia 13: 259–271
Cleland P G, Lawande R V, Onyemelukwe G, Whittle H C 1982 Chronic amebic meningoencephalitis. Archives of Neurology 39: 56–57
Commission on Classification and Terminology of the International League Against Epilepsy 1985 Proposal for classification of epilepsies and epileptic syndromes. Epilepsia 26: 268–278
Costa J M, Mineo R, Livramento J A, Camargo M E 1985 Detecção pelo teste imunoenzimático ELISA de anticorpos IgM anti-cysticercus cellulosae no líquido cefalorraqueano na neurocisticercose. Arquivos de Neuro-Psiquiatria 43: 22–28
Daroff R B, Deller J J, Kastl A J, Blocker W 1967 Cerebral malaria. Journal of the American Medical Association 202: 679–682
De Guetaldi L D, Norman R M, Douville A W 1983 Cerebral cysticercosis treated biphasically with dexamethazone and praziquantel. Annals of Internal Medicine 99: 179–181
Delgado-Escueta A V, Wasterlain C G, Treiman D M, Porter R J 1982 Management of status epilepticus. New England Journal of Medicine 306: 1337–1340
Dennert G 1981 Schistosomiasis. In: Braude A I, Davis C E, Fierer J (eds) Medical microbiology and infectious diseases. Saunders, Philadelphia, p 1093–1105
Dennis J 1978 Neonatal convulsions: aetiology, late neonatal status and long-term outcome. Developmental Medicine and Child Neurology 20: 143–158
De Pasquet E G, Pietra M, Gaudin E S 1972 Etiología de la epilepsia tardía. Acta Neurologica Latinoamericana 18: 256–275
De Pasquet E G, Pietra M, Bonnevaux S, Silva N P, Gomensoro J B, Tenzer M 1976 Estudio epidemiológico de 500 epilépticos adultos procedentes de una población hospitalaria. Acta Neurologica Latinoamericana 22: 50–65
Desmonts G, Couvreur J 1974 Congenital toxoplasmosis: a prospective study of 378 pregnancies. New England Journal of Medicine 290: 1110–1116
Dias J C P, Cançado J R, Chiari C A 1983 Doença de Chagas. In: Neves J (ed) Diagnóstico e tratamento das doenças infectuosas e parasitárias. 2nd edn. Guanabara-Koogan, Rio de Janeiro, p 694–725

Diwan A R, Coker-Vann M, Brown D et al 1982 Enzyme-linked immunosorbent assay (ELISA) for the detection of antibody to cysticerci of taenia solium. American Journal of Tropical Medicine and Hygiene 31: 364–369
Duma R J, Rosemblum W I, McGehee R F, Jones M, Nelson E C 1971 Primary amoebic meningoencephalitis caused by naegleria: two new cases. Response to amphotericin B and a review. Annals of Internal Medicine 74: 861–869
Dumas M, Breton J C, Alexandre M P, Girard P L, Giordano C 1985 Etat actuel de la thérapeutique de la trypanosomiase humaine africaine. La Presse Médicale 14: 253–256
Duque O 1978 Meningoencephalitis amebiana. In: Toro G, Vergara I, Saravia J, Poser C M (eds) Infecciones del sistema nervioso central. Fondo Educativo Interamericano, p 332–339
Egdell H G, Stanfield J P 1972 Paediatric neurology in Africa: Ugandan report. British Medical Journal 1(789): 548–552
Escobar A 1983 The pathology of neurocysticercosis. In: Palacios E, Rodriguez-Carbajal J, Taveras J M (eds) Cysticercosis of central nervous system. Thomas, Springfield, p 27–54
Espinal C A 1982 Drogas antimaláricas. Série de notas técnicas nº. 7 Instituto Nacional de Salud. Bogotá
Espinal C A, Toro G 1986 Malaria. In: Chalem F, Escandon J E, Campos J, Esguerra R (eds) Medicina Interna. Editorial Norma, Bogotá, p 278–288
Espinal C A, Lopez C E 1987 La medicina tropical: un reto para la salud pública y la práctica privada. Acta Médica Colombiana 2: 65–84
Espinal C A, Cortes G T, Gerra P, Arias A E 1985 Sensitivity of Plasmodium falciparum to antimalarial drugs in Colombia. American Journal of Tropical Medicine and Hygiene 34: 675–680
Fabiani A, Trebini F, Torta R 1980 Brain hydatidosis: report of two cases. Journal of Neurology, Neurosurgery and Psychiatry 43: 91–94
Facure N O, Facure J J, Nicci A 1978 Aspecto tumoral da cisticercose intracraniana. Abordagem cirurgica. Arquivos de Neuro-Psiquiatria 36: 200–209
Faria M A M, Goldbaum M, Castilho E, Barros e Silva E 1976a Prevalência de manifestações clínicas e eletrocardiográficas em pacientes chagásicos epilépticos. Arquivos Brasileiros de Cardiologia 29: 303–307
Faria M A M, Assis L M, Silva G R, Camargo M E 1976b Infecção chagásica crônica e síndromes epilépticas. Revista do Instituto de Medicina Tropical de São Paulo 18: 173–181
Feldman H A 1958 Toxoplasmosis, review article. Pediatrics 22: 559–574
Ferreira F S C, Rocha L A C 1982 Tripanossomíase africana. In: Veronesi R (ed) Doenças infecciosas e parasitárias 7th edn. Guanbara-Koogan, Rio de Janeiro, p 713–723
Fishman R A 1980 Cerebrospinal fluid in diseases of the nervous system. Saunders, Philadelphia, p 384
Frenkel J K 1971 Toxoplasmosis. In: Marcial Rojas R A (ed) Pathology of protozoal and helmintic disease. Williams and Wilkins, Baltimore, p 254–290
Frenkel J K 1978 Toxoplasmosis. In: Toro G, Vergara I, Saravia J, Poser C M (eds) Infecciones del sistema nervioso central. Fondo Educativo Interamericano, Bogotá, p 284–301
Gabaldon A 1968 Duration of attack measures in a malaria eradication program. American Journal of Tropical Medicine and Hygiene 17: 1–12
Gastaut H, Gastaut J L 1976 Computerized transverse axial tomography in epilepsy. Epilepsia 17: 325–336
Gelfand M 1948 Cysticercosis of the brain in the African of Rhodesia. East African Medical Journal 25: 110–112
Gelfand M 1973 Neurologic complication of parasitic disease. In: Spillane J D (ed) Tropical neurology. Oxford University Press, London, p 247–258
Gilles H M 1981 Malaria. Medicine 1: 153–155
Girardelli M A 1969a Electroencefalografía y enfermedad de Chagas crónica. Boltein Chileno de Parasitologia 24: 32–35
Girardelli M A 1969b Evolución electroencefalográfica en niños y adultos jóvenes con infección chagásica crónica tratados con BAY 2502. Boletin Chileno de Parasitologia 24: 35–38
Grisolia J S, Wiederholt W C 1982 CNS cysticercosis. Archives of Neurology 39: 540–544
Groll E 1981 Cisticercosis humana y praziquantel: una apreciación panorámica de las primeras experiencias clínicas. Boletin Chileno de Parasitologia 36: 29–37
Grossi-Bianchi M L, Pistone F M 1968 Hypsarrythmia syndrome caused by congenital toxoplasmosis cured by pyrimethamine. Minerva Pediatrica 20: 2345–2347
Hall A P 1976 The treatment of severe falciparum malaria. Transactions of the Royal Society of Tropical Medicine and Hygiene 71: 367–369
Horowitz S L, Bentson J R, Benson F, Davos I, Pressman B, Gottlieb M S 1983 CNS toxoplasmosis in acquired immuno-deficiency syndrome. Archives of Neurology 40: 649–652
Jardim E, Takayanagui O M 1981 Epilepsia e doença de Chagas crônica. Arquivos de Neuro-Psiquiatria 39: 32–41

Jerusalem C, Polder T, Kubat K, Wijers-Rouw M, Trinh P 1984 Brain edema in cerebral malaria: a comparative clinical and experimental intrastructural and histochemical study. In: Gok G., Baethmann A J (eds) Recent progress in the study and therapy of brain edema. Plenum Press, New York, p 127–135
Julião O, Corredor A, Moreno G S 1983 Toxoplasmosis en Colombia. Estudio Nacional de Salud. Ministério de Salud. Instituto Nacional de Salud. Associación Colombiana de Facultades de Medicina, Bogotá.
Krich J A, Remington J S 1978 Toxoplasmosis in adult. An overview. New England Journal of Medicine 298: 550–553
Lange O 1940 Síndrome liquórica da cisticercose encefalo-meningéia. Revista de Neurologia e Psiquiatria 6: 35–41
Lingam S, Marshall W C, Wilson J, Gould J M, Reinhardt M C, Evans D A 1985 Congenital trypanosomiasis in a child born in London. Developmental Medicine and Child Neurology 27: 670–674
Leite J P M, Tsanacus L M, Markourakis T, Bittencourt P R M 1987 Doses-carga de carbamazepina e definil-hidantoína: utilização em pacientes de alto risco. Arquivos de Neuro-Psiquiatria 45: 281–287
Levy L F, Baldachin B J, Clain D 1975 Intracranial bilharzia. Central African Journal of Medicine 21: 76–84
Levy R M, Bredesen D E, Rosemblum M L 1985 Neurological manifestations of the acquired immunodeficiency syndrome (AIDS): experience at VCSF and review of the literature. Journal of Neurosurgery 62: 475–495
Livramento J A, Costa J M, Machado L R, Nóbrega J P S, Spina-França A 1985 ELISA (IgG e IgM) no LCR e soro na neurocisticercose em tratamento com praziquantel. Comparação com Reações de Fixação do Complemento e Imunofluorescência 43: 267–274
Lombardo L, Alonso P, Arroyo L S, Saenz L, Brandt H, Mateos J H 1964 Cerebral amebiasis: report of 17 cases. Journal of Neurosurgery 21: 704–708
Lombardo L, Vasconcelos D, Cruz-Segura H 1983 Tratamiento de la cisticercosis con praziquantel. Informe preliminar de diez casos. Gaceta Medica de Mexico 119: 17–22
Loo L, Braude A 1982 Cerebral cysticercosis in San Diego; a report of 23 cases and review of the literature. Medicine 61: 341–359
Looareesuwan S, Warrell D A, White N J et al 1983 Retinal hemorrhage. A common sign of prognostic significance in cerebral malaria. American Journal of Tropical Medicine and Hygiene 32: 911–915
Looareesuwan S, Phillips R E, White N J et al 1985 Quinine and severe falciparum malaria in late pregnancy. Lancet 11: 4–8
Lópes-Hernandez A, Garaizar C 1982 Childhood cerebral cysticercosis: clinical features and completed tomographic findings in 89 Mexican children. Canadian Journal of Neurological Sciences 9: 401–407
Luft B J, Brooks, R G, Conley F K, McCabe R E, Remington J S 1984 Toxoplasmic encephalitis in patients with acquired immune deficiency syndrome. Journal of the American Medical Association 252: 913–917
Lumsden W H R 1972 Trypanosomiasis. British Medical Bulletin 28: 34–38
Lumsden W H R 1981 Trypanosomiasis. In: Braude A I, Davis C E, Fierer J (eds) Medical microbiology and infectious diseases. Saunders, Philadelphia, 1287–1292
Lyon E 1966 Late damages from malaria. Medizinische Klinik 61: 1579–1582
McGucken R B 1975 Letter: epilepsy in Nigerian children. Developmental Medicine and Child Neurology 17: 119
Manreza M L G 1982 Neurocisticercose na infância: aspectos clínicos e do diagnóstico. Revista Hospitalar Clínica da Faculdade de Medicina de São Paulo 37: 206–211
Marques-Assis L, Ortiz F L 1972 A epilepsia na neurocisticercose. Arquivos de Neuro-Psiquiatria 30: 297–304
Mazer S, Antoniuk A, Ditzel L F S, Araújo J C 1983 The computed tomographic spectrum of cerebral cysticercosis. Computerized Radiology 7: 373–378
Medical Letter 1986 28: 9–18
Memoranda 1984 Immunology of Chagas' disease. Bulletin of the World Health Organization 50: 459–472
Migasena S 1983 Hypoglicemia in falciparum malaria. Annals of Tropical Medicine and Parasitology 77: 323–324
Minguetti G, Ferreira M V C 1983 Computed tomography in neurocysticercosis. Journal of Neurology, Neurosurgery and Psychiatry 46: 936–942
Monteiro de Barros O, Giannoni F G, Marigo C, Frizzo F J 1956 Cor pulmonale e miocardite esquistossomóticos. Considerações clínico-patológicas a propósito de dois casos. Arquivos dos Hospitais da Santa Casa de São Paulo 2: 1–40
Navia B A, Petito C K, Gold J W M, Cho E S, Jordan B D, Price R W 1986a Cerebral toxoplasmosis complicating the acquired immune deficiency syndrome: clinical and neuropathological findings in 27 patients. Annals of Neurology 19: 224–238

Navia B A, Jordan B D, Price R W 1986b The AIDS-Dementia complex: I. clinical features. Annals of Neurology 19: 517–524
Neva F A, Sheagren J N, Shulman R N, Canfield C J 1970 Malaria: host defence mechanisms and complications. Annals of Internal Medicine 73: 295–306
Neves J 1983 Trypanosomiase africana. In: Neves J (ed) Diagnóstico e tratamento das doenças infecciosas e parasitárias 2nd edn. Guanabara-Koogan, Rio de Janeiro, p 725–731
Neves J, Souza D W C 1983 Infecções causadas por tramatódeos sanguíneos. In: Neves J (ed) Diagnóstico e tratamento das doenças infecciosas e parasitárias 2nd edn. Guanabara-Koogan, Rio de Janeiro, p 887–917
Oficina Sanitária Panamericana (Boletin) 1986 Control de la malaria en las Américas. Análises Crítico 101: 522–539
Osuntokum B O 1983 Malaria and the nervous system. African Journal of Medical Sciences 12: 165–172
Pamir M N, Akalan N, Ozgen T, Erbengi A 1984 Spinal hydatid cysts. Surgical Neurology 21: 53–57
Pawlowski Z S 1981 Platyhelminthes. In: Braude A I, Davis C E, Fierer J (eds) Medical microbiology and infectious diseases. Saunders, Philadelphia, p 726–738
Pelley R P, Warren K S, Jordan P 1977 Purified antigen radioimmunoassay in serological diagnosis of schistosomiasis mansoni. Lancet 2: 781–783
Penne P, Mojon M, Garin J P, Coulaud J P, Rossignol J F 1982 Albendazole: a new broad spectrum anthelmintic: double-blind multicenter clinical trial. American Journal of Tropical Medicine and Hygiene 31: 263–266
Perez-Tamayo R, Brandt H 1971 Amebiasis. In: Marcial-Rojas R A (ed) Pathology of protozoal and helmintic diseases. Williams and Wilkins, Baltimore, p 145–181
Peters W 1982 Antimalarial drug resistance: an increasing problem. British Medical Bulletin 38: 187–192
Phillips R E, Warrell D A 1986 The pathophysiology of severe falciparum malaria. Parasitology Today 2: 271–282
Ping Li, Jun L, Xun D S 1985 Praziquantel in treatment and investigation with abdominal hydatidosis. Preliminary report of animal experiments and evaluation of 101 clinical cases. Abstracts, XIII Congresso Internacional de Hidatidologia, p 206
Pitella J E H, Lana-Peixoto M A 1981 Brain involvement in hepatosplenic schistosomiasis mansoni. Brain 104: 621–632
Queiros A C 1973 Tumor-like lesion of brain caused by trypanosoma cruzi. American Journal of Tropical Medicine and Hygiene 22: 473–476
Queiros A C 1974 O envolvimento do sistema nervoso central na esquistossomose mansônica. Revista de Patologia Tropical 3: 255–261
Queiros A C 1978a Estudo das alterações encefálicas em casos humanos agudos da doença de Chagas. Revista de Patologia Tropical 7: 13–22
Queiros A C 1978b Estudo anatomopatológico do encéfalo na forma crônica da doença de Chagas. Revista de Patologia Tropical 7: 135–145
Rabielle-Cervantes M T, Rivas Hernandez A, Rodriguez-Ibarra J, Castillo-Medina S, Cancino F M 1982 Anatomopathological aspects of human brain cysticercosis. In: Flisser A, Willms K, Laclette J P, Larralde C, Ridamra C, Beltran F (eds) Cysticercosis: present state of knowledge and perspectives. Academic Press, New York, p 179–200
Ramirez G 1986 Imunologia de la cisticercosis. Acta Neurológica (Colombia) 2: 7–8
Restrepo A, Alvarez L, Restrepo M 1980 Estudio in vivo de la resistencia del Plasmodium falciparum a la cloroquina en Colombia. Descripción de la resistencia III. Acta Médica Colombiana 5: 367–379
Riikonen R 1978 Cytomegalovirus infection and infantile spasms. Developmental Medicine and Child Neurology 20: 570–579
Riikonen R, Donner M 1979 Incidence and aetiology of infantile spasms from 1969 to 1976: a population study in Finland. Developmental Medicine and Child Neurology 21: 333–343
Rodriguez-Carbajal J, Salgado P, Gutierrez-Alvarado R, Escobar-Izquierdo A, Aruffo C, Palacios E 1983 The acute encephalitic phase of neurocysticercosis: computed tomographic manifestations. American Journal of Neuroradiology 4: 51–55
Rosen L 1981 Cerebral angiostrongyliasis. In: Braude A I, Davis C E, Fierer J (eds) Medical microbiology and infectious diseases. Saunders, Philadelphia, p 1300–1303
Rothenberg G, Schubert S 1982 Assessment of late complications of malaria in travelers to the tropics. Zeitschrift für die Gesamte Innere Medizin 13: 46–47
Ruskin J, Remington J S 1976 Toxoplasmosis in the compromised host. Annals of Internal Medicine 84: 193–199
Saravia J 1986 Toxoplasmosis. In: Chalem F, Escandon J, Campos J, Esguerra R (eds) Medicina Interna. Editorial Norma, Bogotá, p 288–293
Saus A B, Gaudin E S, de Mirabal M P, Iñiguez R A 1973 Hydatid cyst of the brain as an epileptogenic factor. Acta Neurologica Lationo-Americana 19: 78–88

Schantz P M 1984 Echinococcosis (hydatidosis). In: Warren K S, Mahmoud A A F (eds) Tropical and geographical medicine. McGraw-Hill, New York, 487–493
Scrimgeour E M, Gadjusek D C 1985 Involvement of the central nervous system in *Schistosoma mansoni* and *S. haematobium* infection. Brain 108: 1023–1038
Senga P, Mayanda H F, Nzingoula S 1985 Profile of seizures in infants and young children in Brazzaville (Congo). Annales de Pediatrie 32: 477–480
Simanjuntak G M, Margono S S, Sachlan R, Harjono C, Rasidi R, Sutopo B 1977 An investigation of taeniasis and cysticercosis in Bali. Southeast Asian Journal of Tropical Medicine and Public Health 8: 494–497
Simon R P 1985 Management of status epilepticus. In: Pedley T A, Meldrum B S (eds) Recent advances in epilepsy, 2. Churchill Livingstone, Edinburgh, p 137–160
Snider W D, Simpson D M, Nielson S, Gold J W M, Metroka C E, Posner J B 1983 Neurological complications of acquired immune deficiency syndrome: analysis of 50 patients. Annals of Neurology 14: 403–418
Sotelo J, Escobedo F, Rodriguez-Carbajal J, Torres B, Rubio-Donnadieu F 1984 Therapy of parenchymal brain cysticercosis with praziquantel. New England Journal of Medicine 310: 1001–1007
Spina-França Neto A 1961 Síndrome liquórica da neurocisticercose. Arquivos de Neuro-Psiquiatria 19: 287–292
Spina-França A, Nóbrega J P S, Livramento J A, Machado L R 1982 Administration of praziquantel in neurocysticercosis. Tropenmedizin und Parasitologie 33; 1–4
Stern H, Elek S D, Booth J C, Fleck D G 1969 Microbial causes of mental retardation. The role of prenatal infections with cytomegalovirus, rubella virus and toxoplasma. Lancet 2: 443–448
Takayanagui O M, Jardim E 1983 Aspectos clínicos da neurocisticercose. Arquovos de Neuro-Psiquiatria 41: 50–63
Tiberin P, Hellbronn Y D, Hirsch M, Brarmeir E 1984 Giant cerebral echinococcus cyst with galactorrhea and amenorrhea. Surgical Neurology 21: 505–506
Toro G, Vergara I 1978 Malaria cerebral. In: Toro G, Vergara I, Saravia J, Poser C M (eds) Infecciones del sistema nervioso central. Fondo Educativo Interamericano, Bogotá, p 302–315
Toro G, De Onatra S M, Sanin L H 1976 Encefalopatia malarica: una forma de vasculomielinopatia diseminada. Estudio de 19 casos. Acta Médica Colombiana 1: 173–184
Toro G, Roman G, Navarro de Roman L 1983a Paludismo. In: Toro G, Roman G, Navarro de Roman L (eds) Neurología tropical: aspectos neuropatológicos de la medicina tropical. Editorial Printer Colombiana, Bogotá, p 106–113
Toro G, Roman G, Navarro de Roman L 1983b Toxoplasmosis. In: Toro G, Roman G, Navarro de Roman L (eds) Neurología tropical: aspectos neuropatológicos de la medicina tropical. Editorial Printer Colombiana, Bogotá, p 113–117
Toro G, Roman G, Navarro de Ramon L 1983c Amebiasis cerebral. In: Toro G, Roman G, Navarro de Roman L (eds) Neurologia tropical: aspectos neuropatológicos de la medicina tropical. Editorial Prints Colombiana, Bogotá, p 120–122
Torrealba G, Del Villar S, Tagle P, Arriagada P, Kase C S 1984 Cysticercosis of central nervous system: clinical and therapeutic considerations. Journal of Neurology, Neurosurgery and Psychiatry 17: 784–790
Uribe H, Solarte N, Bojanini E, Restrepo A, Zuluaga H 1969 Malaria Hallazgos clínicos. Hematológicos y hepáticos su tratamiento. Antioquia Médica 19: 157–165
Warrell D A, Looareesuwan S, Warrell M J et al 1982 Dexamethazone proves deleterious in cerebral malaria. New England Journal of Medicine 306: 313–319
White N J 1986 Pathophysiology. In: Malaria. Clinics in Tropical Medicine and Communicable Diseases 1: 55–89
White N J, Looareesuwan S, Warrell D A et al 1983a Quinine loading dose in cerebral malaria. American Journal of Tropical Medicine and Hygiene 32: 1–5
White N J, Warrell D A, Chanthavanich P et al 1983b Severe hypoglicemia and hyperinsulinemia in falciparum malaria. New England Journal of Medicine 309: 61–66
Whittle H C, Greenwood B M, Bidwell D E, Bartlett A, Voller A 1977 IgM and antibody measurement in diagnosis and management of Gambian trypanosomiasis. American Journal of Tropical Medicine and Hygiene 26: 1129–1134
Wilson C B, Remington J S, Stagno S, Reynolds D W 1980 Development of adverse sequelae in children born with subclinical congenital toxoplasma infection. Pediatrics 66: 767–774
Winslow D J, Connor D H, Sprinz H 1971 Malaria. In: Marcial-Rojas R A (eds) Pathology of protozoal and helmintic diseases. Williams and Wilkins, Baltimore, p 195–224
Woodhouse E, Flisser A, Larralde C 1982 Seroepidemiology of human cysticercosis in Mexico. In: Flisser A, Willms K, Laclette J P, Larralde C, Ridaura C, Beltran F (eds) Cysticercosis: present state of knowledge and perspectives. Academic Press, New York, p 11–23
World Health Organization Malaria Action Programme 1986 Severe and complicated malaria. Transactions

of the Royal Society of Tropical Medicine and Hygiene 80 (Suppl 22)
Zavala J T 1983 Etiology of cysticercosis. In: Palacios E, Rodriguez-Carbajal J, Taveras J M (eds) Cysticercosis of the central nervous system. Thomas, Springfield, p 18–26
Zuluaga H, Botero D, Restrepo M 1984 Otras amebiasis extraintestinales. In: Botero D, Restrepo M (eds) Parasitosis humanas. Ediciones Corporación para Investigaciones Biológicas. Medellín, p 50–52

# 8. New antiepileptic drugs: prospects for improved treatment of seizures

*R. J. Porter*

## THE NEED FOR NEW ANTIEPILEPTIC DRUGS

The vast majority of patients with recurrent cerebral seizures (epilepsy) are dependent on medical therapy — medications — for control of their attacks. The medications used, known collectively as antiepileptic drugs, are effective in most patients, many of whom lead essentially normal lives. A sizable minority, however, perhaps 20–25% of the total number of patients, respond poorly and are chronically refractory to medications. Although a limited number of such patients may be candidates for surgical intervention, most live in hope of new, more effective drugs. The actual number of patients with uncontrolled epilepsy is quite remarkable. Approximately 1% of the population of the United States has active epilepsy (Commission 1978). Although reports of the worldwide incidence of epilepsy vary, Hauser et al (1983) maintain that there is no firm proof of genuine geographic variation. Differences in terminology and inclusion criteria may be largely responsible for the apparent discrepancies. If a 1% incidence rate and a global population of 4.8 billion are assumed, then 48 million of the world's people suffer from epilepsy. As the vast majority of patients are necessarily dependent on medication for their seizure control, the effective use of currently marketed drugs is clearly critical for optimal seizure control (Porter 1986b). Therapy with existing antiepileptic drugs has been reviewed in detail (Porter 1984, Porter & Pitlick 1986).

This chapter will begin with a brief review of the history of antiepileptic drug development in order to explain older strategies for drug discovery. Newer concepts in preclinical screening will then be considered. Drugs which show promise in preclinical studies must be evaluated in humans, and a considerable portion of the chapter will evaluate clinical trial methodology for antiepileptic drugs. Finally, the status of new potentially useful compounds will be considered.

## HISTORY OF ANTIEPILEPTIC DRUG DEVELOPMENT

### Early advances in antiepileptic drug development

During the mid-1800s, a number of inorganic bromide salts were reported to produce good sedative effects and were accepted into medical practice. Potassium bromide, used by Locock (1857) to treat catamenial seizures, largely replaced earlier drugs when it was found to reduce seizure frequency in many patients after other forms of therapy had failed. Although it was used regularly during the next 50 years, it caused severe skin eruptions and psychosis, prompting a search for less toxic drugs.

The modern history of antiepileptic drugs marketed in the US (Table 8.1) begins in 1912 with the introduction of phenobarbital, a synthetic sedative-hypnotic drug

**Table 8.1** Antiepileptic drugs marketed in the United States (from Swinyard 1982)

| Year introduced | International nonproprietary name | US trade name | Company |
|---|---|---|---|
| 1912 | Phenobarbital | Luminal | Winthrop |
| 1935 | Mephobarbital | Mebaral | Winthrop |
| 1938 | Phenytoin | Dilantin | Parke–Davis |
| 1946 | Trimethadione | Tridione | Abbott |
| 1947 | Mephenytoin | Mesantoin | Sandoz |
| 1949 | Paramethadione | Paradione | Abbott |
| 1950 | Phethenylate[a] | Thiantoin | Lilly |
| 1951 | Phenacemide | Phenurone | Abbott |
| 1952 | Metharbital | Gemonil | Abbott |
| 1952 | Benzchlorpropamide[b] | Hibicon | Lederle |
| 1953 | Phensuximide | Milontin | Parke–Davis |
| 1954 | Primidone | Mysoline | Ayerst |
| 1957 | Methsuximide | Celontin | Parke–Davis |
| 1957 | Ethotoin | Peganone | Abbott |
| 1960 | Aminoglutethimide[c] | Elipten | Ciba |
| 1960 | Ethosuximide | Zarontin | Parke–Davis |
| 1968 | Diazepam[d] | Valium | Roche |
| 1974 | Carbamazepine | Tegretol | Geigy |
| 1975 | Clonazepam | Clonopin | Roche |
| 1978 | Valproic acid | Depakene | Abbott |
| 1981 | Clorazepate dipotassium[d] | Tranxene | Abbott |

[a] Withdrawn in 1952
[b] Withdrawn in 1955
[c] Withdrawn in 1966
[d] Approved by the FDA as an adjunct

which was shown to reduce seizure frequency (Hauptmann 1912). As it proved to be more effective and less toxic than potassium bromide, phenobarbital soon became the drug of choice in the treatment of epilepsy. Since the barbituric acid molecule is easily modified, many analogues of phenobarbital were synthesized, of which approximately 50 were marketed in the first 35 years of this century. One of these analogues, mephobarbital, demonstrated good antiepileptic activity and was marketed in the US in 1935 (Porter et al 1984).

In the absence of experimental models of seizures that could be used to test anticonvulsant activity, the discovery of the antiepileptic effect of bromide and phenobarbital was serendipitous. Later, with the development of seizure models, the search for new antiepileptic drugs was based on scientific screening programs.

One of the earliest models of epilepsy was developed in 1882, when seizures were elicited in dogs by direct faradic stimulation of the motor cortex and used to test chemicals for anticonvulsant activity (Albertoni 1882). Later, other seizure models involving convulsant chemicals were developed, including the naturally occurring picrotoxin, bicuculline, and strychnine and the synthetic compound, pentylenetetrazol. The early use of systemic chemical convulsants as experimental models has been well described (Stone 1972).

The year 1937 marked the beginning of the experimental evaluation of promising anticonvulsant chemicals prior to clinical use. Using a seizure model based on a new electroshock technique for producing convulsions in animals (Spiegel 1937), Merritt & Putnam (1938a,b) screened a group of compounds supplied to them by Parke–Davis and discovered the anticonvulsant properties of phenytoin, then called diphenylhydantoin. Because phenytoin was well tolerated by laboratory animals, it was subjected to clinical trials in 1938 and marketed that same year. The absence of sedative effects and the dramatic control of seizures observed when phenytoin was added to barbiturate therapy were the key factors in its rapid marketing. In addition, its entry into the market was not delayed by regulatory requirements, since at that time the introduction of new drugs was still regulated by the Federal Food and Drugs Act of 1906, which required only that drugs be accurately labeled without requiring proof of safety or efficacy (Federal Food & Drug Administration Act 1906).

The reliability and quantitative capacity of Merritt's method demonstrated the feasibility of testing new chemicals for anticonvulsant activity (Porter et al 1984). Administration to humans, a more costly, time-consuming, and risky procedure, was reserved for the most effective experimental compounds that emerged from such testing programs. In addition, the process through which phenytoin came onto the market demonstrated that academic investigators could work successfully with the pharmaceutical industry, encouraging a relationship that flourished for the next 20 years.

Several pharmaceutical firms began molecular modification of phenytoin and its analogues, and numerous hydantoins were synthesized and tested during this period. In addition, investigators from the pharmaceutical industry as well as academic researchers began to explore new and improved methods of provoking seizures (Porter et al 1984).

In 1944, Richards and Everett reported that trimethadione, a potent analgesic compound that was to become the first anti-absence drug, prevented pentylenetetrazol-induced threshold seizures in rodents. They also showed that these seizures were prevented by phenobarbital, but not by phenytoin (Richards & Everett 1944). Goodman et al (1953) confirmed these results and showed that phenytoin and phenobarbital modified the pattern of maximal electroshock seizures while trimethadione did not. These findings demonstrated the varying anticonvulsant actions of these drugs and the qualitative difference between threshold and maximal seizures (Porter et al 1984).

Between 1945 and 1950, several investigators conducted tests with a variety of seizure models, but failed to find one in which all drugs were active. However, these tests uncovered profiles of anticonvulsant activity which, with few exceptions, correlated well with clinical efficacy and specificity (Swinyard 1949). In 1951, Chen et al investigated the anticonvulsant activity of approximately 65 phenylsuccinimides and found that among the most potent antipentylenetetrazol compounds were phensuximide and methsuximide. Phensuximide was approved for treatment of absence seizures in 1953; methsuximide, in 1957. A third succinimide, ethosuximide, was introduced for the same purpose in 1960 (Porter et al 1984).

During the same period (1938–1960), two analogues of phenytoin (mephenytoin and ethotoin), two of phenobarbital (metharbital and primidone), and one of trimethadione (paramethadione) were marketed in the US. Each had a spectrum of activity comparable to that of its parent drug and was marketed for similar use (Porter et al 1984).

Three other drugs, phethenylate, benzchlorpropamide, and aminoglutethimide, were also introduced during this period. However, both phethenylate and benzchloropropamide were withdrawn by 1960, as the former was associated with a high incidence of hepatic necrosis and the latter demonstrated toxic effects with long-term use in experimental animals. Aminoglutethimide was withdrawn in 1966 after it was linked to a high incidence of goiter (Porter et al 1984).

Interestingly, all antiepileptic drugs developed from 1912 to 1960 were based on a simple heterocyclic ring structure (Fig. 8.1). During this period, genuinely novel

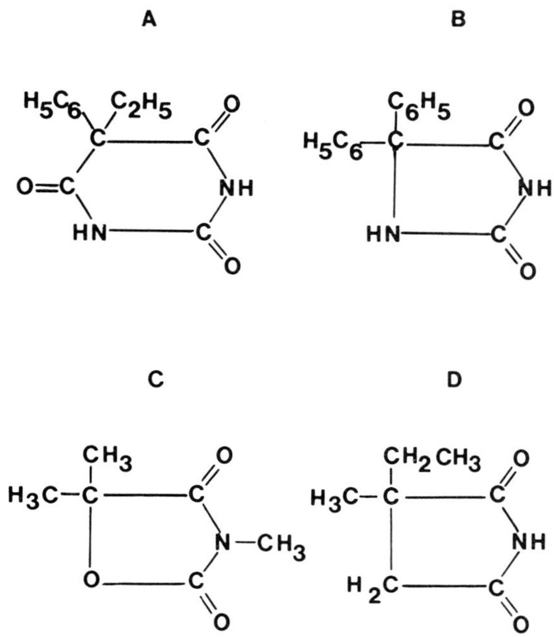


**Fig. 8.1** Chemical structures of (A) phenobarbital; (B) phenytoin; (C) trimethadione; and (D) ethosuxmide. (From Porter 1986b.)

structures were ignored in the development of antiepileptic drugs. Instead, attention centered on the hydantoins, barbiturates, oxazolidinediones, succinimides, and acetylureas (Porter et al 1984).

After 1938, marketing of all drugs in the United States was regulated by the Federal Food, Drug, and Cosmetic Act which required proof of safety in addition to the 1906 labeling provisions. Definitive questions about efficacy usually were not resolved until after a new drug was marketed (Porter et al 1984).

**Decline in antiepileptic drug development**

The highly productive era of antiepileptic drug development in the 1940s and 1950s was followed by a dormant period lasting 12 years, from 1961 to 1973, during which the only new drug of interest was diazepam, an adjunctive drug used mostly in status epilepticus (Table 8.1). What were the reasons for this sudden and dramatic decline in antiepileptic drug development in the United States? Citing the seemingly abundant supply of existing drugs, some clinicians felt that new antiepileptic agents would be superfluous, even though many patients remained uncontrolled or suffered toxic side effects on existing medications. The pharmaceutical industry in the early 1960s was turning its attention to other areas of the central nervous system, especially after the remarkable financial success of tranquilizers and sedative-hypnotic drugs (Porter et al 1984).

Perhaps the major reason for the sudden decline in antiepileptic drug development, however, was the passage in 1962 of the Drug Amendments Act. Known as the Kefauver–Harris amendment, this legislation revised the 1938 Federal Food, Drug, and Cosmetic Act to require not only accurate labeling and proof of safety, but also proof of efficacy before a new drug could be marketed. Up until this time, evidence that a drug was actually efficacious was obtainable only long after the drug had been marketed. The Kefauver–Harris amendment placed the burden and expense of proving a drug's efficacy squarely on the pharmaceutical industry. Not surprisingly, industry was loath to accept this responsibility for antiepileptic drugs, which offered a relatively small financial return and whose efficacy is notoriously difficult to prove. Clinical trials of potential antiepileptic drugs were hampered by the lack of a sizeable population of patients with well-defined seizure types and by ethical considerations (Porter 1986a). By the late 1960's, very few innovative antiepileptic drugs were under development (Porter 1986b).

In an effort to reverse this trend, the Epilepsy Branch of the National Institute of Neurological and Communicative Disorders and Stroke, in collaboration with other investigators, began in 1968 to conduct controlled clinical trials of seven drugs, many of which were already marketed abroad (Porter et al 1984). Between 1974 and 1978, three of these drugs — carbamazepine, clonazepam, and valproic acid — were approved as primary antiepileptic agents; clorazepate dipotassium was marketed in 1981 as an adjunctive drug. These efforts by the Epilepsy Branch became known as the Antiepileptic Drug Development (ADD) Program. Since its inception, this program has encouraged the search for new antiepileptic drugs by conducting and/or funding screening programs for new compounds, toxicity testing for advanced and promising preclinical compounds, and clinical trials. As a result, the waning interest in the US in new medical therapies for epilepsy has been replaced by a productive coalition of government, industry, and academia (Porter 1986b).

## STRATEGIES IN THE DEVELOPMENT OF NEW ANTIEPILEPTIC DRUGS

In the mid 1940's and early 1950's an especially fruitful experimental approach to the development of antiepileptic drugs was being developed by Goodman and Swinyard and their colleagues at the University of Utah (Swinyard 1982). Beginning with an attempt to duplicate the Putnam and Merritt electroshock model, these investigators observed that phenytoin's effect was to shorten the duration of the seizure, suggesting that the effect was not related to its ability to elevate seizure threshold but rather to its ability to prevent seizure spread. Such observations led to standardization of the maximal electroshock seizure (MES) in rodents as a test of this particular antiepileptic effect. During this same period a threshold test was also standardized using subcutaneous pentyleneterazol (PTZ) (Porter & Nadi 1987).

All drugs currently in use have some effect in one or both of the above tests, even though many were not discovered by experimental means. Furthermore, drugs tend to profile clinically as a function of their effectiveness in these two models.

Phenytoin, which is effective in partial and generalized tonic-clonic seizures, is effective against MES but not against PTZ (when used as a threshold test). Ethosuximide, which is effective against absence seizures in humans, has more effectiveness against PTZ. These two tests — considered by some to represent together the final common pathway for many epileptic seizures — have been further refined and used to screen more than 12 000 compounds in the ADD program of the Epilepsy Branch (Porter et al 1984). The screening is performed in a progressively more sophisticated manner, eliminating less promising compounds at each step (Porter & Nadi 1987).

The use of MES and PTZ to discover new antiepileptic drugs is not above criticism. One major argument is that such a program will develop new drugs which are just like the drugs already available. A counter argument, however, can be made using carbamazepine as an example. This drug is approximately equally effective as phenytoin against MES and is generally effective against the same human seizure types, but its toxicologic profile is extraordinarily different from phenytoin and its addition to the pharmacy has helped millions of patients with epilepsy. It may be used in combination with phenytoin for added effectiveness (without sedation) in a number of patients (Porter 1984, Porter & Nadi 1987).

Another argument against the use of MES and PTZ is that the mechanisms by which drugs work against these rather empirical tests are obscure. It is argued that we might find better, more effective drugs using basic and more rational approaches. The counter argument is that we simply do not sufficiently understand the basic mechanisms of epileptic seizures to be certain which drug effect to seek or whether any effect — once documented — is in fact a mechanism of action. Even when a potential drug is developed by rational methods, additional problems arise regarding clinical testing, as one cannot predict in which subgroup of the epileptic syndromes one should test the new drug. On the other hand, the discovery of a clinically effective drug which is *ineffective* in MES and PTZ screening would open a whole new avenue for basic and clinical investigation (Porter & Nadi 1987).

In the past decade, however, avenues for the rational development of new antiepileptic drugs have been pursued. This development has progressed through two fundamental phases. The earliest of these phases was the search for drugs that act, by various mechanisms, to enhance neuronal inhibition. The second and more recent phase of rational approaches to antiepileptic drug development has been the effort to find drugs that diminish neuronal excitation. The following two paragraphs summarize the more detailed review by Meldrum (1986).

In the normal neuron, neuronal inhibition is presumably a function of inhibitory synaptic activity directly affecting the neuronal membrane. Most studies of such inhibition have been directed toward gamma-amino-butyric acid (GABA), the most important central inhibitory neurotransmitter. A number of mechanisms are at least theoretically available for enhancement of GABA-mediated inhibition, and a number of these have been thoroughly investigated, even to the point of clinical studies of drugs which are potentially active in the GABA system. A GABA agonist, muscimol, has been tested in humans but appears to be too toxic. A GABA prodrug, progabide, has shown sufficient activity to be marketed in France. Benzodiazepines may act by enhancement of GABA efficacy, and barbiturates by direct action on the chloride ionophore. Inhibition of the catabolic enzyme, GABA-transaminase, is accomplished by gamma-vinyl GABA; its potential toxicity presents special problems. In spite of more than a decade of investigation, no striking, highly potent new antiepileptic drug has come from investigations on enhancement of brain inhibition.

Neuronal excitation, like inhibition, is presumably modulated by neurotransmitters acting at synapses. Most of the investigative activity has centered on diminishing the effects of glutamate or aspartate, or both. Drugs currently under clinical investigation may act by decreasing synaptic release (e.g. lamotrigine) or by decreasing post-synaptic action (e.g. MK 801). Other mechanisms of diminishing excitatory amino acid transmission include decreasing maximal rate of synthesis or enhancing reuptake of excitatory neurotransmitters (Meldrum 1986).

Approaches other than synaptic neurotransmitter alteration have been considered in the search for new antiepileptic drugs. These investigations include neurophysiologic approaches such as membrane stabilization and effects on neuronal synchrony. Although substantive progress has been made in our understanding of such phenomena, these advances have not been translated into potential new antiepileptic drugs of any note.

One might reasonably ask how the decision is made to submit a particular chemical compound to clinical testing. No single, simple answer is sufficient. Some compounds advance purely on their preclinical capabilities in the oldest screening tests. Others advance almost exclusively on the basis of a proposed rational approach. A few compounds satisfy both criteria. Given the uncertainty of finding the best drugs using the available methods, such as multiplicity of approaches is not unreasonable.

## THE CLINICAL TESTING OF NEW ANTIEPILEPTIC DRUGS

A potential drug must successfully undergo a variety of clinical studies before being approved for general use in patients. These studies may include early tolerance and pharmacologic trials in normal volunteers as well as pilot studies of potential efficacy, but the controlled trial to evaluate efficacy is usually the most difficult and the most important. In any clinical trial, the peculiarities of the disorder being treated must be examined. Clinical trials of drugs in epilepsy, therefore, must be designed to deal with the characteristics of that complex disorder. Of primary importance is the realization that many different syndromes are included in the epilepsies. To be meaningful, data must be collected from a differentiated group of epileptic persons. Patients are usually categorized according to clinical seizure type. Fortunately, this categorization is based upon very empirical information and correlates well with the various therapeutic measures. Clinical seizure types are usually classified according to the 1981 International Classification of Epileptic Seizures (Commission 1981), and the resulting data serve as a first step in obtaining a modicum of homogeneity in the patients included in the clinical trial (Porter 1986a). A number of critical variables are worthy of discussion with regard to controlled clinical trials of antiepileptic drugs. These are further considered in the following sections.

### The patients

A clinical trial must be based upon a patient population that is both sufficiently large and sufficiently homogeneous to test the new drug effectively. Seizure classification allows investigators to identify patients with a shared seizure type. Preclinical testing determines which human seizure type is most likely to respond to the new compound. Obviously, a minimum number of patients with the targeted seizure type must be available for the study to be performed. It is pointless to test the effect of a drug on a seizure type that is unavailable in sufficient quantities to demonstrate the drug's efficacy (Porter 1986a). On those few occasions when a drug is especially effective against a rare seizure type, the therapeutic effect may become immediately apparent, eliminating the necessity for a large patient sample. The dramatic effect of valproate on certain unusual myoclonias provides a case in point (Porter 1984). Such observations are unfortunately only likely to be made after the drug has been marketed for a different indication. In the vast majority of cases, large numbers of patients or seizures are required to demonstrate unequivocal efficacy (Porter 1986a).

The seizure frequency of patients must also be considered. This frequency must be high enough for a new compound to have an effect that can be reliably measured. Including too many patients with infrequent seizures can expand the clinical trial to enormous proportions, either in numbers of patients or duration of study (Porter 1986a). Inadequate seizure frequency presents a problem in many clinical trials using generalized tonic-clonic seizures.

The three types of attacks most frequently considered for clinical trials are absence, generalized tonic-clonic and partial seizures. Studies of atonic seizures are difficult because these attacks are inherently heterogeneous, there is no reliable EEG correlate, and the patients must be continuously observed as self-reporting is rarely possible. Furthermore, preclinical testing has failed to establish any animal model for predicting effectiveness against atonic seizures (Porter 1986a).

Clinical trials for absence seizures involve a pediatric patient population since the disorder is largely limited to children. The absence seizure has a very high frequency relative to other seizures and has a direct electrographic (EEG) correlate. Although there is always some concern about possible harm to the patient as a result of poor control during a clinical trial, this anxiety is lower for absence seizures than for other seizure types. As a result of these characteristics, clinical trials for absence seizures can be shorter, use objective EEG measurements as a criterion for drug effect, and limit the overall exposure of each patient. However, suitable patients are not always readily available, and the exact criteria for 'typical' and 'atypical' absences are controversial (Holmes et al 1987, Porter 1986a).

The generalized tonic-clonic seizure has a major advantage is being relatively easy to record. Moreover, a large segment of the population of patients with epilepsy has generalized tonic-clonic attacks. The impressive numbers, however, are rather misleading since many of these patients have only a single generalized tonic-clonic attack, are never treated, and are, therefore, unavailable for clinical trials. Many other patients with generalized tonic-clonic seizures have attacks which are easily controlled on available medications. Pharmacologic therapy using phenytoin or carbamazepine is highly effective in a very considerable number of these patients (Porter 1984, Mattson et al 1985). For obvious ethical reasons, a patient whose seizures are well controlled must be excluded from clinical trials. In the case of generalized tonic-clonic seizures, anxiety about poor control is considerable, and maximal conventional therapy seems most appropriate at all times (Porter 1986a).

Partial seizures in adults are the third commonly studied seizure type. These attacks are relatively easy to record, although some observation is required in most patients. A substantial number of patients with epilepsy have partial seizures that are poorly controlled with available medications even when these drugs are optimally prescribed. Partial seizures are the most common uncontrolled seizure type in adults. Partial seizures are often recurrent, lessening the investigators' problem of inadequate seizure frequency. Anxiety about uncontrolled partial seizures is not as high as for generalized tonic-clonic seizures although higher than for absence attacks. Patients are, therefore, relatively easy to find and recruit. With-in group heterogeneity can cause difficulties in clinical trials for partial seizures, especially if simple partial and complex partial attacks are studied together. An additional disadvantage is the need for a rather prolonged study. A patient having three partial seizures per month would need to be studied for 8 or 9 months. Assuming this rate of frequency, 50 or 60 patients would constitute an adequate patient sample (Porter 1986a).

**Exclusion criteria**

Having indicated the major advantages and disadvantages of clinical trials using three common seizure types, it must be noted that seizure type is not the only criterion for inclusion in clinical trials. Certain patients are ineligible for trials in epilepsy for reasons that go beyond their seizure classification. For example, age and weight limits are imposed in most clinical trials. Children and adolescents require special permissions before they can be studied (Porter 1986a). A typical (and actual) list of exclusions for a study of a new compound for complex partial seizures is shown in Table 8.2. The ideal patient is one in whom the seizures are frequent but not

**Table 8.2** Exclusion criteria. (From Porter & White 1986.)

*The following patients were not considered suitable for participation in an actual trial of a new antiepileptic drug in partial seizures:*

1. Patients with treatable causes of seizures, e.g. patients whose seizure etiology is metabolic, neoplastic, or infectious. A CT scan within the last 6 years is required to confirm absence of a treatable lesion, e.g. tumor, together with no new neurologic signs since the CT scan.
2. Patients who have received an investigational antiepileptic drug within 3 months before the beginning of baseline.
3. Patients who are abusers of other drugs (e.g. narcotics) including alcohol.
4. Patients with progressive neurological disorders.
   Patients with a history of generalized tonic-clonic status epilepticus within 3 months before baseline, while receiving antiepileptic drug therapy.
5. Patients who have other serious medical or psychiatric disorders (e.g. cardiac disease requiring drug therapy; a need for tranquilizers and psychotherapeutic agents; renal or hepatic disease).
6. Patients with gastrointestinal abnormalities potentially capable of affecting drug pharmacokinetics.
7. Patients receiving chronic therapy with non-antiepileptic drugs, including OTC ('over the counter') drugs. Vitamins and mineral supplements are permitted.
8. Patients having cancer with metastatic potential (does not include, e.g. skin cancer).
9. Patients with a history of poor compliance with past antiepileptic drug therapy, as judged by the principal investigator.
10. Patients with abnormal laboratory values. For entrance, a white count greater than 3000 $mm^3$ with granulocytes greater than 50% will be considered normal. Patients should also be within their laboratory's upper limit for white count. Platelet counts are to be greater than 150 000 $mm^3$.
11. Patients with elevated SGOT, SGPT, and alkaline phosphatase levels (up to two times the upper limit of normal) will be permitted to enter the study. However, if more than one baseline level doubles during the study, the patient must be removed. Patients may be retained in the study when one of these values is doubled, but if this value reaches three times baseline, the patient must be removed.
12. Patients incapable of signing an informed consent.
13. Patients unable to be hospitalized for a period of 2 weeks.

severe, and whose seizures are likely to be drug-responsive. Such patients, of course, are quite rare (Porter 1986a).

**Concomitant medications**

Most clinical drug trials are designed to test a new compound against either a placebo or against a drug that has already been proven effective. In testing antiepileptic drugs, however, compromises are required because of (1) the potential harm to the patient from uncontrolled seizures and (2) the realization that currently marketed compounds exert at least some effectiveness for virtually all patients. Institutional review boards have become increasingly sensitive to ethical considerations when asked to approve clinical trials. This more stringent standard of 'what is permissible' makes approval of epilepsy research protocols especially difficult (Cereghino & Penry 1982). The clinical trial that proved the effectiveness of valproate against absence seizures (Sato et al 1982) affords a good example. Originally, a simple crossover design had been planned. However, for ethical reasons it was decided that patients who were fully controlled on ethosuximide could not be crossed over to valproate and vice versa. The result was a much more complicated response-conditional study. Even though anxiety over poor control of absence seizures is relatively low, no patient in this study went untreated at any time. Furthermore, the test compound, valproate, had already demonstrated unequivocal efficacy against absence seizures in both pilot and foreign trials and could therefore be used as a sole therapy in the study (Porter 1986a).

Most clinical trials in epilepsy face more severe limitations than those in the example just cited. The seizure type to be studied may be too severe to risk uncontrolled attacks; the efficacy of the test drug may not have been sufficiently proven in preliminary trials, or both impediments may exist. Consequently, in most initial trials of a new antiepileptic drug, the test compound is 'added on' to one or more already marketed drugs. Establishing a homogeneity of concomitant medication in both the active and the control group helps to avoid such puzzling variables as drug–drug interactions (Porter 1986a).

The actual choice of concomitant medication can be very difficult. Having singled out the human seizure type most likely to respond to the test drug, investigators must consider the various possible concomitant therapies. For example, in planning a study of a new drug for complex partial seizures, one must decide which concomitant regimens are most appropriate. Marketed drugs that have shown a prominent drug–drug interaction with the test compound in preclinical or pilot pharmacological data should be eliminated if at all possible. Primidone and phenobarbital, two currently marketed drugs for complex partial seizures, would be relatively contraindicated if the new compound has sedative side effects. In trials involving complex partial seizures, the usual concomitant drugs are carbamazepine, phenytoin, or a combination of both (Porter 1986a).

If the control drug or drugs are *too* effective, the patients will not have enough seizures on which to test the new compound. Patients having a tolerable but high seizure frequency (a state that is obviously difficult to define) on a single concomitant medication such as carbamazepine or phenytoin are ideal for the best, most uncomplicated design (Porter 1986a). Patients are always eliminated from the study if their needs run counter to the research protocol. For example, if excessive seizures occur in a patient on carbamazepine in the middle of a study and the attending physician decides that the addition of phenytoin might be of benefit, the patient's regimen would be altered even though he or she would be lost to the study. The problem of 'excess seizures' during a clinical trial is less severe if the patients are already being treated with maximal therapy. If, in a trial for complex partial seizures, both phenytoin and carbamazepine are used as concomitant medications, then maximal seizure control efforts are in force, and investigator anxiety over both patient safety and possible intervention in the trial is greatly lessened. The major disadvantages of including multiple concomitant drugs are the heightened probability of drug–drug interactions and the extremely high standard which the new compound must surpass to prove its efficacy. In the trial cited above, the test compound must exert an efficacious effect over and above that already provided by two drugs — both of which are somewhat effective against partial seizures. A new drug of modest efficacy may be lost in such a trial (Porter 1986a).

**The dose of the test compound**

How much of the test drug to administer to patients is a problem that is often underestimated in planning a clinical trial. It is naive to think that *any* dose will be effective. Too often a drug is judged ineffective without having been tested at anywhere near the maximal tolerated dose, i.e. that dose which reliably produces dose-related side effects. To have its best chance of success, a new compound should be administered near the maximal tolerated dose especially in a trial in which concomitant medications are being used. To do otherwise is to expect miracles and may result in a failure to detect the drug's efficacy and the waste of an expensive clinical trial.

There is little merit to the argument that one should not approach the maximal tolerated dose because of possible unknown toxicity. Although one must approach dose-related side effects slowly and carefully, there are several reasons why this maximally tolerated dose should be achieved. Once an antiepileptic drug is marketed, it is 'pushed to toxicity' in many patients by many physicians. For the well-being of all patients with epilepsy, it is imperative that side effects be detected and documented before the drug becomes widely available. For this reason, physicians conducting the clinical trial should already be alerted to known side effects that have been recognized in pilot studies. Patients participating in the controlled clinical trial are closely and carefully supervised; every effort is made to assure their safety. A clinical trial affords the logical opportunity to increase the amount of critical information about dose-related side effects (Porter 1986a).

**Bias control**

Perhaps the most important single feature of a controlled clinical trial is the management of extraneous variables that may influence the outcome. The goal of a clinical trial is to answer a question; it is not to confirm a pre-existing opinion regarding the efficacy and safety of a mode of diagnosis or therapy. More than one question may be asked by a single clinical trial, but the complexities of conducting trials with more than one outcome variable are great, and most of the best trials are those in which simple, unambiguous outcome variables are defined. The most important outcome variable of most controlled clinical trials of antiepileptic drugs is whether the compound causes a persistent decrement in seizure frequency. Other variables, such as seizure severity and absence of deleterious adverse effects are important, but seizure frequency should be the major outcome variable of most clinical trials as (1) it is a primary quantification of a drug's effectiveness and (2) although it is usually *not easy* to measure, it is the *easiest* outcome variable to measure. Difficulties involving this outcome measure have already been discussed for certain seizure types.

Given that a clinical trial is designed to answer a question, and that in a clinical trial of an antiepileptic drug the question is how effective the compound is against epileptic seizures, then the next concept of importance is the planning of a trial in which one can measure this effect in an unambiguous manner. This task is surprisingly difficult, not so much in the architecture of a rigorous design but in finding compulsive neurologists who are enthusiastic about applying the onerous restrictions of such a trial in an unyielding manner.

*Randomization*

Randomization is an attempt to make 'experimental' and 'control' groups as similar as possible for both known and unknown factors that could influence the outcome of the study. The need for scientific rigor, such as is provided by randomization and blinding has been well documented, but especially germane is the analysis by Chalmers et al (1983) of 145 trials of treatment for myocardial infarction. Chalmers divided the trials, in which the outcome variable (case fatalities) was similar in all cases, into those studies in which randomization and blinding were an integral part of the study, those which were unblinded but randomized, and those in which the study was conducted without randomization or blinding. The analysis showed (as have other such analyses) that studies which are not randomized are extraordinarily likely to reject the null hypotheses, i.e. the trial is likely to be 'positive' in 58% of cases. If the simple additional rigor of randomization is added, the likelihood of rejection of the null hypothesis falls dramatically: only 24% of the trials yielded what one might consider 'positive' results. The blinded and randomized studies found a difference between treatment and control groups in an astoundingly low 9%! Many possible reasons exist for this remarkable discrepancy, but most can be reduced to the desire of all who participate in the trial — the pharmaceutical company, the investigators, the technical staff, and even the patients — to have the enormous effort of the trial come to what is viewed as 'fruition.' Fruition is unavoidably defined as a 'positive' result (in the case of antiepileptic drug trials, the drug proves to be effective) rather than the really desirable outcome which is to *answer the question* of whether the trial is 'positive' or 'negative.' It is well accepted that no human being who is goal-oriented (and all clinical investigators have a heavy dose of this trait) can, on a continuous basis, accurately distinguish between conscious desire for a good study and the conscious and unconscious desire for the study to be 'positive'. It is for this reason that external control (bias control), such as randomization (which also implies either multiple groups or multiple periods with control groups or periods) is mandatory to decrease the likelihood of such bias. No reason exists to suggest that less bias control is needed for studies of antiepileptic drugs than for myocardial infarction.

*Blinding*

Randomization is, in itself, insufficient. Even though control of the accession of patients into the trial may be taken away from the investigator by randomization, the desire to influence the trial toward a 'positive' outcome remains undiminished. Blinding is necessary to control further erosion of the goal of answering the question of drug efficacy. An example (which occurs frequently) may suffice:

> In a randomized but *unblinded* trial of partial seizures, seizure frequency was the major outcome variable. During an analysis period (i.e. a period during the trial in which seizure occurrence — or lack thereof — has a direct effect on the outcome of the trial), the patient has an event at home which is atypical but witnessed by a relative. The investigator is then asked by his staff to decide whether or not this event is or is not a 'seizure.' Since the investigator knows whether the patient is on active or control medication, the investigator is in a unique position to influence the trial toward a 'positive' result. By calling the event a 'seizure' if the patient is on control medication or by calling the event a 'non-seizure' if the patient is on active medication, bias may be directly introduced. In many trials (especially those with small numbers) remarkably few such decisions can dramatically alter the trial result.

It is not possible for the investigator to be objective in this kind of decision unless the study is 'double-blind," i.e. the patients and the persons involved in the decisions which may unfavorably influence the major goal of the trial are unaware of the group or period in which the patient resides. If, in the above case, the study were double-blind, the investigator could comfortably make the best available decision independent of any desire, conscious or unconscious, to make the trial a 'positive' event.

*The half-controlled trial*

One of the worst scenerios that clinical investigators inflict upon themselves is the half-controlled trial. The trial is designed so that the aura of bias control is established but the unconscious desires of the investigators are, in subtle but effective ways, allowed to influence the results. The example just cited of a trial with randomization but without appropriate blinding typifies such a trial. The probability of a 'positive' result (desired by everyone) soars, and one more drug is deemed effective in a 'controlled' trial. Years of effort and great sums of money are wasted on such trials, and even more effort and money are required to undo the damage wrought. Another unfortunate consequence of such trials is the gradually increasing cynicism about the results of 'controlled' trials, especially when the details regarding the conduct of the study are not fully available — hence the desire of the Federal Food and Drug Administration to have *all* the records. A final unfortunate, but seemingly inescapable, conclusion is that a 'negative' study is more likely to be an accurate reflection of the truth than a 'positive' study, since lack of adequate bias control almost always influences the trial in a 'positive' direction. Cynicism about 'positive' results is heightened, of course, by the fundamental observation that many proposed treatments eventually prove ineffective.

*Bias control: when should it be introduced?*

Although a case can be made for a continuum of clinical trials — from pilot studies to rigidly controlled trials — we would all be better served by viewing trials of efficacy of new antiepileptic drugs as *either* pilot studies or definitive, controlled studies. Any study which does not adhere to the highest standards of bias control is to be termed a *pilot* effort, yielding only 'suggestive' data. Since efficacy is hard enough to measure in a controlled trial (let alone a pilot study), all drugs which have any promise should advance quickly to a controlled trial for early definitive decisions. This approach would eliminate the misleading of pharmaceutical companies with 'promising' results of compounds of no value and would hasten to market those drugs that are useful.

*Bias control: summary*

These concepts of bias control are not really new. On the other hand, since we all know the rules, why do we continuously break them? The answer is clearly the difficulty in executing a rigidly controlled trial; the answer is rarely couched in these terms, however. Instead, explanations are given for the unnecessity or impracticality of such bias control. However, as Kurtzke (1986) reminds us, 'the gold standard for therapeutic trials . . . has properly become the randomized, double-blind, placebo-controlled design.'

The choice of an appropriate statistical design for the clinical evaluation of a new antiepileptic agent requires consideration of at least three competing viewpoints: clinical, pharmacological, and statistical. Figure 8.2 gives a summary of the most important

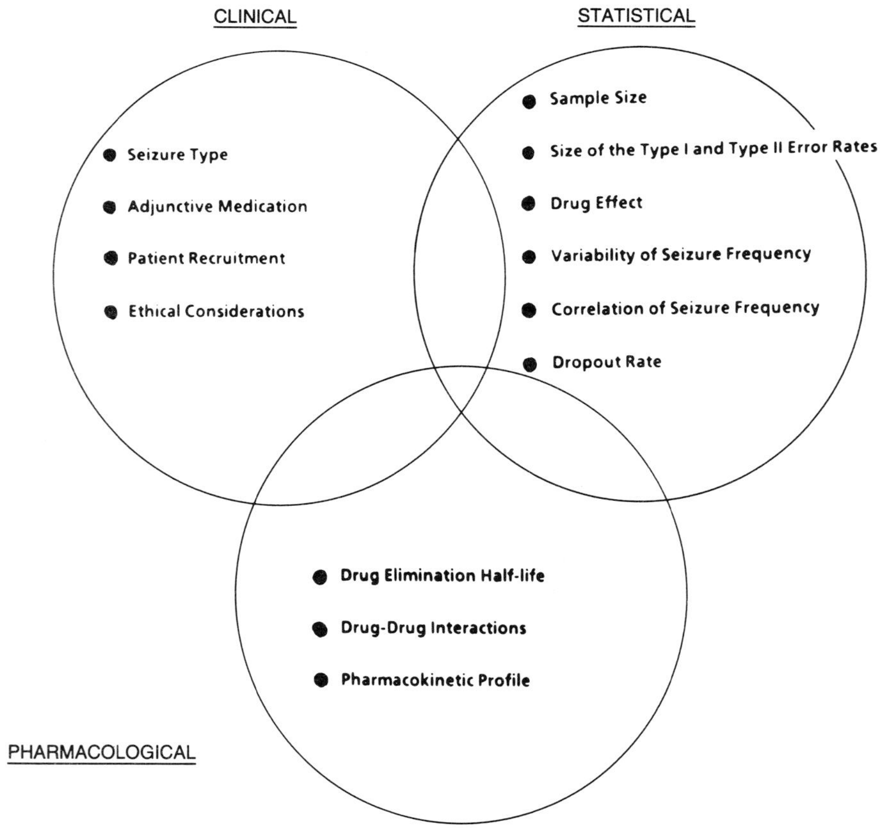


**Fig. 8.2** Considerations for selection of the appropriate design for the evaluation of a new antiepileptic drug. (From Porter & White 1986.)

concepts within each of these three broad areas. A full review of study designs is beyond the scope of this chapter; such a review has recently been published (Porter & White 1986). Other considerations related to design strategies are critically discussed by van Belle & Tempkin (1983).

## PROSPECTIVE ANTIEPILEPTIC DRUGS

In this decade, numerous compounds have reached various stages of preclinical and clinical investigation. Each of these compounds has had some claim to being antiepileptic. Summarizing the status of such compounds is a difficult task. First, the data are not easy to obtain, especially for preclinical compounds in which the pharmaceutical company has little to gain by providing information. Some potential preclinical compounds have recently been described (Meldrum & Porter 1986). Secondly, the information can very quickly become out-of-date, especially as toxic effects eliminate drugs from further clinical exposure. Finally, since the routes by which compounds are evaluated are heterogeneous, the developmental state of a particular compound can be difficult to ascertain. This section will summarize data on selected compounds that are, or have been, in clinical studies. In-depth, although somewhat less current, information is available in the volume by Meldrum & Porter (1986). For those compounds in which studies have ceased, limited information is provided here. These data reflect activity and available information as of April, 1987. The compounds are listed in alphabetical order.

### Felbamate

Felbamate is a dicarbamate that is closely related to meprobamate, a sedative-hypnotic compound. Unlike meprobamate, felbamate in higher doses does not present clinically with sleepiness. Its clinical side effects are nausea and vomiting, suggesting that felbamate has a nonsedative central action. The drug has been developed primarily on the basis of its activity against maximal electroshock activity in rodents. This activity is approximately four times less potent than phenytoin or carbamazepine, but the drug is exceedingly nontoxic, and adult patients can often tolerate 3000 mg per day.

Two randomized, double-blind trials are underway. One, a multicenter study, involves the University of Virginia and the University of Minnesota. Patients with partial seizures are being evaluated in a two-period crossover design. The study is scheduled for completion in late 1987. The second study is being conducted at the National Institutes of Health in Bethesda, Maryland. More severely affected patients with partial seizures are participating in a three-period crossover design. This second study should be completed in 1988. Since neither study included plans for an interim analysis, meaningful efficacy data will not be available until the studies are complete. Additional data on felbamate are available (Perhach et al 1986).

### Flunarizine

Flunarizine is a difluorinated piperazine derivative that was originally introduced for vertigo and migraine. It has the intriguing effect, and possible mechanism of action, of being a calcium channel blocker. This drug has an extraordinary half-life of more than 2 weeks in many patients.

The drug has been studied clinically in epileptic patients since 1978. Following pharmacokinetic studies at UCLA, the Epilepsy Branch of the National Institutes of Health, Bethesda, Maryland plans a large multicenter parallel design study that is scheduled to begin in late 1987. For this study, patients must have uncontrolled partial seizures. The concomitant medications will be phenytoin or carbamazepine. Additional data on flunarizine are available (Vanden Bussche et al 1986).

**Gabapentin**

Although a GABA-related amino acid that moves through the blood-brain barrier, gabapentin is thought to exert its antiepileptic effect by interfering with the action of excitatory amino acids such as aspartate. It should be noted, however, that only limited data are available describing the drug's mechanism of action. Furthermore, seizure type specificity is difficult to determine from the available preclinical data.

Numerous studies of this drug are underway, both in Europe and in the United States. Many of these studies are controlled, and efficacy data should emerge within the next several years. Additional data on gabapentin are available (Bartoszyk et al 1986).

**Lamotrigine**

Lamotrigine is a phenyltriazine derivative that was developed in an effort to find antifolate drugs. Such a search was based on the hypothesis that compounds that interfere with folate metabolism may be antiepileptic. Although lamotrigine has only weak antifolate activity, the drug is effective against maximal electroshock in rodents.

Several controlled trials in Europe are complete, and the data are encouraging. A five-center controlled study is underway in the United States; long-term studies are planned. If the drug proves effective, marketing might occur within 5 years in the United States. Additional data on lamotrigine are available (Miller et al 1986).

**Milacemide**

Milacemide is metabolized to glycine in the brain. It is most effective against bicuculline-induced seizures. The drug has been widely studied clinically, but initial efficacy data were not very promising, and studies in the United States have been discontinued by the pharmaceutical company. Additional data on milacemide are available (Roba et al 1986).

**MK-801**

MK-801 began as one of the most promising preclinical compounds of the decade. It is more potent than phenytoin in maximal electroshock, it is nonsedative, and it has the additional advantage of having a rational mechanism for its proposed action: MK-801 is an antagonist of the excitatory amino acid receptor, N-methyl-D-aspartate (NMDA).

Clinical studies were conducted at UCLA and elsewhere. Unfortunately, promising efficacy data were not obtained and studies in epilepsy have been discontinued. Additional data on MK-801 are available (Troupin et al 1986).

**Nafimidone**

Nafimidone is an imidazole derivative that has activity against maximal electroshock. In clinical studies, its lack of efficacy and its toxicity profile caused it to be abandoned as an active potential antiepileptic compound. Further data are available on nafimidone (Buhles et al 1986).

**Org 6370**

Org 6370 is an amino-benzobicyclononene derivative with activity against both maximal electroshock and pentylenetetrazol models in rodents. The drug has an active metabolite that is likely of considerable significance in its activity.

Early clinical studies in Europe and in at least two centers in the United States demonstrate the safety of the compound. Controlled clinical trials are planned. Additional data on Org 6370 are available (de Graaff et al 1986).

**Oxcarbazepine**

Oxcarbazepine is closely related to carbamazepine. However, its mechanism of action does not include an epoxide metabolite. Oxcarbazepine may therefore be less toxic. Large clinical trials are nearing completion in Europe, but because of the limited differences between this drug and carbamazepine, no studies are currently planned in the United States. Additional data are available on oxcarbazepine (Gram & Philbert 1986).

**Progabide**

Progabide acts by direct stimulation of the GABA receptors. Its acid metabolite shows similar activity. Although usually referred to as a GABA agonist, progabide is considered by some to be a GABA prodrug.

Early clinical trials of progabide were promising, and sufficient data were accumulated to allow for the marketing of the drug in France. Applications are pending in several other European countries, and clinical studies have been initiated in Japan. Two multicenter studies in the United States, however, suggested a limited benefit/risk ratio, and studies in this country have been discontinued. Additional data on progabide are available (Morselli et al 1986).

**Vigabatrin**

Vigabatrin, gamma-vinyl GABA, is an irreversible inhibitor of GABA-transaminase and increases brain GABA concentrations in animals. Its mechanism, therefore, is presumably one of increased inhibitory synaptic activity.

Numerous clinical studies have been initiated in the United States and in Europe, and initial efficacy data are encouraging. However, because of white matter lesions in the brains of animals, additional studies in the United States have been stopped by the Federal Food and Drug Administration. Trials continue in Europe as the significance of these lesions remains uncertain. Additional information is available on vigabatrin (Schechter 1986).

**Zonisamide**

Zonisamide is a benzisoxazole with minimal carbonic anhydrase activity. It is active against maximal electroshock in rodents. Its mechanism of action is thought to be similar to that of phenytoin.

Zonisamide was very advanced in its development with efficacy well documented in multiple controlled clinical trials. The unexpected appearance of renal calculi caused the compound to be abandoned by the pharmaceutical sponser. Additional information on zonisamide is available (Taylor et al 1986).

**Other new compounds in clinical trials**
A number of new compounds currently in clinical trials have not been reviewed in this chapter either because activity with the compound is proceeding slowly or because inadequate new information is available. Some data are available for clobazam, denzimal, eterobarb, flupirtine, and stiripentol in individual chapters of Meldrum & Porter (1986).

## SUMMARY

The development of new antiepileptic drugs is a prolonged process. Its history is filled with both science and serendipity. The advent of renewed interest by pharmaceutical companies, coupled with rigorous standards for clinical evaluation, allows promise and hope for the future of millions of patients with uncontrolled epilepsy.

## REFERENCES

Albertoni P 1882 Untersuchungen uber die Wirkung einiger Arzneimittel auf die Erregbarkeit des Grosshirns nebst Beitragen zur Therapie der Epilepsie. Arch Exp Pathol Pharmakol 15: 248–288
Bartoszyk G D, Meyerson N, Reimann W, Satzinger G, von Hodenberg A 1986 Gabapentin. In: Meldrum B S, Porter R J (eds) New anticonvulsant drugs. Libbey, London, p 147–163
Buhles W C Jr, Wallach M B, Chaplin M D, Treiman D M 1986 Nafimidone. In: Meldrum B S, Porter R J (eds) New anticonvulsant drugs. Libbey, London, p 203–214
Cereghino J J, Penry J K 1982 Testing of antiepileptic drugs in humans: clinical considerations. In: Woodbury D M, Penry J K, Pippenger C E (eds) Antiepileptic drugs, 2nd edn. Raven Press, New York, p 141–157
Chalmers T C, Celano P, Sacks H S, Smith H 1983 Bias in treatment assignment in controlled clinical trials. New England Journal of Medicine 309: 1358–1361
Chen G, Portman R, Ensor C R, Bratton A C Jr 1951 The anticonvulsant activity of a-phenyl succinimides. J Pharmacol Exp Ther 103: 54–61
Commission for the Control of Epilepsy and Its Consequences 1978 Plan for nationwide action on epilepsy. Vol I DHEW Publication No. (NIH) 78–276 US Department of Health Education and Welfare, Washington, DC
Commission on Classification and Terminology of the International League Against Epilepsy 1981 Proposal for revised clinical and electroencephalographic classification of epileptic seizures. Epilepsia 22: 489–501
de Graff J S, Redpath J, Sam A P, Sitsen J M A, Timmer C J, van der Waart M 1986 Org 6370. In: Meldrum B S, Porter R J (eds) New anticonvulsant drugs. Libbey, London, p 215–227
Drug Amendments Act of 1962 Public Law 87–781, 21 USC 355
Federal Food and Drugs Administration Act of 1906 Public Law 384, 59th Congress
Federal Food, Drug, and Cosmetic Act of 1938 Public Law 717, 75th Congress
Goodman L S, Grewal M S, Brown W C, Swinyard E A 1953 Comparison of maximal seizures evoked by pentylenetetrazol (Metrazol) and electroshock in mice, and their modification by anticonvulsants. J Pharmacol Exp Ther 108: 168–176
Gram L, Philbert A 1986 Oxcarbazepine. In: Meldrum B S, Porter R J (eds) New anticonvulsant drugs. Libbey, London, p 229–235
Hauptmann A 1912 Luminal bei Epilepsie. Munch Med Wochensehr 59: 1907–1909
Hauser W A, Annegers J F, Anderson V E 1983 Epidemiology and the genetics of epilepsy. In: Ward A A Jr, Penry J K, Purpura D (eds) Epilepsy. Raven Press, New York, p 267–294
Holmes G L, McKeerer M, Adamson M 1987 Absence seizures in children: clinical and electroencephalographic features. Annals of Neurology 21: 268–273
Kurtzke J F 1986 Neuroepidemiology: assessment of therapeutic trials. Annals of Neurology 19 (no 4): 311–319
Locock C 1857 Discussion of paper by E H Sieveking: analysis of 52 cases of epilepsy observed by the author. Lancet 1: 527
Mattson R H, Cramer J A, Collins J F et al 1985 Comparison of carbamazepine, phenobarbital, phenytoin, and primidone in partial and secondarily generalized tonic-clonic seizures. New England Journal of Medicine 313: 145–151
Meldrum B S 1986 Pharmacological approaches to the treatment of epilepsy. In: Meldrum B S, Porter R J (eds) New anticonvulsant drugs. Libbey, London, p 17–30

Meldrum B S, Porter R J 1986 New anticonvulsant drugs. Libbey, London
Merritt H H, Putnam T J 1938a A new series of anticonvulsant drugs tested by experiments on animals. Arch Neurol Psychiatry 39: 1003–1015
Merritt H H, Putnam T J 1938b Sodium dipheny hydantoinate in the treatment of convulsive disorders. JAMA 111: 1068–1073
Miller A A, Sawyer D A, Roth B et al 1986 Lamotrigine. In: Meldrum B S, Porter R J (eds) New anticonvulsant drugs. Libbey, London, p 165–177
Morselli P L, Bartholini G, Lloyd K G 1986 Progabide. In: Meldrum B S, Porter R J (eds) New anticonvulsant drugs. Libbey, London, p 237–253
Perhach J L, Weliky I, Newton J J, Sofia R D, Romanyshyn W M, Ardnt W F Jr 1986 In: Meldrum B S, Porter R J (eds) New anticonvulsant drugs. Libbey, London, p 117–123
Porter R J 1984 Epilepsy: 100 elementary principles. Saunders, London
Porter R J 1986a Clinical trials relating to epilepsy. In: Proceedings of the 13th World Congress of Neurology. Springer-Verlag, Berlin, p 305–312
Porter R J 1986b Antiepileptic drugs: efficacy and inadequacy. In: Meldrum B S, Porter R J (eds) New anticonvulsant drugs. Libbey, London, p 3–15
Porter R J, Nadi N S 1987 Investigations in the pharmacotherapy of the focal epilepsies. In: Weiser H G, Speckmann E H, Engel J (eds) The epileptic focus. Libbey, London, p 175–191
Porter R J, Pitlick W H 1986 Antiepileptic drugs. In: Katzung B G (ed) Basic and clinical pharmacology, 3rd edn. Lange Medical, Los Altos, p 262–278
Porter R J, White B G 1986 Evaluation in man. In: Meldrum B S, Porter R J (eds) New anticonvulsant drugs. Libbey, London, p 49–61
Porter R J, Cereghino J J, Gladding G D et al 1984 Antiepileptic drug development program. Cleveland Clinic Quarterly 51: 293–305
Richards R K, Everett G M 1944 Analgesic and anticonvulsive properties of 3,5,5-trimethyloxazolidine-2,4-dione (Tridione). Fed Proc 3: 39
Roba J, Cavalier R, Cordi A et al 1986 Milacemide. In: Meldrum BS, Porter R J (eds) New anticonvulsant drugs. Libbey, London, p 179–190
Sato S, White B G, Penry J K, Dreifuss F E, Sackellares J C, Kupferberg H J 1982 Valproic acid versus ethosuximide in the treatment of absence seizures. Neurology 32: 157–163
Schechter P J 1986 Vigabatrin. In: Meldrum B S, Porter R J (eds) New anticonvulsant drugs. Libbey, London, p 265–275
Spiegel E A 1937 Quantitative determination of the convulsive reactivity by electric stimulation of the brain with the skull intact. J Lab Clin Med 22: 1274–1276
Stone W E 1972 Systemic chemical convulsants and metabolic derangements. In: Purpura D P, Penry J K, Tower D B, Woodbury D M, Walter R D (eds) Experimental models of epilepsy — A manual for the laboratory worker. Raven Press, New York, p 407–432
Swinyard E A 1949 Laboratory assay of clinically effective antiepileptic drugs. Journal of the American Pharmaceutical Association 38: 201–204
Swinyard E A 1982 Introduction. In: Woodbury D M, Penry J K, Pippenger C E (eds) Antiepileptic drugs, 2nd edn. Raven Press, New York, p 1–9
Taylor C P, McLean J R, Bockbrader H N et al 1986 Zonisamide: AD-810, CI-912. In: Meldrum B S, Porter R J (eds) New anticonvulsant drugs. Libbey, London, p 277–294
Troupin A S, Mendius J R, Cheng F, Risinger M W 1986 MK-801. In: Meldrum B S, Porter R J (eds) New anticonvulsant drugs. Libbey, London, p 191–201
van Belle G, Tempkin N 1983 Design strategies in the clinical evaluation of new antiepileptic drugs. In: Pedley T A, Meldrum B S (eds) Recent advances in epilepsy — 1. Churchill Livingstone, Edinburgh, p 93–112
Vanden Bussche G, Wauquier A, Ashton D, de Beukelaar F 1986 Flunarizine. In: Meldrum B S, Porter R J (eds) New anticonvulsant drugs. Libbey, London, p 125–133

# 9. Corpus callosotomy in the treatment of intractable seizures

*S. S. Spencer*

## INTRODUCTION

Conservatively, 300 000 epileptic patients in the United States alone are uncontrolled by optimal medical management. These patients represent a spectrum of seizure types and of associated neurological syndromes. Some patients are neurologically normal and fully functional because their seizures are mild or relatively infrequent, and others may be devastated mainly by their associated neurological deficits. The great majority, however, may have some neurological deficit but are mostly disabled by their seizures which are of considerable frequency and severity. In this group, treatment alternatives involving risks and unknown factors are often an acceptable, and someties the only, possibility for improved quality of life. The choices are experimental drug protocols and epilepsy surgery.

Few operative procedures for epilepsy have withstood the test of time. Stereotactic lesions of various structures including H fields, reticular formation, and thalamic nuclei, and cerebellar stimulation are examples of this evanescence. Presently accepted surgical options for uncontrolled epilepsy are confined to resective procedures, hemispherectomy, and corpus callosum section (Spencer 1986).

Resective procedures are preferred whenever possible since they offer the possibility of cure with usually predictable and often minimal neurological sequelae. This approach requires definition of a single localizable epileptic focus as the site of habitual seizure origin and its location in a resectable region of brain. Hemispherectomy is the most extreme resective procedure and is applicable to patients with severe cerebral damage and significant motor impairments who have multifocal seizures of unilateral origin (Goodman et al 1985).

Although the majority of operations performed for uncontrolled epilepsy are resective procedures, such approaches will be unsuccessful if the focus is poorly defined (multifocal or unlocalized) or if the region involved is only partially resectable. This situation commonly arises with extratemporal foci (Spencer & Spencer 1985, Spencer 1986). In some patients who are not candidates for a resective procedure, for whatever reason, the only surgical possibility is corpus callosum section (CCS).

The first 31 corpus callosum sectioned patients at Yale will form the basis for a discussion of the (few) agreements and (multitudinous) controversies which continue to surround the use of this procedure for uncontrolled epilepsy of focal or multifocal origin without a definable or resectable focus.

## DEVELOPMENT

It is likely that over the last century thousands of animals in laboratories across the globe have undergone section of the cerebral commissures including or confined to the corpus callosum in the course of anatomical and physiological studies. The application of these experimental models to epilepsy began in 1940 with Erikson. Because of the variability in (1) commissural connections in different species, (2) surgical technique and methods of verification of section among basic investigators, (3) appropriate chronic animal models of human epilepsy, and (4) outcome including at least some experiments in which disruption of normal commissural connections seemed to exacerbate seizures, it is perhaps fortunate that VanWagenen and Herren, simultaneous with the initiation of the early animal studies, applied the technique to epileptic humans, based on clinical rationale, without the knowledge of experimental results in animals (VanWagenen & Herren 1940).

Clinical experience had not shown significant deficits when neurosurgical procedures involved at least partial section of the corpus callosum, and anatomical reasoning dictated that such an interruption of interhemispheric electrical discharges might help patients who were devastated by generalized seizures. Indeed, VanWagenen and Herren's trials of this procedure were prompted by patients with fortuitous disconnection secondary to other processes which seemed coincidentally to afford some relief of seizures. Despire its success in some patients, however, criteria for cerebal commissurotomy were not developed and the procedure did not develop as many other newly described, successful techniques. The desired effect on seizures in early patients was overshadowed by an unacceptably high complication rate. In 1962, Bogen and Vogal reported a case of epilepsy treated by commissurotomy, but it was not until 1975 that any single center reported more than 10 patients in detail with attempts to synthesize the indications for this procedure. Donald Wilson at Dartmouth deserves the credit for giving the current impetus to use commissurotomy for epilepsy, which is reflected now in ever growing numbers of reported cases (see Fig. 9.1) (Wilson

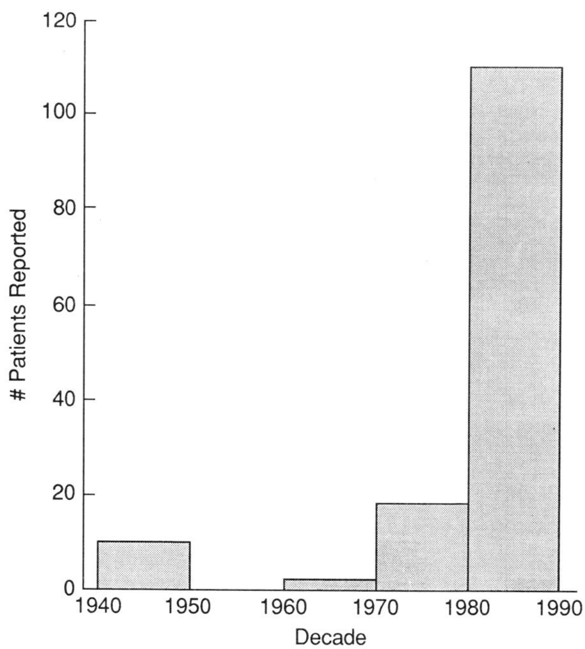


**Fig. 9.1** Reported cases of callosotomy by decade.

et al 1977, 1978, 1982). He and his colleagues' contributions included the careful analysis of complications of the procedure itself, especially ventriculitis, hydrocephalus, and meningitis, with subsequent revision of the procedure from *complete commissurotomy* (section of the corpus callosum, anterior commissure, 1 fornix, and the hippocampal commissure) to *frontal commissurotomy* (section of the rostral half of the corpus callosum, anterior commissure, and 1 fornix) to *central commissurotomy* (section of the corpus callosum and hippocampal commissure). They established that there was no significant difference in the effects on seizures among these various procedures, but there was a clear decline in the rate and severity of postoperative complications using the modified central commissurotomy technique. The final modification was to stage the procedure so that part of the corpus callosum (usually the posterior half in the early series) was sectioned first and then the callosotomy was completed at a second operation (Harbaugh et al 1983). This staging was found to reduce the duration of the postoperative disconnection syndrome characterized by abulia, incontinence, and apraxia of the nondominant hand (Ross et al 1984).

The exact procedure used for cerebral commissurotomy has continued to evolve. Other centers instituted anterior section of the corpus callosum alone, demonstrating it to be as effective as total section in some patients, particularly those with frontal lobe seizure foci (Avila et al 1980, Wada & Moyes 1983, Marino 1985, Marino & Ragazzo 1985). Lack of strict criteria for when partial section might be sufficient has resulted in the policy presently followed at Yale. We perform a two-stage central commissurotomy in which demonstrated failure after the initial portion of the section is the prerequisite for completion of the section (Spencer et al 1987b,c). In fact, completion of the section is required in at least half of our patients, and this number is increasing with time. The anterior portion is usually sectioned first because most of our patients have frontal lobe seizure foci, but on occasions when EEG criteria suggest more posterior seizure onset, the initial section is posterior. Further modifications at other centers include anterior callosal section combined with limited frontal cortical resection, a procedure which is certainly effective as reported but confuses clinical studies designed to clarify the most appropriate technique for the individual patient (Bouvier et al 1983, St Hilaire et al 1985), and section of various portions of the corpus callosum alone as dictated by EEG abnormalities (Marino 1985).

For simplicity and consistency herein, the exact operation will be designated by the term initially applied to it in these early reports. These terms are indeed logical, although other names have been applied in a haphazard fashion. Table 9.1 gives the acceptable terminology including synonyms and structures sectioned. In this review, the term corpus callosum section (CCS) implies section of the corpus callosum and hippocampal commissure; it is synonymous with the term central commissurotomy, and represents the usual present day approach.

A full description of operative technique(s) is beyond the scope of this chapter, but unfortunately the reader cannot be referred to any single authoritative source. Wilson's initial intentions in modifying the technique stemmed from a desire to avoid entering the ventricular system which he deemed responsible for the high rate of complications seen in complete and frontal commissurotomy (Harbaugh et al 1983, Wilson et al 1978, 1982). His modified technique for section of corpus callosum and hippocampal commissure, still practiced at Dartmouth (Roberts 1985), involves a two-stage section through anteriorly and posteriorly situated trephines with minimal

**Table 9.1** Terminology for commissurotomy procedures

| Procedure name | Structures sectioned |
|---|---|
| Complete commissurotomy | Corpus callosum, hippocampal commissure, anterior commissure, 1 fornix |
| Frontal commissurotomy | Rostral 1/2 of corpus callosum, anterior commissure, 1 fornix |
| Central commissurotomy (commonly called callosotomy or corpus callosum section) | Corpus callosum and hippocampal commissure |
| Anterior callosotomy (or anterior callosal section) | Rostral portion (variable amount) of corpus callosum |
| Posterior commissurotomy (or posterior callosotomy) | Caudal portion (variable amount) of corpus callosum and hippocampal commissure |

exposure. At Yale, although the structures intended for section are the same, adequate intraventricular exposure enables visualization of the foramen of Monroe (felt to be essential to assure complete section of the rostrum), and the fornices (to assure complete section of the hippocampal commissure). Ventricular access is thus intentional in this approach, and no appreciable complication rate has been observed. A recent spate of papers emphasizing less than complete section of corpus callosum by MRI after supposed complete section underlines the relevance of this issue (Gazzaniga et al 1985, Gates et al 1987, Sussman et al 1987).

## EXPECTATIONS

The expectation voiced by VanWagenen and Herren in 1940 remains the rationale for the use of CCS in 1987: division of the main interhemispheric pathway should prevent seizures from generalizing from one hemisphere to the other, and (implicitly) from one side of the body to the other. Despite increasing clinical experience, sophisticated anatomical mapping studies, intensive study of laboratory models, and careful EEG analyses, the pathophysiological basis for this logic is still not established. A consistent dichotomy between the lack of generalization of the clinical seizure and the continued generalization of at least some of the paroxysmal EEG discharges has been established in both animals and man after CCS (Torres & French 1973, Spencer et al 1987a, Spencer et al 1985, Gates et al 1985). Animal data establish the existence of pathways both through the corpus callosum and through diencephalic/brainstem structures which are utilized in the generalization of the EEG discharge from a unilateral focus (Kopeloff et al 1950, Mattson & Bickford 1961, Marcus & Watson 1968, Ottino et al 1971). That the clinical seizure should no longer become generalized is not logical but true, and accounts for our continuing use of this technique. The goals of the operation remain explicitly the same: the elimination of clinical seizure generalization in patients with secondary generalized seizures.

VanWagenen and Herren also knew that division of the corpus callosum in the relatively intact neurosurgical patient was not associated with detectable neurological deficit. This observation has subsequently been substantiated in patients with third ventricular lesions which are resected through a trans-callosal approach (Long & Chou 1973, Shucart & Stein 1978). Unfortunately chronic epileptic patients are not relatively intact, as they often have a significant history of early cerebral injury which has infinite possibilities for unusual cerebral reorganization. Nevertheless, the neurological function of these patients after CCS is not generally significantly altered (but see further on). The goal thus remains completion of CCS with a minimum of neurologic sequelae. Since we lack the means to determine the extent of cerebral functional reorganization, the effects of disconnection must remain speculative in certain patients.

## JUDGING OUTCOME

The perspective of goal is critical in judging outcome. If the goal of CCS is the elimination of clinically generalized seizures, then accomplishment of this goal should represent a perfect outcome. Unfortunately many reports judge outcome in terms of percentage reduction of all seizure types, which contradicts the intended result.

More difficult to assimilate in judging outcome are the other changes in seizures which may occur after CCS. Patients may cease to have generalized seizures but may have increased numbers of partial seizures (Rayport et al 1983, 1985, Spencer et al 1984, 1987a, Gates et al 1987). Should deterioration in control of partial seizures nullify the 'perfect' result?

The neurologic sequelae of CCS may also affect perceived outcome. Clearly the marked increase in reports of CCS parallel a decreasing operative complication rate and growing perception that the procedure is 'safe'.

Nonetheless the degree to which neurologic function is reported to be different postoperatively varies widely (see below), and many combine with changes in seizure frequency and type to produce widely differing functional results.

## THE YALE EXPERIENCE

The Yale series is presented first because I have personally analysed the data and have personal knowledge of the patients. Thirty-one patients have had CCS since 1979, including 15 with total section of the corpus callosum and hippocampal commissure, and 16 with anterior corpus callosum section alone. These patients have been only partially reported before (Spencer et al 1987b, c, Sass et al 1987).

### Seizure frequency

1. 80% had complete cessation of generalized seizures (including tonic, atonic, and tonic-clonic types) and falls after total CCS, while 50% stopped having generalized seizures and falls after partial (anterior) corpus callosum section.
2. About 50% had no further complex partial seizures after total section.
3. Two patients had no further seizures of any type but remain on medications.
4. About 25% of our patients developed more intense partial seizures (simple or complex), at times with a prolonged latency (up to 4 years). This occurred after either partial or total section.
5. In patients with limited intellectual capacity, the more intense partial seizures were a poor trade-off for control of generalized seizures because of fear due to retained consciousness during seizures.

### EEG findings

1. Most patients had a decrease in bisynchronous EEG discharges which were replaced by focal, often alternating, spikes (Figs. 9.2, 9.3).

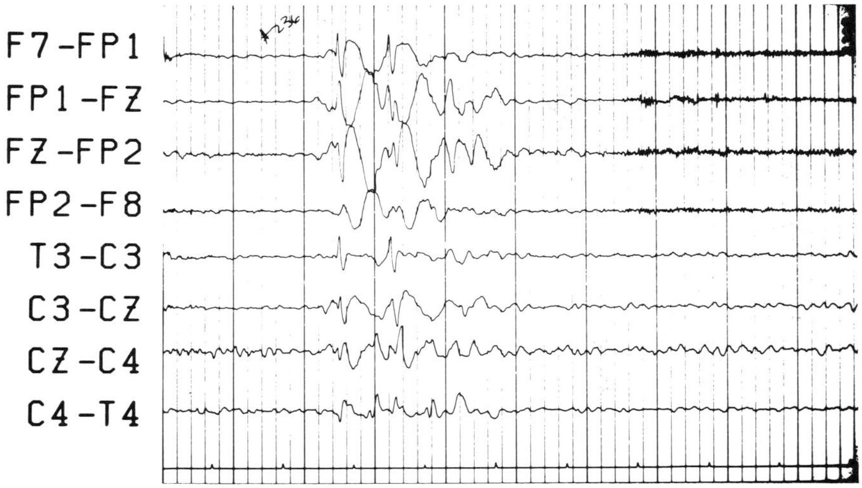


**Fig. 9.2** Preoperative EEG, shows bilaterally synchronous bursts of sharp and slow wave discharge.

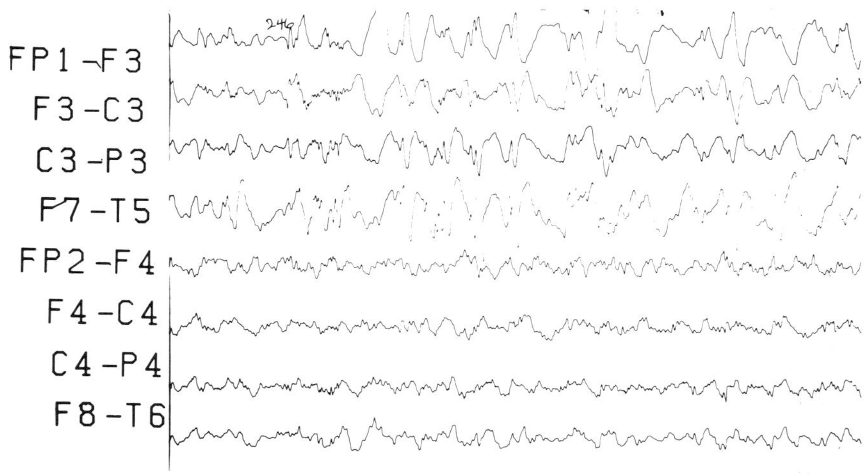


**Fig. 9.3** Same patient as Figure 9.2, postoperatively, shows strictly left-sided paroxysmal activity with same sharp and slow wave morphology.

2. There was an occasional increase in frequency of focal EEG discharges, surpassing the preoperative frequency of bilateral discharges. These were poorly correlated with development of more intense focal seizures.

3. It was rare for EEG bisynchrony to be completely eliminated.

4. Some patients showed clear EEG lateralization of ictal onset after CCS, despite bilateral ictal onset before surgery (Figs. 9.4, 9.5).

**Operative complications**

1. Previously reported operative complications of ventriculitis, meningitis, and hydrocephalus were not seen.

2. Five patients had severe and frequent focal seizures immediately postoperatively which resolved over several weeks.

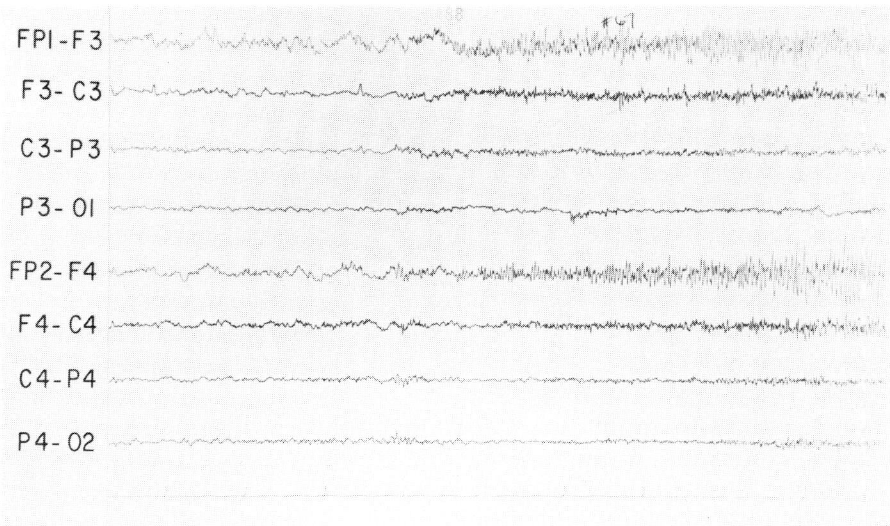


**Fig. 9.4** Preoperative seizure with bilateral simultaneous low voltage high frequency onset.

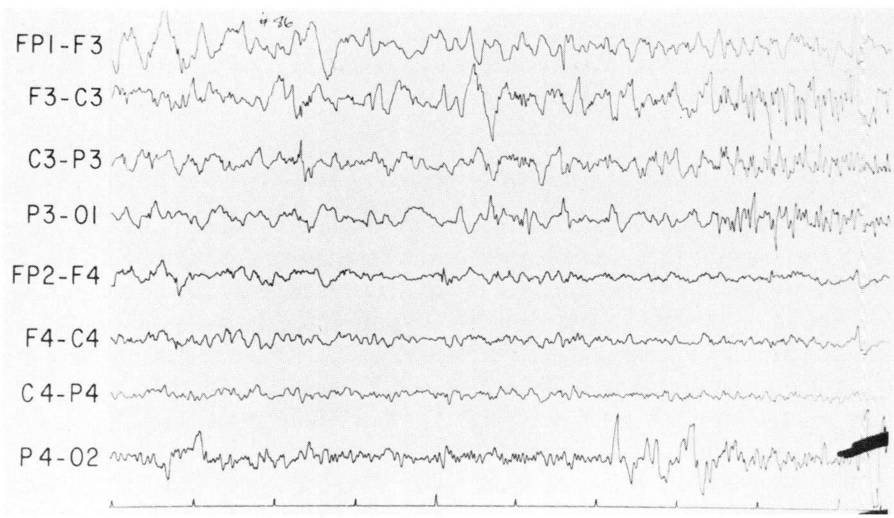


**Fig. 9.5** Seizure in same patient as Figure 9.4, postoperatively, which has clearly identifiable left central seizure onset with high frequency low voltage spiking.

3. Disconnection syndrome could occur after partial or complete section, but was minimal in severity and length after staged procedures.

*Neurologic function*

1. New motor deficits usually represented an exacerbation of pre-existing weakness, and improved to baseline or nearly so within the first 6 postoperative months.
2. Noticeable cognitive deficits were rare.
3. Language impairments predictably and exclusively followed CCS in patients

with opposite hemispheres controlling speech and handedness (e.g. right handed, right hemisphere dominant or left handed, left hemisphere dominant individuals).

4. Preoperative aggressive behavior disorders were occasionally more pronounced.

Analysis of predictor variables to enable selection of patients with the greatest benefit to risk ratio has revealed no perfect criteria, but multiple trends. Patients with low IQ (less than 45) were more likely to have persistent generalized seizures; patients with bilateral (usually frontal) independent foci were most likely to develop more intense focal seizures; and patients with well localized (but unresectable) seizure foci were most likely to be cured of complex partial seizures. With respect to neurological outcome, the model proposed by Novelly & Lifrak (1985) was most applicable: CCS might reinstate earlier deficits which were partially resolved by interhemispheric co-operation. Thus, patients who sustained severe unilateral cerebral damage before 6 years of age had few neurological defecits since recovery was presumably due to assumption of functions by the intact hemisphere. On the other hand, patients with only moderate degrees of damage, or damage occurring later in life, whose recovery would more likely involve interhemispheric mechanisms to utilize some portions of the damaged hemisphere, were more likely to exhibit increased deficits in motor, cognitive, and behavioral spheres. This was particularly evident in language function, since patients with impaired language after CCS consistently had contralateral speech and handedness representation, thus requiring the two hemispheres to communicate for language-related tasks. More often, deficits after CCS did not arise de novo, but represented an increase in an existing liability.

## COMPARISON OF YALE RESULTS WITH OTHER CENTERS

The Yale results to date form a basis for comparison with other published reports. Table 9.2 juxtaposes the basic elements of the cumulative experiences with cerebral commissurotomy. When single centers published multiple reports on the same groups of patients, only the report with the most detailed information was used in this table to avoid overrepresentation of the experience at any one institution. Only basic information categories were selected for inclusion in the table, and are those which appear to offer the most promise of developing criteria for patient selection. Since reports and centers vary in the amount of information presented or obtained, details are not strictly comparable, but information is generally sufficient for valid comparisons.

### Areas of agreement

Most compelling is the disparity in the data. A particular patient with any IQ score, any neurological examination, and EEG pattern, or any seizure characteristics or frequencies, might have an excellent response to CCS. Similarly, almost any combination of preoperative characteristics might be associated with increased postoperative neurological deficit and no appreciable change in seizure frequency or seizure type. Nevertheless, these reports are in agreement on some important observations: (1) A significant majority of patients with secondary generalized seizures responded to central commissurotomy with marked decrease or elimination of tonic-clonic, tonic and atonic seizures. This eliminated falls. (2) Patients with a history of frequent episodes of status epilepticus usually had few or no further attacks of status.

**Table 9.2** Review of literature on cerebral commissurotomy.

| Author | | Diagnosis | Procedure | Seizure change | Neurological change | EEG change |
|---|---|---|---|---|---|---|
| Amacher (1976) | 1 | L hemiplegia, unknown etiology | Complete commissurotomy (see text) | Full control of GTC, marked ↓ focal szs | None persistant, some better (data for all 4 patients lumped) | No data |
| | 2 | Encephalitis | Complete commissurotomy | Full control of GTC, 50% ↓ akinetic and focal szs | | No data |
| | 3 | Encephalitis | Complete commissurotomy | 90% ↓ GTC, no akinetic szs | | No data |
| | 4 | Hypoxia | Complete commissurotomy | Cured of GTC and akinetic spells | | No data |
| Blume (1984) | 1–8 | No data | Anterior callosotomy | 3 with less szs and falls (all IQs >64), 3 with no change (all IQs <66), 2 with equivocal results | No permanent sequelae | No data |
| Bogen & Vogel (1975) (see also Bogen 1965, Bogen & Vogel 1962, Zaidel & Sperry 1974) | 1 | Trauma | Complete commissurotomy (see text) | Elimination of GTC and status, persistant SP and CP | Apractic L hand | No data |
| | 2 | Calcification on skull X-ray | Complete commissurotomy | No szs on meds | None | ↓ LT focus |
| | 3 | Anoxia | Complete commissurotomy | ↓ ↓ GTC spells, persistant tonic szs | L hand apraxia and mutism | No data |
| | 4 | Birth trauma | Complete commissurotomy | Poor data | L leg spasticity | No data |
| | 5 | Birth trauma | Complete commissurotomy | Continued R adversive szs | Mute for 3 m; aggressive | No data |
| | 6 | Birth trauma | Complete commissurotomy | No GTC; rare SP | None | No data |
| | 7 | Trauma | Complete commissurotomy | Rare SP and GTC | None | No data |
| | 8 | Unknown etiology | Complete commissurotomy | ↓ Frequency but persistant GTC | None | No data |
| | 9 | Unknown etiology | Complete commissurotomy | Only brief CP and much less frequent | L hand apraxia | No data |
| | 10 | Trauma | Complete commissurotomy | No GTC while on meds, ↓ ↓ frequency CP | L hand apraxia | No data |
| Bouvier et al (1983) (see also St Hilaire et al 1982) | 1 | No data | Frontal corticectomy and 4 cm anterior callosotomy | Cured | Better | Better |
| | 2 | No data | 8 cm anterior callosotomy | 90% ↓ in szs | Slight improvement | No change |
| | 3 | No data | 8 cm anterior callosotomy | 85% ↓ in szs | No change | No change |
| | 4 | No data | Frontal corticectomy and 4 cm anterior callosotomy | Cured | No change | Improved |
| | 5 | No data | 6 cm anterior callosotomy | 85% ↓ in szs | No change | No change |
| | 6 | No data | Frontal corticectomy and 4 cm anterior callosotomy | 95% ↓ in szs | Marked ↓ in function | Better |
| | 7 | No data | 6 cm anterior callosotomy | 90% ↓ in szs | Marked ↓ in function | Better |
| | 8 | No data | 6 cm anterior callosotomy | 90% ↓ in szs | Improved | Better |
| | 9 | No data | 8 cm anterior callosotomy | 60% ↓ in szs | No change | No change |
| | 10 | No data | 6 cm posterior callosotomy | 90% ↓ in szs | Improved | Better |

**Table 9.2** (*cont.*)

| Author | | Diagnosis | Procedure | Seizure change | Neurological change | EEG change |
|---|---|---|---|---|---|---|
| Gates et al (1987) | 1 | Unknown etiology | Total central commissuorotomy, 1 stage (see text) | ↓ ↓ Tonic, atonic, CP; no more SP or GTC | No data | No more bisync. |
| | 2 | Encephalitis | Total central commissurotomy, 1 stage | Elimination of GTC, tonic, atonic; ↑ CP | No data | ↓ ↓ Bisync. |
| | 3 | Birth trauma | Total central commissurotomy, 1 stage | Elimination of tonic, atonic, GTC, CP; new SP | No data | No more bisync. |
| | 4 | Birth trauma | Total central commissurotomy, 1 stage | ↓ ↓ Tonic, atonic; elimination of GTC and CP | No data | No more bisync. |
| | 5 | Unknown etiology | Total central commissurotomy, 1 stage | Elimination of tonic, atonic, GTC, CP; new SP | No data | No change |
| | 6 | Neuroblastoma | Total central commissurotomy, 1 stage | Elimination of GTC, no change in tonic or atonic, ↑ CP | No data | No more bisync. |
| | 7 | Birth trauma | Total central commissurotomy, 1 stage | ↓ ↓ Tonic, atonic, GTC; no change in CP | No data | No data |
| | 8 | Encephalitis | Total central commissurotomy, 1 stage | ↓ ↓ Tonic, atonic, GCT; ↑ CP | No data | No data |
| | 9 | Birth trauma | Total central commissurotomy, 1 stage | ↓ ↓ Tonic, atonic; slight ↑ CP | No data | No data |
| | 10 | Birth trauma | Total central commissurotomy, 1 stage | Elimination of GTC; ↓ ↓ tonic, atonic, CP | No data | No data |
| | 11 | Unknown etiology | Total central commissurotomy, 1 stage | Elimination of tonic, atonic, CP, GTC; new SP | No data | No data |
| | 12 | Trauma | Total central commissurotomy, 1 stage | Elimination of tonic, atonic, CP | No data | No data |
| | 13 | Birth trauma | Total central commissurotomy, 1 stage | ↓ ↓ Tonic, atonic, CP | No data | No data |
| | 14 | Encephalitis | Total central commissurotomy, 1 stage | ↓ ↓ Tonic, atonic, GTC; ↑ CP | No data | No data |
| | 15 | Unknown etiology | Total central commissurotomy, 1 stage | Elimination of tonic, atonic, ↓ CP | No data | No data |
| | 16 | Trauma | Total central commissurotomy, 1 stage | ↓ Tonic, atonic, GTC | No data | No data |
| | 17 | Encephalitis | Total central commissurotomy, 1 state | ↓ ↓ Tonic, atonic, less ↓ CP, no more GTC | No data | No data |
| | 18 | Birth trauma | Total central commissurotomy, 1 stage | No change in tonic, atonic; ↑ CP | No data | No data |
| | 19 | Unknown etiology | Total central commissurotomy, 1 stage | ↓ ↓ Tonic, atonic, less decrease CP, no more GTC | No data | No data |
| | 20 | Unknown etiology | Total central commissurotomy, 1 stage | ↓ Tonic, atonic | No data | No data |
| | 21 | Unknown etiology | Total central commissurotomy, 1 stage | Elimination of GTC, ↓ ↓ tonic, atonic | No data | No data |
| | 22 | Unknown etiology | Total central commissurotomy, 1 stage | Elimination of tonic, atonic, CP | No data | No data |

**Table 9.2** (*cont.*)

| Author | | Diagnosis | Procedure | Seizure change | Neurological change | EEG change |
|---|---|---|---|---|---|---|
| Gates et al (1987) | 23 | Trauma | Total central commissurotomy, 1 stage | ↓ ↓ Tonic, atonic, GTC; new CP | No data | No data |
| | 24 | Unknown etiology | Total central commissurotomy, 1 stage | ↓ ↓ Tonic, atonic, GTC; no change in CP | No data | No data |
| Geoffrey et al (1983) | 1 | Unknown etiology, retarded | Total central commissurotomy, 1 stage (see text) | Cured of GTC and absence, still myoclonic | ↑ Cooperation ↑ Function | Less paroxysmal |
| | 2 | Premature | Total central commissurotomy, 1 stage | Still GTC, new focal | ↑ Awareness and speech | ↓ Generalization |
| | 3 | Retarded unknown etiology | Total central commissurotomy, 1 stage | No more absence and akinetic, still myoclonic | ↑ Awareness | ↓ Generalization |
| | 4 | Congenital hydrocephalus | Total central commissurotomy, 1 stage | Akinetic cured new focal szs | ↑ Arousal and coordination | No generalization |
| | 5 | Cytomegalovirus infection | Total central commissurotomy, 1 stage | Absence cured, still akinetic | ↑ Control | More focal |
| | 6 | Prenatal encephalopathy | Total central commissurotomy, 1 stage | No more GTC, new akinetic | ↑ Equilibrium | ↓ ↓ Bisync. |
| | 7 | Microcephaly, retarded | Total central commissurotomy, 1 stage | Eliminated GTC, new focal szs | ↑ Control and coordination | Bilateral independent |
| | 8 | Neonatal encephalopathy | Total central commissurotomy, 1 stage | Eliminated GTC, new focal szs | ↑ Contact and grasp | More focal |
| | 9 | Congenital hydrocephalus | Total central commissurotomy, 1 stage | Eliminated GTC, absence and akinetic; new focal szs | ↑ Cooperation and equilibrium | More focal |
| Luessenhop et al (1970) | 1 | Infantile hemiplegia and retardation | Complete commissurotomy (see text) | Very rare generalized szs, marked ↓ in frequency | Very impaired preop,? no change | L spikes, no change |
| | 2 | Neonatal szs, slow development | Complete commissurotomy | ↓ Frequency, only focal szs | No change | RF spikes, no change |
| | 3 | Progressive encephalopathy from infancy | Complete commissurotomy | No GTC, ↓ focal szs | No change, (maybe better) | More lateralized |
| | 4 | Neonatal onset, retarded | Complete commissurotomy | No change | No change, (very impaired to start) | No data |
| Marina et al (1982) (see also Avila et al 1980) | 1–5 | Generalized epilepsy | Not specified for individual groups but included 14 with anterior 1/3 callosotomy, 2 with section of trunk only, 2 with | ↓ ↓ Or elimination of absence, less improvement in other seizure types | Improved attention | Marked disruption in bisynchrony |
| | 6–14 | Lennox Gastaut syndrome | section of callosum sparing only splenium, and 2 with section of rostral | Important improvement in seizure frequency, especially absence | No data | Partial disruption of bisynchrony |
| | 15 | Sturge Weber | callosum plus frontal cortical re- | Marked improvement | No data | ↓ ↓ In bisynchrony |
| | 16 | L parietal lesion | section | | | |
| | 17 | Porencephaly | | | | |
| | 18 | Petit mal | | No change | No data | 3 Hz spike/wave with no change |
| | 19 | Adversive szs | | ↓ Frequency, SP only | No data | No data |
| | 20 | Myoclonus | | Resolution of myoclonus | No data | No data |

**Table 9.2** (*cont.*)

| Author | | Diagnosis | Procedure | Seizure change | Neurological change | EEG change |
|---|---|---|---|---|---|---|
| Rayport et al (1982, 1983) | 1 | Classical absence and GTC | Central commissurotomy, 2 stage | Four-fold ↓ in absence, no change in GTC | ? None | No data |
| | 2–9 | No data | Central commissurotomy, 2 stage | No more drop attacks in two ↓ szs of at least 1 type in 7; ↑ szs of at least 1 type in 2 | 1 severe split brain syndrome, 3 with impaired language | No data |
| Roberts et al (1983) | 1 | No data | Total central commissurotomy, 2 stage (see text) | No change | No data | Bilateral Independent (↓ bisync) |
| | 2 | No data | Total central commissurotomy, 2 stage | No absence, still CP | No data | No change |
| | 3 | No data | Total central commissurotomy, 2 stage | ↓ Akinetic | No data | Bilateral independent (↓ bisync) |
| | 4 | No data | Total central commissurotomy, 2 stage | Too soon | No data | ↓ Bisync |
| | 5 | No data | Total central commissurotomy, 2 stage | ↓ Frequency, absence and GTC | No data | Bilateral independent |
| | 6 | No data | Total central commissurotomy, 2 stage | ↓ GTC, new blinking spells | No data | Bilateral independent |
| Spencer (1987) | 1 | Infantile hemiplegia | Central commissurotomy, 1 stage (see text) | More intense CP and SP, ? any GTC | Nasty, ↑ R weakness | Less bisync |
| | 2 | Birth trauma | Central commissurotomy, 1 stage | Only SP now and no CP | ↑ IQ | No change |
| | 3 | Unknown etiology | Central commissurotomy, 1 stage | ↓ SP and ↓ CP and no more falls | Quick temper, ↓ memory and VIQ | More unilateral |
| | 4 | Perinatal injury | Central commissurotomy, 1 stage | Only SP now | Nasty, irritable, paranoid | ↓ ↓ Bisync |
| | 5 | Rasmussen's syndrome | Central commissurotomy, 1 stage | Minimal SP, no falls, no status | Improved strength and VIQ | Less bisync |
| | 6 | Unknown etiology | Central commissurotomy, 2 stage | GTC, tonic eliminated; only SP | No declines. ↑ memory and PIQ | Less bisync |
| | 7 | Unknown etiology | Anterior callosotomy | ↓ Frequency and only SP | None | ↓ ↓ Bisync |
| | 8 | Infantile hemiplegia | Central commissurotomy, 2 stage | Only SP | ↑ Speech, ↑ visual memory, ↑ verbal memory | No change |
| | 9 | AVM (R frontal) | Anterior callosotomy | Sz free on medication | None | Normal |
| | 10 | Intra uterine injury | Central commissurotomy, 2 stage | Persistent GTC, tonic, CP | ± ↓ L weakness, irritable, headaches | ↓ Bisync |
| | 11 | Rasmussen's syndrome | Central commissurotomy, 2 stage | No GTC but persistent CP and SP | Mutism, ↑ hemiparesis | No change |
| | 12 | Unknown etiology | Central commissurotomy, 2 stage | Less falling; still GTC, CP, tonic | ↓ Writing | ↓ Bisync spike/wave |
| | 13 | Electrical injury | Anterior callosotomy | Only SP but still falls | ↓ Writing, R side weak | ↓ ↓ Bisync spike/wave |
| | 14 | Unknown etiology | Central commissurotomy, 2 stage | No more GTC or falls, just SP | ↓ R arm function ↑ L side function | ↓ ↓ Bisync |
| | 15 | Trauma | Anterior callosotomy | No more drops, still GTC, CP | Poor behavior, ↓ memory | More focal, R |
| | 16 | Trauma | Anterior callosotomy | Persistent GTC and CP, mild ↓ frequency | None | Less bilateral |
| | 17 | Unknown | Central commissurotomy, 2 stage | Rare GTC, moderate ↓ CP | ↓ Writing, memory; violent | More focal |
| | 18 | ? Anaphylaxis | Anterior callosotomy | Falls, CP, and SP all ↓ by 50% | None | No change |

**Table 9.2** (*cont.*)

| Author | | Diagnosis | Procedure | Seizure change | Neurological change | EEG change |
|---|---|---|---|---|---|---|
| Spencer (1987) | 19 | Rasmussen's syndrome | Anterior callosotomy | No appreciable change | ↓ ↓ Spontaneous speech | No bisync |
| | 20 | Infantile hemiplegia | Central commissurotomy, 2 stage | No GTC but many CP and SP | None? (poor follow-up) | ↑ Focal spikes |
| | 21 | Unknown | Anterior callosotomy | Only SP, alternating sides, just as frequent | All motor functions improved | ↓ Bisync |
| | 22 | Trauma | Anterior callosotomy | ↓ ↓ GTC for 2 years, now ↑ again, still CP, new dizzy spells | ↑ Rages, ↓ memory | No change |
| | 23 | Perinatal injury and febrile szs | Anterior callosotomy | CP ↓ for 1 year, now same | Irritable, headaches | No change |
| | 24 | Unknown | Central commissurotomy, 2 stage | No GTC but now drops, same CP | ↓ Memory, ↓ R motor much better | No data |
| | 25 | Birth trauma | Anterior callosotomy | Marked ↓ GTC, (rare, nocturnal only), no falls, no CP | ↓ Spontaneity of speech, stiff on L | No data |
| | 26 | Perinatal injury | Anterior callosotomy | Still rare GTC, ↓ frequency CP and SP, no falls | ↓ R dexterity and strength, improved speech | ↓ bisync |
| | 27 | Trauma | Anterior callosotomy | ↓ Frequency but persistent CP, GTC | ↑ Verbal memory | No change LF spikes |
| | 28 | Perinatal injury | Central commissurotomy, 2 stage | ↓ ↓ Falls, ↑ focal szs | Rages, ↓ verbal memory | No data |
| | 29 | Perinatal injury | Anterior callosotomy | None since surgery | Poor writing, lazy | More focal |
| | 30 | Perinatal injury | Anterior callosotomy | No change, persistent CP szs | Stuttering, irritable, ↓ PIQ | No data |
| | 31 | Trauma | Anterior callosotomy | Still GTC, CP, tonic but nocturnal and ↓ frequency | More alert, ↓ L grip | No data |
| Van Wagenen & Herren (1940) | 1 | Perinatal injury, R hemiatrophy | Partial central commissurotomy (see text) | No GTC | No change | Not given |
| | 2 | Trauma | Partial central commissurotomy | Still GTC | No change | Not given |
| | | | Completed | No more GTC | | |
| | 3 | Birth injury | Partial central commissurotomy | Still GTC | No change | Not given |
| | | | Completed | No GTC | | |
| | 4 | L hemiparesis, perinatal injury | Partial central commissurotomy | Blank spells only | No change | Not given |
| | 5 | Unknown etiology, gradual deterioration | Partial central commissurotomy | Still GTC | No change (better) | Not given |
| | 6 | Unknown etiology, switched hands | Partial central commissurotomy | Still GTC | No change | Not given |
| | 7 | Unknown etiology | Partial central commissurotomy | Only partial seizures | No change | Not given |
| | 8 | R temporal astrocytoma | Partial central commissurotomy | 'Petit mal' only | No change | Not given |
| | 9 | Trauma | Complete central commissurotomy | Many szs with secondary generalization | Unclear | Not given |
| | 10 | Diphtheria, L hemiparesis | Complete central commissurotomy | Focal only | No change | Not given |
| Wilson (1977, 1982) (see also Reeves & O'Leary 1985) | 1 | Hemiatrophy | Complete commissurotomy | Less than 3 szs/year | None | ↓ ↓ Bisync |
| | 2 | Unknown etiology and normal exam | Complete commissurotomy | Changed from GTC to CP at 1/week | ↓ ↓ Memory | ↓ ↓ Bisync |

**Table 9.2** (*cont.*)

| Author | | Diagnosis | Procedure | Seizure change | Neurological change | EEG change |
|---|---|---|---|---|---|---|
| Wilson (1977, 1982) (see also Reeves & O'Leary 1983) | 3 | Unknown etiology and normal exam | Complete commissurotomy | 50% ↓ GTC and CP | None noted | ↓ Bisync |
| | 4 | Unknown etiology and normal exam | Frontal commissurotomy | 50% ↓ GTC, CP, atonic | None | ↓ Bisync |
| | 5 | Unknown etiology and normal exam | Frontal commissurotomy | Less than 3 szs/year | None | Normal |
| | 6 | Unknown etiology and normal exam | Frontal commissurotomy | 50% ↓ CP and GTC | Not noted | Minimal change, less sync |
| | 7 | Unknown etiology and normal exam | Frontal commissurotomy | No change, only CP | Marked ↓ cognitive ability | More unilat |
| | 8 | Unknown etiology and normal exam | Frontal commissurotomy | Postoperative death | — | — |
| | 9 | Herpes encephalitis | Central commissurotomy, 1 stage | Only occasional CP | None | Unilat |
| | 10 | Febrile seizures | Central commissurotomy, 1 stage | Some GTC | Not noted | Unilat |
| | 11 | L frontal astrocytoma | Central commissurotomy, 1 stage | Some GTC and absence | Dull | Improved |
| | 12 | Mumps encephalitis | Central commissurotomy, 1 stage | None | Brighter | More unilat |
| | 13 | Unknown etiology | Central commissurotomy, 1 stage | None | Language deficit | Min change |
| | 14 | Etiology unknown; dysphasic | Central commissurotomy, 1 stage | Persistent GTC, absence, SP | Very impaired to start | Marked lateralization |
| | 15 | Unknown etiology | Central commissurotomy, 2 stage | 50% ↓, still GTC, CP | None | Marked lateralization |
| | 16 | Perinatal injury | Central commissurotomy, 2 stage | Less than 3 szs/year | None | ↓ Bisync |
| | 17 | L hemisphere dysfunction, unknown etiology | Central commissurotomy, 2 stage | ↓, but persistent GTC, CP | Dull | More lateralized |
| | 18 | Measles encephalitis | Central commissurotomy, 2 stage | Many GTC and CP | Retarded, more manageable | More lateralized |
| | 19 | Perinatal injury | Central commissurotomy, 2 stage | ↓ but still absence and CP | Borderline | Complete lateralization |
| | 20 | Febrile seizures | Central commissurotomy, 2 stage | No more akinetic, still GTC | Dull | More asymmetric |

bisync, bisynchrony; R, right; L, left; min, minimal; ↑, increased; ↑↑, markedly increased; ↓, decreased; ↓↓, markedly decreased; sz(s), seizure(s); GTC, generalized tonic clonic; SP, simple partial; CP, complex partial; meds, medications; mos, months; uni, unilateral.

Partial section alone (anterior or posterior) gave good results in only a minority of patients. Anterior section in patients with strictly frontal lobe foci was more often successful. (4) Since benefit from partial section cannot be predicted with certainty, and since staged commissurotomy reduces postoperative complications and shortens convalescence, it is reasonable to perform CCS as a two stage procedure with the second stage delayed sufficiently to determine success or failure after the initial phase. Completion of the section can be done at any time without significant decrement in the ultimate response. (5) Results after central commissurotomy are comparable by all reports to those of complete commissurotomy, and it is therefore the operation of choice since it carries less risk to critical structures.

**Areas of controversy**

The list of controversial issues is much longer, and undoubtably accounts for the hesitancy of many centers to include corpus callosotomy among surgical options offered to patients with refractory epilepsy. Each item in this list will be addressed separately with sufficient citations to available literature to permit the topic to be explored in greater depth as desired.

*Mechanism of action*

The resolution of this very basic issue should provide answers to multiple questions in the following discussion. The corpus callosum connects neocortical areas while the anterior commissure connects olfactory structures (anterior portion) and portions of the middle and inferior temporal gyri (posterior portion) (Brodal 1983, Carpenter & Sutin 1983). The hippocampal commissure, which shows decreasing size with advancing phylogeny (and about which some controversy exists in humans), is likely to connect at least some homologous hippocampal areas. Recent studies have also shown that the corpus callosum has both homotopic and heterotopic connections with terminations in deeper layers of neocortex (Goldman-Rakic & Schwartz 1982, Schwartz & Goldman-Rakic 1982). The corpus callosum maintains anatomical integrity with respect to the location of axons connecting particular cerebral areas within its struc ture, such that fibers from rostral frontal lobe traverse the genu; fibers from remaining frontal lobe and parietal lobe, the body; and fibers from temporal and occipital regions, the splenium. Within this framework, then, it is reasonable to assume that section of the corpus callosum and hippocampal commissure would effectively interrupt interhemispheric transmission in certain regions and achieve the desired antiepileptic effect if the sectioned fibers were serving as pathways of spread from the seizure focus to the contralateral hemisphere. Since most seizure foci are contained in neocortical or hippocampal locations and thus connected to the contralateral hemisphere by the corpus callosum and hippocampal commissure, section of these commissural fibers alone would be expected to eliminate bilateral spread of epileptic discharge, and by implication, of clinically secondarily generalized seizures. Thus, Wilson's demonstration that central commissurotomy is as effective as complete commissurotomy would be predicted.

If all interhemispheric communication occurred by these routes, then explanation of the effects of transection of the corpus callosum and hippocampal commissure would be clearcut. However, experimental studies have established that focal epileptic discharges generalize using pathways both across the corpus callosum and down through diencephalic/mesencephalic structures (Kopeloff et al 1950, Mattson & Bickford 1961, Ottino et al 1971). This is supported in humans by the persistence of some (although considerably fewer) bisynchronous discharges in the EEGs of patients after CCS (Spencer et al 1985, Gates et al 1985). If additional pathways for generalization of interictal EEG discharge exist, it might be expected that generalization of the clinical seizure would also utilize other routes. Yet the clinical results of CCS dispute such a contention: central commissurotomy is definitely effective in preventing secondarily generalized seizures of any type in most patients. Clearly, generalization of the clinical seizure is a phenomenon somewhat different from generalization of the interictal EEG discharge. The explanation of this dichotomy is unknown, but may relate to disparate factors modulating the manifestation of clinical seizures and the spread of EEG discharges.

*Complex partial seizures*

The clinical studies outlined show inconsistent but not infrequent reduction in complex partial seizures by commissurotomy. Complex partial seizures are cured or altered to simple partial spells in about 50% of patients undergoing total section of the corpus callosum and hippocampal commissure (with or without other commissural pathways).

The aforementioned outline of anatomical connections predicts that complex partial seizures arising in any cerebral lobe should be eliminated if generalization of seizure discharge is required for their manifestation (also an unresolved issue). The lack of response in at least half the patients is unexplained. Analysis of our patients for preoperative criteria that might predict response of complex partial seizures showed that more focal and definitely unilateral seizure onset favored a good outcome after CCS. One hypothesis to explain these observations might be that discharging of bilateral seizure foci, despite their isolation from one another by CCS, continues to produce effective bilateral functional abnormalities which lead to loss of consciousness akin to that created by the spread of epileptic discharge from one hemisphere to the other. Against this hypothesis are the results from patients with bilateral independent foci who have only simple partial seizures after CCS, and other patients with unilateral foci who continue to have complex partial seizures.

Another hypothesis to explain the variable response of complex partial seizures to CCS is dependent upon the physiological basis of the complex partial seizure. If a complex partial seizure can sometimes occur with strictly unilateral cerebral epileptic involvement in the ictal pattern, then those patients should continue to have complex partial seizures after CCS. Patients whose complex partial seizures require bilateral spread of the ictal discharge in order to be manifest should be expected to stop having complex partial seizures after CCS. Although this issue is not entirely resolved, and although some patients with strictly unilateral seizure discharge may experience a classical clinical complex partial seizure with altered consciousness, this is unusual, and certainly does not account for 50% of patients with complex partial seizures. Thus, this hypothesis seems unlikely.

To my mind, the most likely explanation for the variable response of complex partial seizures to CCS was mentioned by Demeter et al based on animal studies of the ventral and dorsal hippocampal commissures (Amaral et al 1984, Demeter et al 1985). The dorsal hippocampal commissure connects parahippocampal and neocortical areas and is likely to be sectioned during CCS because it is closely applied to the corpus callosum. On the other hand, the ventral hippocampal commissure may well be spared in the usual CCS, particularly if the ventricles are not entered. If the ventral hippocampal commissure connects homologous hippocampal areas in the human (as it does in the experimental animal) variable responses of complex partial seizures should be observed after CCS depending on how much, if any, of the ventral hippocampal commissure is actually sectioned in patients with seizure onset in the hippocampus. This hypothesis is only viable if an effective hippocampal commissure exists in humans, an issue of some controversy (Lieb & Babb 1986, Lieb et al 1986). A recent study of seizure propagation from unilateral temporal foci demonstrated variable spread from one hippocampus, sometimes first to ipsilateral neocortex, and sometimes initially to contralateral hippocampus without involvement of contralateral neocortex. It was concluded that such patterns are consistent with the existence of a functional hippocampal commissure in humans (Spencer et al 1987d). This hypothesis does not, however, account for the observed greater likelihood of control of complex partial seizures in patients with more localized seizure onset.

*More intense focal seizures (MIFS)*

A corollary series of observations on complex partial seizures after CCS showed an increase in severity, frequency, or type of partial seizure in about 25% of patients. This has been described at Yale and several other centers (Rayport et al 1983, 1985, Spencer et al 1984, Gates et al 1987). These patients usually (but not always) had bilateral (usually frontal) independent seizure foci preoperatively. We proposed this might be due to decreased inhibitory influence from the contralateral hemisphere, which might be enhanced in patients with bilateral seizure foci. Alternatively, the interictal contralateral discharge might itself be a reflection of increased inhibition and not a true independent focus, which would explain why not all patients with bilateral independent foci have MIFS. The level of activity of the interictal discharging focus, and the exact location of the primary or secondary focus may also have important bearing on the final outcome. Although MIFS may be distressing, particularly to those patients with minimal understanding of the process, most patients are happy to exchange generalized seizures for partial seizures, no matter how intense.

Interestingly, some patients have a postoperative increase in focal interictal spiking at a frequency greater than the preoperative bilateral discharge rate. These are not, however, always the patients who exhibit MIFS (Spencer et al 1984, 1985). Thus, changes in clinical seizures and EEG abnormalities exhibit parallel phenomena suggesting a very real role for the contralateral hemisphere in inhibition; however the phenomena are, to some extent, dichotomous in individual patients. Just as for generalized seizures and generalized EEG discharges, this suggests that the clinical seizure and the EEG activity are somehow independent or modulated by different factors which remain so far undefined.

*Primary generalized epilepsy*

The cerebral structures underlying generation of primary generalized epileptic disturbances are unknown. Experimental data have shown that the corpus callosum and cerebral hemispheres with bilateral foci are sufficient to produce typical generalized 3 per second spike/wave abnormalies on EEG and accompanying seizures bearing resemblance to absence seizures (Marcus & Watson 1966, 1967, 1968, Marcus et al 1968). At least in the feline model of generalized penicillin epilepsy, Musgrave & Gloor (1980) demonstrated that the corpus callosum was solely responsible for the inter-hemispheric bisynchrony of EEG discharges. Occasionally, however, patterns resembling typical 3 per second spike and wave activity, and clinical seizures bearing strong resemblance to classical absence spells, may result from a single epileptogenic focus, usually mesial frontal, with rapid spread causing secondary bilateral synchrony (Tükel & Jasper 1952). Careful audiovisual/EEG analysis is usually sufficient to make the distinction in questionable cases. CCS is presently recommended only for patients with secondary generalized seizures. The question arises, however, whether the procedure might be applicable to patients with uncontrolled primary generalized epilepsy. If generalization of seizure discharge on EEG is somewhat independent of generalization of the clinical seizure (see preceding discussion), the latter being modulated by factors at a presumably cortical level, then CCS might be expected to alter the clinically generalized seizure of primary epilepsy regardless of its mechanism of generation. Since such patients presumably do not have a localized area of cerebral discharge, they might be considered good candidates for CCS because they would be spared the possible occurrence of MIFS. Also, because they presumably do not have underlying cerebral pathology, they should be spared increased neurological deficits which represent exacerbation of a partially recovered previous insult. Nonetheless, the various uncertainties involved, as well as the rationale upon which CCS was initiated and continues to be based, have not yet permitted patients with primary epilepsy to be considered as candidates for CCS. Table 9.2 indicates only two patients in the literature who clearly had petit mal EEG and seizure patterns. One had a significant decrease in absence episodes with persistent tonic-clonic seizures, and the other did not fare well at all. Anecdotal results of patients at other centers suggest similar results. Insufficient data should not prevent an appropriate research study of CCS as a surgical alternative in those rare patients with incapacitating primary generalized epilepsy uncontrolled by standard medical management.

*Longterm changes in seizures*

Since the incidence of seizure recurrence increases over time in patients who initially had complete seizure control from resective procedures, it is appropriate to be concerned about the permanence of beneficial effects of CCS. In Bogen's and Wilson's patients, some with longterm followup, a good response seems to endure (Zaidel & Sperry 1974, Harbaugh et al 1983). The Yale experience likewise suggests that beneficial response of secondarily generalized seizures after total CCS is permanent. However, MIFS may appear with a latency of up to four years, and partial seizure types may continue to change with time after CCS, whether partial or total. Some patients who underwent partial (anterior) CCS had temporary relief of generalized seizures, which then recurred, usually within six to twelve months; they required completion of the section for persistent elimination of generalized seizures. Finally, a not significant number of patients have had a gradual improvement in seizure control following partial CCS to the point that they became nearly seizure free within the first postoperative year. This phenomenon has not been reported previously and is important, since it means that longer observation may be warranted between the first and second stages of callosotomy, even if the initial response to the first stage seems poor. Generally, 12 months has been the outside limit for improvement to occur.

The change in partial seizure character over time has not been studied, nor has it been reported by other centers. It is interesting to speculate that such changes involve reorganization of the projections from neurons in the primary focus. Alternatively, the change might be due to structural alterations in the neurons of the more normal cerebral hemisphere whose connections have been severed by CCS. Such changes might then exert a modifying influence on the seizure focus. After section of the corpus callosum in rats, neurons in the basal nuclei hypertrophy bilaterally; after unilateral lesions, ipsilateral basal nucleus neurons shrink and their contralateral counterparts hypertrophy (Pearson et al 1985). These neurons represent the major cholinergic input to rat neocortex. Different transmitters and neuronal populations in the human may be important to this concept which has yet to receive significant attention.

## *Selection criteria*

### IQ

Wilson et al (1977, 1978, 1982) instigated a series of controversies by stating that patients with low IQ were poor candidates for CCS, a conclusion supported by Blume (1984) and by the Yale group (Spencer et al 1987c), yet Geoffroy et al (1983) showed a definite favorable response in a group of nine retarded children. They made a plea for continued consideration of low IQ individuals, since their patients' lives and the lives of their families were significantly improved when generalized seizures decreased. Furthermore, developmental abilities also seemed to improve (Geoffroy et al 1983). It may be that such patients need early operation before their lives are irreversibly affected by multiple seizures, episodes of status epilepticus, falls, injuries, and lack of development for which no compensation can later be achieved. The discrepant results in the different reports may reflect differing goals or variably compulsive analysis of preoperative seizures. Patients with low IQ in our series have had poor results reflected by continued generalized seizures and prominent MIFS. These patients have known bilateral cerebral damage, and presumed bilateral foci, a factor which seems to promote the development of MIFS. These patients follow the general rules for predicting seizure responses to CCS, but the overall change in lifestyle may not be nearly as good as in other patients because of the prominent MIFS superimposed upon limited ability to cope with preserved consciousness during seizure of any sort. Patients with Lennox–Gastaut syndrome and its variants can be included in this group.

### BILATERAL INDEPENDENT FOCI

Despite the increase risk of MIFS in patients with bilateral independent EEG foci, CCS seems to be a reasonable consideration in such patients and often produces gratifying results. Relatively normal IQ and functional abilities correlate with better outcome in this group as in other patients.

### INFANTILE HEMIPLEGIA

Some analyses of CCS results have assessed responses according to diagnosis. The best outcome occurred in patients with infantile hemiplegia (Williamson 1985). Previously such patients were considered for hemispherectomy, and the question of which operation is the preferred one has been raised (Goodman et al 1985). Complications of hemispherectomy have decreased with modified operations, and CCS cannot prevent focal seizures. Logic dictates, then, that if the motor deficit is severe, and partial seizures are frequent, modified hemispherectomy is preferred. However, when generalized seizures predominate and manual dexterity is preserved, CCS is a satisfactory alternative.

## *Neurological deficits*

### MEMORY

The occurrence of memory deficits as a significant complication of CCS remains unresolved. Although Zaidel & Sperry (1974) reported consistently impaired memory in Bogen's patients after complete commissurotomy, their conclusions are open to question because no preoperative memory testing was available for comparison. Most centers report an occasional patient with memory decline which has been attributed by one group to impaired attention and concentration (Beniak et al 1985).

### LANGUAGE

At least 8 patients have had persistent mutism or language impairment after CCS (Sussman et al 1983, Rayport et al 1984, Sass et al 1987). Our analysis has strongly correlated contralateral representation of handedness and speech (right handed, right hemisphere dominant or left handed, left hemisphere dominant) with postoperative language impairment (Sass et al 1987). The deficit occurs with partial or total CCS, but it is usually more prominent after total CCS. Preoperative amobarbital testing for side of cerebral dominance (Wada test) is strongly recommended, with subsequent exclusion of high-risk patients or at least, detailed preoperative counselling as to the possible effects.

### MOTOR

Apraxia and/or paresis of the nondominant hand or leg have been reported (Bogen & Vogel 1975, Wilson et al 1977, 1978, 1982, Sass et al 1987). These, together with decreased language production and incontinence, comprise a transient disconnection syndrome seen almost uniformly after total one stage CCS and to lesser degrees after two stage procedures (Ross et al 1984). In some patients, components of the syndrome may persist. Although traction on the nondominant parasagittal region has been suggested as the mechanism for these deficits, different centers have reported similar deficits after only anterior or posterior section, procedures which do not involve traction on the same anatomical areas (Rayport et al 1984, Sass et al 1987, Spencer et al 1987a). The current literature is not clear about which hemisphere was retracted in individuals with the most severe post-operative deficits. Considering the different procedures, however, it is unlikely that retraction is the only explanation, and disconnection of important interhemispheric connections is probably important. If interhemispheric synergy has been an important compensatory mechanism for a previously significant cerebral injury, motor impairment is more likely (Novelly & Lifrak 1985, Sass et al 1987). More extensive unilateral injury, particularly early in life, suggests that the contralateral hemisphere has assumed functions of the damaged area in entirely, providing the explanation of why infantile hemiplegia epitomizes the ideal candidate in this respect.

### BEHAVIOR

Only minimal data are available regarding behavioral alterations after CCS, except for the vary rare split brain syndrome (Ferguson et al 1985). Patients experiencing this complication suffer from persistent and debilitating hemispheric antagonism which may interfere with activities of daily living. Although the syndrome usually improves, it may not fully clear with time.

Four of our patients, had increased aggression postoperatively (all of whom had severe preoperative behavior disturbances). It is not established whether improved altertness and functional abilities in these patients promoted more effective aggressivity with no appreciable change in affect, or whether indeed CCS had some more basic effect. All these patients, however, had low IQ, bilateral independent seizure foci, and prominent behavioral disorders before CCS.

PARTIAL VS. TOTAL CCS

There is a tendency to recommend partial section in patients known to be at risk for neurological complications assuming (or hoping) that this will avoid such complications. Yet no data exist to support this contention. In our series, language, motor, and cognitive deficits appeared after partial *or* total section and were predictable by the same guidelines (Spencer et al 1987b). (Note that anterior section at Yale is extensive, however, and encompasses at least 2/3 and often 4/5 of the corpus callosum.) Deficits in patients who later had completion of the section increased even further. Other centers have not reported neurological sequelae after uncomplicated partial section. However, information may not be directly comparable, since procedures at many centers are always total one stage or only anterior. At Yale, preoperative evaluations, prediction of possible deficits, and patient counseling are done without regard to extent of CCS.

*Use for localization*

Several centers have suggested that CCS, by decreasing the rapidity of contralateral spread and generalization of the epileptic discharge, may permit definitive localization of a resectable focus that was not previously possible (Bouvier et al 1983, St Hilaire et al 1985). Particularly in frontal lobe epilepsy, where cortical discharges so rapidly involve bifrontal areas that even lateralization of onset is often obscure, such an approach is reasonable (See Fig. 9.4, 9.5). Many of these patients have stereotyped partial seizures and thus have the potential for a curative resective procedure if an elusive focus can be adequately localized. Personal experience with this approach has been unsatisfactory but limited, and more data are needed.

*Use in children*

It seems logical that generalization of seizures and EEG discharges is more likely to involve subcortical structures when myelination of the corpus callosum is incomplete, and that the cortical-cortical modulation of the secondarily generalized clinical seizure is not fully operational in the immature brain (Salamy 1978). Is CCS then a reasonable option in young children? Our experience is limited although our youngest patients were indeed among the poorest responders. In contrast, Luessenhop (1970), Amacher (1976), and Geoffroy et al (1983) describe the beneficial effects from CCS in children as young as 1 year. Will these patients be more likely to develop altered seizure types because of the greater potential for cerebral reorganization as well as continued development of cerebral connections? No answers to these questions are yet available, and the few children reported should be reanalyzed periodically to address them.

## SUMMARY

Section of the corpus callosum and hippocampal commissure is an accepted palliative procedure for secondary generalized uncontrolled seizures. Tonic, atonic, and tonic-clonic seizures are permanently relieved in 80% of these patients. Use of CCS in primary epilepsy is not established, but probably should be attempted in a controlled investigation. More intense focal seizures may occur postoperatively, especially in patients with bilateral foci. Complex partial seizures are sometimes relieved, particularly in patients with unifocal disease. Neurological sequelae are variable, and there is continuing controversy as to the best selection criteria. Despite the dearth of published information, risk versus benefit can be optimized and gratifying results obtained if appropriate attention is paid to details of the preoperative evaluation.

## REFERENCES


Amacher A L 1976 Midline commissurotomy for the treatment of some cases of intractable epilepsy. Child's Brain 2: 54–58

Amaral D G, Insausti R, Cowan W M 1984 The commissural connections of the monkey hippocampal formation. Journal of Comparative Neurology 224: 307–336

Avila J O, Radvany J, Huck F R et al 1980 Anterior callosotomy as a substitute for hemispherectomy. Acta Neurochirurigica Supplement 30: 137–143

Beniak T E, Gates J R, Risse G L 1985 Comparison of selected neuropsychological test variables pre- and postoperatively on patients subjected to corpus callosotomy. Epilepsia 26: 534

Blume W T 1984 Corpus callosum section for seizure control: rationale and review of experimental and clinical data. Cleveland Clinic Quarterly 51: 319–332

Bogen J 1965 Cerebral commissurotomy. A second case report. Journal of the American Medical Association 194: 1328–1329

Bogen J E, Vogel P J 1962 Cerebral commissurotomy in man: preliminary case report. Bulletin of the Los Angeles Neurological Society 27: 169–172

Bogen J, Vogel P J 1975 Neurologic status in the longterm following complete cerebral commissurotomy. In: Michel F, Schott B (eds) Hopital Neurologique, Lyon, p 227–251

Bouvier G, Mercier C, St Hilaire J M, Giard N, Labrecque R, Beique R A 1983 Anterior callosotomy and chronic depth electrode recording in the surgical management of some intractable seizures. Applied Neurophysiology 46: 52–56

Brodal A 1983 Neurological anatomy in relation to clinical medicine. Oxford University Press, New York

Carpenter M B, Sutin J 1983 Human neuroanatomy. Williams and Wilkins, Baltimore

Demeter S, Rosene D, VanHoesen G W 1985 Interhemispheric pathways of the hippocampal formation, presubiculum, and entorhinal and posterior parahippocampal cortices in the rhesus monkey: the structure and organization of the hippocampal commissures. Journal of Comparative Neurology 233: 30–47

Erickson T E 1940 Spread of the epileptic discharge: an experimental study of the afterdischarge induced by electrical stimulation of the cerebral cortex. Archives of Neurology and Psychiatry 43(3): 429–452

Ferguson S M, Rayport M, Corrie W S 1985 Neuropsychiatric observations on behavioral consequences of corpus callosum section for seizure control. In: Reeves A G (ed) Epilepsy and the corpus callosum, ch. 28. Plenum, New York, p 501–514

Gates J R, Leppik I E, Yap J, Gumnit R J 1984 Corpus callosotomy: clinical and electroencephalographic effects. Epilepsia 25: 308–316

Gates J R, Mireles R, Maxwell R, Sharbrough F, Forbes G 1986 Magnetic resonance imaging, electroencephalogram, and selected neuropsychological testing in staged corpus callosotomy. Archives of Neurology 43: 1188–1191

Gates J, Rosenfeld W, Maxwell R E, Lyons R 1987 Response of multiple seizure types callosotomy. Epilepsia 28: 28–34

Gazzaniga M S, Holtzman J D, Deck M D F, Lee B C P 1985 MRI assessment of human callosal surgery with neuropsychological correlates. Neurology 35: 1763–1766

Geoffroy G, Lassonde M, Delisle F, Decarie M 1983 Corpus callosotomy for control of intractable epilepsy in children. Neurology (Cleveland) 33: 891–897

Goldman-Rakic P S, Schwartz M L 1982 Interdigitation of contralateral and ipsilateral columnar projections to frontal association cortex in primates. Science 216: 755–757

Goodman R N, Williamson P D, Reeves A G et al 1985 Interhemispheric commissurotomy for congenital hemiplegia with intractable epilepsy. Neurology 35: 1351–1354

Harbaugh R E, Wilson D H, Reeves A G, Gazzaniga M S 1983 Forebrain commissurotomy for epilepsy: review of 20 consecutive cases. Acta Neurochirurgica 68: 263–275

Kopeloff N, Kennard M A, Pacella B L, Kopeloff J M, Chusid J G 1950 Section of corpus callosum in experimental epilepsy in the monkey. Archives of Neurology and Psychiatry 63: 719–727

Ledoux J E, Risse G L, Springer S P, Wilson D W, Gazzaniga M S 1977 Cognition and commissurotomy. Brain 100: 87–104

Lieb J P, Babb T L 1986 Interhemispheric propagation time of human hippocampal seizures. II. Relationship to pathology and cell density. Epilepsia 27: 294–300

Lieb J P, Engel J, Babb T L 1986 Interhemispheric propagation time of human hippocampal seizures. I. Relationship to surgical outcome. Epilepsia 27: 286–293

Long D M, Chou S N 1973 Transcallosal removal of craniopharyngiomas within the third ventricle. Journal of Neurosurgery 39: 563–567
Luessenhop A J 1970 Interhemispheric commissurotomy: (the split brain operation) as an alternate to hemispherectomy for control of intractable seizures. American Surgeon 36: 265–268
Luessenhop A J, dela Cruz T C, Fenichel G M 1970 Surgical disconnection of the cerebral hemispheres for intractable seizures: results in infancy and childhood. Journal of the American Medical Association 213(10): 1630–1636
Marcus E M, Watson C W 1966 Bilateral synchronous spike wave electrographic patterns in the cat. Archives of Neurology 14: 601–610
Marcus E M, Watson C W 1967 Bilateral symmetrical epileptogenic foci in cerebral cortex of the monkey. Electroencephalography and Clinical Neurophysiology 23: 77–97
Marcus E M, Watson C W 1968 Symmetrical epileptogenic foci in monkey cerebral cortex: mechanisms of interaction and regional variations in capacity for synchronous discharges. Archives of Neurology 19: 99–116
Marcus E M, Watson C W, Simon S A 1968 An experimental model of some varieties of petit mal epilepsy. Electrical behavioral correlations of acute bilateral epileptogenic foci in cerebral cortex. Epilepsia 9: 233–248
Marino Jr R 1985 Surgery for epilepsy. Selective partial microsurgical callosotomy for intractable multiform seizures: criteria for clinical selection and results. Applied Neurophysiology 48: 404–407
Marino Jr R, Ragazzo P C 1985 Selective criteria and results of selective partial callosotomy. In: Reeves A G (ed) Epilepsy and the corpus callosum, ch 13. Plenum, New York, p 281–301
Mattson R H, Bickford R G 1961 Firing patterns of strychnine spikes in the cortex of the cat. Electroencephalography and Clinical Neurophysiology 13: 144–148
Musgrave J, Gloor P 1980 The role of the corpus callosum in bilateral interhemispheric synchrony of spike and wave discharge in feline generalized penicillin epilepsy. Epilepsia 21: 369–378
Novelly R A, Lifrak M D 1985 Forebrain commissurotomy reinstates effects of preexisting hemisphere lesions: an examination of the hypothesis. In: Reeves A G (ed) Epilepsy and the corpus callosum, ch 27. Plenum, New York, p 467–500
Ottino C A, Meglio M, Rossi G F, Tercero E 1971 An experimental study of the structure mediating bilateral synchrony of epileptic discharges of cortical origin. Epilepsia 12: 299–311
Pearson R C A, Sofroniew M V, Powell T P S 1985 Hypertrophy of cholinergic neurons of the rat basal nucleus following section of the corpus callosum. Brain Research 338: 337–340
Rayport M, Ferguson S M, Corrie W S 1983 Outcomes and indications of corpus callosum section for intractable seizure control. Applied Neurophysiology 46: 47–51
Rayport M, Ferguson S M, Corrie W S 1984 Mutism after corpus callosum section for intractable seizure control. Epilepsia 25: 655
Rayport M, Ferguson S M, Corrie W S 1985 Corpus callosum section for control of clinically and electroencephalographically classified intractable seizures. In: Reeves A G (ed) Epilepsy and the corpus callosum, ch 16. Plenum, New York, p 329–337
Reeves A G, O'Leary P M 1985 Total corpus callosotomy for control of medically intractable epilepsy. In: Reeves A G (ed) Epilepsy and the corpus callosum, ch 12. Plenum, New York, p 269–280
Roberts D W 1985 Corpus callosotomy: surgical technique. In: Reeves A G (ed) Epilepsy and the corpus callosum, ch 11. Plenum, New York, p 259–267
Roberts D W, Allen C D, Allen A H, Reeves A G 1983 Depth electrode recording in patients undergoing corpus callosotomy for intractable epilepsy. Applied Neurophysiology 46: 26–32
Ross M K, Reeves A G, Roberts D W 1984 Post-commissurotomy mutism. Annals of Neurology 16: 114
Saint-Hilaire J M, Giard N, Bouvier G, Labrecque R 1985 Anterior callosotomy in frontal lobe epilepsies. In Reeves A G (ed) Epilepsy and the corpus callosum, ch 14. Plenum, New York, p 303–314
Salamy A 1978 Commissural transmission: maturational changes in humans. Science 200: 1409–1411
Sass K J, Spencer D D, Spencer S S, Novelly R A, Williamson P D, Mattson R H 1988 Corpus callosotomy for epilepsy II: neurological and neuropsychological outcome. Neurology 38: 24–28
Schwartz M L, Goldman-Rakic P S 1982 Single cortical neurones have axon collaterals to ipsilateral and contralateral cortex in fetal and adult primates. Nature 299: 154–156
Shucart W A, Stein B M 1978 Transcallosal approach to the anterior ventricular system. Neurosurgery 3(3): 339–343
Spencer S S 1986 Surgical options for uncontrolled epilepsy. Neurologic Clinics 4: 669–695
Spencer D D, Spencer S S 1985 Surgery for epilepsy. Neurologic Clinics 3: 313–330
Spencer S S, Spencer D D, Glaser G H, Williamson P D, Mattson R H 1984 More intense focal seizure types after callosal section: the role of inhibition. Annals of Neurology 16: 686–693
Spencer S S, Spencer D D, Williamson P D, Mattson R H 1985 Effects of corpus callosum section on secondary bilaterally synchronous interictal EEG discharges. Neurology 35: 1689–1702

Spencer S, Gates J, Reeves A, Spencer D, Maxwell R, Roberts D 1987a Corpus callosum section for uncontrolled epilepsy. In: Engel J (ed) Surgical management of the epilepsies. Raven, New York, p 425–444
Spencer S S, Spencer D D, Sass K J, Novelly R A, Williamson P D, Mattson R H 1987b Partial vs. total callosotomy for epilepsy. Advances in Epileptology (The 16th Epilepsy International Symposium), Vol 16. Raven, New York p 323–325
Spencer S S, Spencer D D, Williamson P D, Mattson R H, Sass K J 1988c Corpus callosotomy for epilepsy I: seizure effects. Neurology 38: 19–24
Spencer S S, Williamson P D, Spencer D D, Mattson R H 1987d Human hippocampal seizure spread studied by depth and subdural recording: the hippocampal commissure. Epilepsia 28: 479–489
Sussman N M, Gur R C, Gur R E, O'Connor M J 1983 Mutism as a consequence of callosotomy. Journal of Neurosurgery 59: 514–519
Sussman N M, Scanlon M, Garfinkle W, Callanan M, O'Connor M J, Harner R N 1987 Magnetic resonance imaging after corpus callosotomy. Neurology 37: 350–354
Torres F, French L A 1973 Acute effect of section of the corpus callosum upon 'independent' epileptiform activity. Acta Neurologica Scandinavia 49: 47–62
Tŭkel K, Jasper H 1952 The electroencaphalogram in parasagittal lesions. Electroencephalography and Clinical Neurophysiology 4: 481–494
Van Wagenen W P, Herren R Y 1940 Surgical division of commissural pathways in the corpus callosum: relation to spread of an epileptic attack. Archives of Neurology and Psychiatry 44: 740–759
Wada J A, Moyes P D 1983 Anterior callosal section in medically refractory generalized seizure patients. Epilepsia 24: 262
Williamson P D 1985 Corpus callosum section for intractable epilepsy: criteria for patient selection. In: Reeves A G (ed) Epilepsy and the corpus callosum, ch 10. Plenum, New York p 243–257
Wilson D H, Reeves A, Gazzaniga M, Culver C 1977 Cerebral commissurotomy for control of intractable seizures. Neurology 27: 708–715
Wilson D H, Reeves A G, Gazzaniga M 1978 Division of the corpus callosum for uncontrollable epilepsy. Neurology 28: 649–653
Wilson D H, Reeves A, Gazzaniga M S 1982 'Central' commissurotomy for intractable generalized epilepsy: series two. Neurology (NY) 32: 687–697
Zaidel E, Sperry R W 1974 Memory impairment after commissurotomy in man. Brain 97: 263–272

# 10. Depression in patients with epilepsy reconsidered

*M. M. Robertson*

## INTRODUCTION

Although the word 'depression' is mentioned frequently in association with epilepsy, few have defined what precisely is meant by this word. This chapter is intended to offer some operational guidelines as to the various definitions and classifications. After having teased out that problem, acknowledging the difficulties, the possible links between epilepsy and depression will be explored, focussing on studies using standardised methods of assessment. In conclusion, recent studies in relevant areas and suggestions for the management of depression in the context of epilepsy will be considered.

### History

The first documentation of depression was by Hippocrates in the fourth century B.C. who stated that 'if fear (phobos) or distress (dysthmia) last for a long time it is melancholic', while the next detailed description comes from Aretæus a physician in the first century A.D. Galen, in the second century, believed that one ought to be well acquainted with the physiology of the brain in order to understand the pathology and treatment of it. He agreed that melancholia depended on a superfluity of black bile 'in the very substance of the brain' (Lewis 1934). During the middle ages there was a dearth of information about depression, but from the eighteenth century to the present time literature has been filled with vivid descriptions of the illness. Recently (Meyer & Meyer 1987) illustrations from the writings of the depressed poet, William Cowper, elegantly describe some of the emotions of a depressed person: 'Day and night I was upon the rack, lying down in horror and rising in despair ... rising cheerless and distressed in the morning, and brightening a little as the day goes on'.

### The meaning of depression

The definition, description and classification of depression have been the subject of much discussion and controversy, as Andreason pointed out in 1982: 'although affective disorders have been recognised for thousands of years, clinicians and researchers have still not reached agreement on the basic concepts of these disorders and the best methods of classifying them'.

Recent ideas about depression stem from the work of Kraeplin who formulated the concept of manic-depressive disease (Kraeplin 1921). This is defined as 'a disorder in which a change of mood is the primary and central feature, mood being raised in the case of mania and lowered in depression' (Hamilton 1982). Hamilton describes the clinical symptoms of depression thoroughly, and makes the point that lowering of mood is not the central feature of minor forms of the illness, and may not occur at all in the controversial category of masked depression. Depressive symptoms are different from depressive illness and may constitute hopelessness, demoralisation, simple unhappiness or bereavement (Frank 1961, Wing et al 1978, Clayton et al 1972). As early as 1959 Lehmann noted that depression has three different meanings, referring to a symptom, a syndrome and a nosological entity. Hamilton (1982) points out that when the illness is severe, the three symptoms of depressed mood, feelings of guilt and suicidal thoughts, generally regarded as central features of the illness, are present; the three most common symptoms, being found in almost every patient are depressed mood, loss of interest and anxiety. Recently Snaith (1987) suggested that 'Anhedonic' depression is the best indicator of melancholia.

The term 'affective disorders' was first used in 1951 in the Standard Veteran's Administration classification and included manic depressive reaction, psychotic depressive reaction and involutional melancholia: in addition the cyclothymic personality was delineated for the first time in a section entitled character and behaviour disorders (Spitzer et al 1977).

Today there are several widely employed nosological systems to guide clinicians and researchers in identifying depressive illness. Thus, the St Louis group (Feighner et al 1972), the Research Diagnostic Criteria (RDC) (Spitzer et al 1978), the third revision of the Diagnostic and Statistical Manual (DSM. III, American Psychiatric Association, 1980) and the International Classification of Diseases, at present in its ninth version (ICD. 9: World Health Organization 1978) have gained credibility and popularity. They not only incorporate *inclusion criteria* (for example as in the case of DSM. III, depressed mood, loss of interest or pleasure, appetite and sleep disturbances, psychomotor agitation or retardation, loss of energy or fatigue, feelings of worthlessness, complaints of diminished ability to concentrate and recurrent thoughts of death or suicide), but also have *exclusion criteria* (for example in DSM. III, mood incongruent delusions or hallucinations, bizarre behaviour, evidence of schizophrenia or due to organic mental disorder or uncomplicated bereavement) and have *duration requirements* (for example 1–2 weeks for RDC, 2 weeks for DSM. III and Feighner criteria).

## The classification of depression

The precise classification of depression is a matter of controversy. Kendell (1976) reviewed the relevant literature and referred to the 'contemporary confusion' which still exists. He succinctly describes the various methods of classification such as simple typologies (using from one to five categories), tiered typologies (with divisions and subdivisions thereof) and finally dimensional systems (both of which address the psychotic-neurotic problem from different angles). The 13 systems of classification mentioned reflect the complexity of the problem. Kendell (1976) traces the origins, pitfalls and positive features of current themes of classification. Debates as to which constitutes an internationally accepted classification continue, but generally there are broad categories to which most authors adhere and which will be used in this chapter.

The St Louis group (Robins et al 1972) distinguished between primary and secondary depression. A primary affective disorder, for example depression, is one in which the first evidence of a diagnosable psychiatric illness is an affective episode; a secondary affective disorder is one which the affective episode was preceded by another diagnosable psychiatric illness (Robins et al 1972). Leonhard (1959) and Perris (1966) described bipolar and unipolar illnesses. Bipolar illness represents bouts of both mania and depression; unipolar illness denotes recurrent mania or depression. Both these classifications are widely accepted.

The area where controversy still reigns is between endogenous (Type A, psychotic, melancholic, retarded) depression and non-endogenous (Type B, neurotic, reactive, exogenous, anxious-tense) depression. It has been pointed out that either type is incapable of definition and often means little more than 'severe' and 'mild' (Bowman & Rose 1951). The Newcastle School (Kiloh & Garside 1963, Carney et al 1965) suggest that patients' depression scores subjected to statistical analysis are bimodally distributed, and that there is a clear-cut boundary between endogenous and reactive depressions. Others (Kendell & Gourlay 1970) view the distribution of depression scores of their patients as unimodal and thus see a psychotic/neurotic continuum. In a later paper from the Newcastle School (Carney & Sheffield 1972) it was felt that a compromise could be reached—that neurotic depression is dimensional, and endogenous depression categorical. This means that the two are not mutually exclusive, and that an individual could have endogenous depression with neurotic features as well. Mendels & Cochrane (1968) suggested that Type A was a pure depressive illness, while Type B depression was mixed, and diluted with other syndromes—'the so-called endogenous factor might represent the core of depressive symptomatology, whereas the clinical features of the reactive factor may represent phenomenological manifestations of psychiatric disorders other than depression which contaminate the depressive syndrome'. Kiloh et al (1972) suggested that Type A or endogenous depression was a disease entity with a biological basis, but Type B simply one facet of the broad spectrum of neurotic reactions to stress. In conclusion, most people accept endogenous depression as a syndrome with certain characteristic clinical features, genetic predisposition and biological abnormalities. At the other end of the distribution are the non-endogenous illnesses, a heterogeneous group of syndromes, most of which have in common the change of mood characteristic of depression.

**The measurement of depression**

For many years clinical acumen was the only available means of diagnosing depression. It is probably still true to say that a thorough history taking and a sound mental status examination are diagnostically and clinically indispensable. However, in areas of research, where one desires to compare data, standardised methods of assessment are essential, resulting in the advent of rating scales, many of which measure aspects of mood. Some, for example, the self rating scales such as the Minnesota Multiphasic Personality Inventory (MMPI), the Bear-Fedio Self Report Personal Inventory, the Middlesex Hospital Questionnaire now known as the Crown Crisp Experiential Index (CCEI) and the physician rated Present State Examination (PSE) measure, when used to screen populations, depressive symptomatology; the self rated Beck Depression Inventory (BDI), the Zung Depression Inventory and Levine Pilowsky Questionnaire (LPD) measure severity of depression, and have cut off points to indicate the transition from depressive symptoms to probable depressive illness. The physician rated Hamilton Depression Rating Scale (HDRS) quantifies severity of depression in persons who have already been diagnosed as clinically depressed, while the physician rated

Newcastle Scale and the LPD distinguish between endogenous and reactive depression. To quantify adequately the severity of depressive illness, patients should first satisfy diagnostic criteria and then be assessed using both a self rating and a physician rated scale. Many of the scales contain items which could be accounted for by distress and somatic disturbances which often rate highly in people with physical illness (Snaith 1987) such as those with epilepsy, and therefore the Hospital Anxiety Depression Scale (Zigmund & Snaith 1983) which measures the severity of depression as opposed to sadness and is not weighted with somatic items is preferable in those with medical illnesses.

## AETIOLOGY OF DEPRESSION IN EPILEPSY

When considering a topic concerned with depression in the setting of epilepsy, the various aetiological theories of depression should be mentioned, as many have been implicated in both disorders. Some may help tease out the links between the two disorders, while others may have treatment implications. Genetic predisposition or vulnerability seems to have been fairly clearly demonstrated in bipolar (manic-depressive) illness and recurrent unipolar depressions, although there is probably some genetic overlap, as the different illnesses can occur in each of the twins (Slater & Cowie 1971, Allen et al 1974, Perris 1966, Bertelsen et al 1977). Various psychosocial models of depression reflecting the dominant schools of thought are presented in Table 10.1 Several of these, such as those involving loss of self esteem, negative cognitive set, loss of reinforcement and loss of role status may well apply to people who have epilepsy. While considering the psychosocial models of depression in people with epilepsy, the questions of stigma, how people with epilepsy perceive themselves, how they think others perceive them and how they function psychosocially should be addressed. This body of work will be discussed in some detail in the following section. Many have reported on the stigma and social prejudice to which people with epilepsy are subject (Bagley 1972, Hauck 1968, Schutte 1968), while others suggest they do not feel totally stigmatised by their illness (Ryan et al 1980).

Danesi et al (1981) interviewed 113 adolescent and adult epileptics, aged 10–60, mean 17 years, attending a neurological clinic about their social problems. On the basis of clinical diagnosis 80% had primary generalised epilepsy. It was reported that half withdrew prematurely from school due to the frequency of their seizures, approximately a third had lost income because of epilepsy, one-sixth had lost friends or spouses and a few had withdrawn from social activities for fear of having an attack in public. It was concluded that most of the problems arose from poor seizure control, due to irregular medication.

Several studies using questionnaires or standardised methods have also addressed the problems which people with epilepsy face. Thus, Beran & Read (1981) reported the results of a pilot study evaluating how 51 epileptic patients attending a neurological clinic saw their condition, their role in society and society's expectations of them, using a locally devised questionnaire. The majority of subjects considered that they, that is people with epilepsy, had an increase in emotional problems and mood swings compared to people without epilepsy, and there was a tendency for epileptics to regard themselves as less well endowed with all attributes other than ambition, reliability at work, absenteeism and a tendency to violence. They saw the community's perception

**Table 10.1** Psychosocial models of depression. (Modified from Akiskal & McKinney 1975)

| School | Date | Proponent | Model | Mechanism |
|---|---|---|---|---|
| Psychoanalytical | 1911<br>1917 | Abraham<br>Freud | Aggression turned inward | Conversion of aggressive instinct into depressive affect |
| | 1955 | Klein | Object relations | Failure to internalise a good object |
| | 1946<br>1952<br><br>1980 | Spitz<br>Robertson & Bowlby<br>Bowlby | Object loss | Separation: disruption of an attachment bond |
| | 1965 | Bibring | Loss of Self-esteem | Helplessness in attaining goals or ego-ideal |
| Psychological and Behavioural | 1955 | Kelly | Personal construct theory | Constriction |
| | 1967 | Beck | Negative cognitive set | Hopelessness |
| | 1972 | Seligman | Learned helplessness | Uncontrollable aversive stimulation |
| | 1968<br>1973<br>1975 | Lazarus<br>Ferster<br>Lewinsohn | Loss of reinforcement | Rewards of 'sick role' substitute for lost sources of reinforcement |
| | 1969 | Burgess | Reduced reinforcement | Subject's response frequency or quality diminishes because of reduced reinforcement |
| | 1977 | Rehm | Self control | Deficits in self control result in insufficient self reward and excessive self punishment |
| Sociological | 1969<br><br>1973 | Paykel et al<br>Brown et al | Life events | Exit and undesirable events precede depression<br>Precipitating events 'bring forward' occurrence of depression |
| | 1978 | Brown & Harris | | Vulnerability factors |
| | 1974 | Bart | Sociological | Loss of role status |
| Existential | 1964 | Becker | Existential | Loss of meaning of existence |

of them in order of frequency of response, as viewing them with ignorance, understanding, indifference, concern, suspicion and fear. A clear-cut majority of people with epilepsy agreed that many people do not understand epilepsy and fear (98%), that job opportunities for epileptic people are very restricted (79%), that many employers who claim not to discriminate against people with epilepsy in fact do so (76%), and that people with epilepsy are treated as a minority group (65%). Britten et al (1984) addressed the question of stigma in 46 patients with early epilepsy (age of onset 0–26 years), of whom 33 (72%) were diagnosed before or during their school years. The cases were identified from the National Survey of Health and Development, and an 'index of social visability' was derived from teachers' reports of survey members' behaviour at the age of 15 years. This index was significantly associated with poorer educational outcomes but not associated with poor occupational achievement: moreover, it did not differentiate between epileptic and non-epileptic children. Subjects with epilepsy were shown to be more at risk for psychiatric disturbance, confirming results of others (Rutter et al 1970), but data from the study indicated that stigma did not affect the lives of those with epilepsy which was not complicated by other pathologies.

Patient perspectives of epilepsy were studied by Danesi (1984) who found that about one-third, despite having seizures, did not accept a diagnosis of epilepsy, and of those who did accept the diagnosis, two-thirds were unwilling to disclose it to other people. In addition, the majority thought that people generally fear epilepsy and avoid contact with people who have epilepsy. Dodrill et al (1984a) evaluated the psychosocial problems among 315 adults with epilepsy in a nationwide study using the self-rating Washington Psychosocial Seizure Inventory (WPSI) and reported that emotional, interpersonal, vocational and financial concerns were commonly found, as well as problems in coping with seizures. In conclusion it would appear that many people with epilepsy are psychosocially disadvantaged.

Hermann (1979) specifically argued the case for epilepsy being a human analogue/paradigm of the 'learned helplessness' theory of depression proposed by Seligman and colleagues (Seligman 1975, Maier & Seligman 1976, Abramson et al 1978) predominantly applied to animal models. Thus Hermann (1979) proposed that epilepsy is a high psychopathological risk disorder, as affected people are constantly exposed to unpredictable, uncontrollable, aversive events, which produce a pattern of emotional, motivational and cognitive disorders initially presenting as anxiety, but if prolonged, depression (Seligman 1975, Maier & Seligman 1976; Abramson et al 1978). Hermann (1979) proposed that epilepsy is supported as a model of learned helplessness in two areas. In the first instance, many would agree that epileptic attacks are unpredictable, uncontrollable, aversive events, although it is accepted that high stress predisposes to attacks (Temkin & Davis 1984). The fact that sudden unexpected death (Leestma et al 1984) is recognised as a consquence of seizures must make the fit or its outcome all the more unpredictable and aversive. Secondly, people with epilepsy suffer discrimination, a higher incidence of employment difficulties, social exclusion, lower marital rates and are predisposed to cognitive impairment due to cerebral damage and/or anticonvulsant medication (Dodrill et al 1984b; Danesi 1984, Broughton et al 1984, Bagley 1972, Dansky et al 1980, Gudmundson 1966). This is seen as more important when one considers that many of these problems, and indeed the reactions by society to the epileptic, are more often than not neither predictable nor under the control of the person with epilepsy (Hermann 1979).

It therefore seems reasonable to conclude that for a variety of reasons people with epilepsy are particularly vulnerable to being psychosocially disadvantaged. Several of the models of the aetiology of depression embraced by the schools of thought documented in Table 10.1 can be seen as significant in altering their mental status.

Although the literature concerning the biological theories of depression is vast, it is important to note that many of the abnormalities documented in depressives, are also found in people with epilepsy. Thus, abnormalities of noradrenaline (Crunelli et al 1981, Schildkraut 1965), dopamine (Goodwin et al 1973, Maynert et al 1975), 5-hydroxytryptamine (Coppen 1972, Wada et al 1972) gamma-aminobutyric acid (Gerner & Hare 1981, Meldrum 1975), and malfunctioning of the hypothalamic-pituitary axis have been implicated in the two conditions. Of particular interest is folic acid. Decreased values of serum folic acid levels have been reported in depression

(Gough et al 1963, Reynolds et al 1966, 1970, Reynolds 1985), in epilepsy (Jensen & Olesen 1969, Mannheimer 1952, Reynolds 1975), in psychiatrically impaired epileptic patients (Bruens 1971, Callaghan et al 1969) and especially epileptic patients with depression (Snaith et al 1970, Trimble et al 1980, Rodin & Schmaltz 1983, Edeh & Toone 1985, Reynolds 1985, Robertson 1986a).

## DEPRESSION IN THE CONTEXT OF EPILEPSY

A relationship between depression and epilepsy has been described since antiquity. Hippocrates obviously thought epilepsy and melancholia were closely related when he commented 'melancholics ordinarily become epileptics and epileptics melancholics: of these two states, what determines the preference is the direction the malady takes; if it bears upon the body, epilepsy, if upon the intelligence, melancholy' (Lewis 1934). Temkin (1971) quotes Aretæus as saying that epileptics were 'languid, spiritless' and dejected, while nearer our own time several authors from Griesinger in 1857 to White (1900), Barham (1907), Baugh (1908) and Jones (1912) have discussed melancholia as specifically interlinked with epilepsy.

Noting the widespread improper use of the word depression, and frequently so in relation to epilepsy, Betts (1981), (see Table 10.2) emphasises that a person may have a depressive reaction, similar to a grief reaction when given the diagnosis of epilepsy. Thereafter epilepsy can bring with it many social, family and interpersonal problems which, if not dealt with or shown to be overwhelming, may also cause the individual to develop a depressive reaction (Betts 1981).

Currently, in keeping with one of the classifications of psychiatric disorders in epilepsy, there are broadly two types of depression: peri-ictal (those relating to the ictus or seizures) and interictal, in which the disturbances are chronic and not directly related to the ictal electrical disturbances. A useful breakdown of the various types of depressive phenomena and their relationships to the ictus is presented by Betts (1981), see Table 10.2.

**Table10.2** Depression and epilepsy. (Adapted from Betts 1981)

| | |
|---|---|
| 1. Depressive reaction to acquiring the label of epilepsy | |
| 2. Depressive reaction to social or family problems of epilepsy | |
| 3. Prodromal depressive feelings (symptoms) before a fit | Ictal |
| 4. Depressive feelings (symptoms) as an aura | |
| 5. Depressive feelings (symptoms) as a ictal experience | |
| 6. Postictal depressive feelings (symptoms) | |
| 7. Depressive twilight state | |
| 8. Epileptic depressive delirium | |
| 9. Depressive illness | Interictal |
| 10. Depressive symptoms in the setting of a paranoid or schizophrenic psychosis | |

### Peri-ictal depression

Not many reports of this condition are available, but lowered mood around the ictus has been noted for some time by clinicians (Reynolds 1861, Mulder & Daly 1952, Weil 1955, 1959, Williams 1956). It can have serious consequences, as Betts (1982) reported a patient who cut his throat during an ictal depressive state. One of the characteristics of the condition is that the alteration of mood lasts longer than usual for an aura or postictal automatism. Prolonged depressive moods have been documented during status epilepticus (Wells 1975), 'petit mal' status (Tucker & Forster 1950, Jaffe 1963) and partial seizure status (Henricksen 1973).

Gupta et al (1983) described the aura in 290 patients with temporal lobe epilepsy and complex partial seizures without documented psychiatric disorders and who were attending epilepsy neurological clinics. The EEG abnormality was clearly lateralised in 250 patients (R = 140; L = 110). Auras were grouped into those with motor-sensory symptoms (n = 37), psychic symptoms (n = 50), and autonomic symptoms (n = 48). By far the most common psychic auras were those with affective symptomatology (n = 39), of which 29 had right sided foci. Greenberg et al (1984) reported four patients with complex partial seizures who had become preoccupied with death in association with their seizures: all four had generalised seizures and were being treated for this as well as cerebral malignant disease. They all experienced unusual states of affect including periods of anxiety, terror, fear, agitation, rage, and depression; in addition they felt that they had died or had an appointment with death. Electroencephalographic and CT scan examination revealed fronto-temporal abnormalities. Clinically, complex partial seizures were diagnosed, and responded to appropriate medication. Laterality of foci was: right = 2: left = 1: bilateral = 1.

Hermann & Chabria (1980) reported two patients with temporal lobe epilepsy who experienced ictal fear. During the interictal period both patients experienced similar episodes of fear which were almost as intense as those followed by seizure activity, and began to associate those feelings not with the epilepsy but with other people becoming suspicious. They became socially isolated and behaved in a fear-related way such as seeking out places of refuge. Such behaviour could be interpreted as indicating depression.

Ficol et al (1984) also reported fear in people with epilepsy, in some as an aura prior to a complex partial seizure, whilst in others the episodic fear was the sole ictal event.

Two patients who presented with depression and who were later shown on electroencephalographic investigation to be in temporal lobe status were described by Robertson (1986a). Both had had previous bouts of depression necessitating treatment; one had a family history of epilepsy (maternal uncle), the other had two aunts who were both treated for depression. One had a left, the other a right temporal abnormality. Both the patients improved with regards to their mental state and EEG status abnormalities, with the introduction of carbamazepine.

Lim et al (1986) described a case of psychotic depression presenting as catatonia as the sole manifestation of non-convulsive status epilepticus in a 67 year old male with no previous psychiatric history and the only relevant history being one seizure 15 years previously, secondary to a head injury. An EEG showed continuous spike and wave complexes originating in the right fronto-central region with some spread to the left hemisphere. A CT scan showed minimal diffuse cerebral atrophy. Both the clinical state and EEG abnormalities responded rapidly after 1 g of intravenous phenytoin.

Graham & Freemon (1982) reported a patient with continuous psychomotor seizures who had presented with, and was diagnosed as having, long standing mental illness, with a 10–15 year history of confusional episodes which were associated with automatisms. His psychiatric problems led to a gradual social deterioration with four divorces and unemployment, and several hospital admissions during which he had been investigated but never received anticonvulsants. After 15 years he was reviewed in a specialised unit, automatisms were noted and a concomitant EEG showed continuous epileptic discharges, predominantly from the temporal leads. Treatment with anticonvulsants resulted in sustained improvement of his mental state.

Blanchet & Frommer (1986), in a specifically designed and controlled prospective study, reported on mood changes preceding seizures in 27 adults with diverse forms of epilepsy who were investigated for a minimum of 56 days, 13 of whom had at least one seizure during the study period. Subjects rated their mood on a modified version of the Standardised Personal Feelings Scales which included the following emotions: depression, anxiety, energy, freedom, thought processes, love, companionship, anger, restraint and moral judgment. Ratings were compared with subjects who suffered from migraine and asthma, with comparable frequency of attacks. Mood ratings for the seven days surrounding each seizure were compared to interictal periods, with the exception of menses and physical illness. The mean ratings of mood on eight of the ten scales decreased before and rose after the seizure, with the ratings of six patients being responsible for most of the reduction. Decline in the ratings (more of the emotions) was most evident on the depression, anxiety, freedom and anger scales. Of particular note is that for 12 of the 13 patients the mean depression scale on the day before the seizure was below the mean on normal interictal days, in four the level being statistically significant. In other words, the patients reported themselves as being more depressed than usual. For all seizures, the most significant decreases in ratings on the Depression Scale occurred on the 2 days preceding the fit, and the most increases the day of and the day following the attack. In addition, a significant increase in negative life events was reported for patients whose mood deteriorated before seizures. Moreover, mood fluctation of the index group differed from the asthma and migraine subjects, suggesting the deterioration in mood was specific to epilepsy and not merely precedent to any acute episodic disorders (Blanchet & Frommer 1986), with the differences being more remarkable for the migraine group. The authors suggested that negative, depressed or dysphoric mood and negative life events may increase the likelihood of seizures in some patients, conceding that the processes were not necessarily dependent on each other.

What is clear from these reports is although the mood changes have been severe, not many would qualify as being *depressive illness*. Having said that, several warranted treatment, which improved the condition. This illustrates several points. Clinical judgment remains an important diagnostic and therapeutic tool. The depression in these cases was secondary to organic brain disease (an ictal episode) and therefore it would not only have been excluded from criteria, but the management involved treatment of the cause, namely ictal activity, with, therefore, anticonvulsants being used.

**Interictal depression**

There are no studies that have directly addressed the question as to whether depression occurs more frequently in people with epilepsy than in those with other conditions. However, some conclusions can be drawn indirectly from the data derived from investigations using standardised rating scales.

Many studies employing the MMPI have indicated that depression is raised in people with epilepsy (Modlin 1960, Guerrant et al 1962, Kløve & Doehring 1962, Meier & French 1965, Matthews & Kløve 1968, Glass & Mattson 1973). Mignone et al (1970) reported the average MMPI scores for all scales of their index epileptic group to be higher than a control population, while the depression scores were higher for those epileptics with later onset fits. In addition, several studies have reported higher MMPI depression scores for patients with psychomotor/temporal lobe epilepsy compared to those with generalised seizures (Stevens 1975, Rodin et al 1976, Hermann et al 1982, Dikmen et al 1983).

Others, using alternatives to the MMPI, have also used rating scales to assess psychiatric symptomatology in people with epilepsy. Standage & Fenton (1975) used the PSE to compare the psychiatric status of patients with chronic epilepsy and an age and sex matched control group with locomotor disorders, who were also matched for duration of illness. 60% of the index group had somatic symptoms of depression compared to 30% of the control group, while depressive mood, occuring in 75% of the index subjects was the most common symptom in the group.

Bear & Fedio (1977) used their own scale of 18 traits taken from the literature which were reported to be characteristic of people with temporal lobe epilepsy, to compare a group of 27 people with temporal lobe epilepsy with 12 normal adults and nine patients with neuromuscular disorders. They noted more depression in the group with epilepsy.

The CCEI was employed by Trimble & Perez (1980a,b) to ascertain the phenomenology and frequency of psychiatric symptoms in a cohort of 281 adult patients with epilepsy who were admitted to a centre for epilepsy for rehabilitation, control of their epilepsy or evaluation of their seizures. The index group scored higher on the anxiety and depression subscales than did a normal control population, with the mean depression score being similar to that reported in psychiatric outpatients. No relationship was found between type of epilepsy and depression.

Kogeorgos et al (1982) assessed the psychopathology of a group of 66 patients with chronic epilepsy who were attending a neurological outpatient clinic and were without any psychiatric history, employing the 'General Health Questionnaire' and the CCEI, comparing them to 50 consecutive neurological control outpatients who satisfied similar criteria. Almost half (45.5%) of the patients with epilepsy were identified as probable psychiatric 'cases' and psychopathology was more prevalent and severe in this index group compared to the controls. Moreover, depression, anxiety and hysterical symptoms were most evident in the psychiatrically impaired group.

Twenty children with epilepsy were compared by Margalit & Heiman (1983) with non-handicapped children and learning disabled children using standardised scales. The children with epilepsy showed significantly higher levels of trait anxiety measured by the Spielberger State-Trait Anxiety Inventory, than either of the control groups, and also more self-dissatisfaction, assessed by the self-concept scale.

Brown et al (1986) assessed 28 patients with temporal lobe (n = 14) and idiopathic tonic-clonic (n = 14) epilepsy using the Standard Psychiatric Interview, and those with TLE complained of more irritability and impaired concentration, and were rated as more depressed and 'slowed up'. In addition, somatic and obsessional symptoms, depression and anxiety occurred in approximately one-quarter of the patients: the authors made the point, however, that this may not be a particularly high figure for a general hospital outpatient population (Brown et al 1986).

Eighty-two adult patients with epilepsy from general practices were investigated by Edeh & Toone (1985) using the standardised Clinical Interview Schedule (CIS), chosen because of its wide use in commmunity morbidity prevalence studies, and its ability to discriminate between anxiety and depression. Those patients who scored 13 or more on the CIS were regarded as 'cases' and each case received a clinical diagnosis according to the International Classification of Diseases, 9th Revision (ICD-9). Each patient was examined and special investigations including blood for vitamin B12, red blood cell (rbc) and serum folic acid, an EEG and CT Scan. Of the 37 patients with psychiatric morbidity, the most common illness was affective disorder, with depressive neurosis (n = 19), followed by anxiety neurosis (n = 11) and affective psychosis (n = 1), accounting for 84% of the diagnoses. Levels of rbc and serum folate were significantly lower in patients on anticonvulsant polytherapy (n = 40) than those on monotherapy. The folate concentrations were also significantly lower in the group with psychiatric morbidity: moreover, the subgroup with depressive neurosis had significantly lower folate than the patients without psychiatric morbidity, whereas the subgroup with anxiety did not.

Fenton (1986) also reported on a study using patients with epilepsy in a general practice population. The CCEI was completed by 182 patients with epilepsy between the ages of 18 and 83 years and a control sample of non-epileptic patients from the same practices, matched for age, sex and social class. The male epileptic patients scored significantly higher on the depression, free floating anxiety and obsessionalism subscales than did the control patients, while the scores of the female patients with epilepsy showed insignificant differences on all subscales when compared to controls. The scores of the index group were then compared to those from a neurotic outpatient population taken from the scores from the CCEI manual, and similar results were obtained; namely, that the male epileptic patients scored significantly higher on the depression, free floating anxiety and obsessionalism subscales. The gender difference was found to be significantly related to seizure frequency (increased seizures, more psychopathology) and a state of unemployment, but not to anticonvulsant polytherapy, high plasma anticonvulsant levels, or the type of epilepsy. The type of neurotic symptoms differed with age in that younger patients exhibited anxiety, while older patients reported more depression.

Whitman et al (1984) conducted a thorough literature search and located all published MMPI investigations of adult patients with (1) epilepsy, and the majority of studies on patients with (2) other neurological disorders and diseases, such as multiple sclerosis, cerebral palsy and localised or diffuse brain damage, and (3) non-neurological chronic physical disorders such as cardiac disease, asthma, renal disease, orthopaedic problems, skin conditions, hyperthyroidism, burns and arthritis. Due to the sophisticated statistical tests to which these were going to be applied, selection criteria had to be met. Ten studies of patients with epilepsy embracing 809 subjects, 22 studies of persons with neurological disorder totalling 870 subjects and 15 studies of people with non-neurological disorders comprising a total of 1107 subjects with the above mentioned conditions were included. The authors used a recognised MMPI sequential diagnostic system to re-analyse the profiles of the above 2786 patients. Results showed that no significant age or sex effects were found. The data suggested that patients with epilepsy run a higher risk for psychopathology than members of the general population. No increase of overall psychopathology was found in patients with epilepsy compared to patients with other chronic disorders, and no difference was found between patients with temporal lobe and generalised epilepsy. Patients with neurological conditions were found to be at significantly greater risk compared to people with epilepsy and other chronic illnesses, although it was acknowledged that the neurological group was extremely heterogeneous. However, data showed that higher levels of 'psychosis' were found in both the epilepsy and the neurological groups, the highest levels being found in those with epilepsy. The question as to whether depression occurs more commonly in people with epilepsy was not asked, but five out of the ten studies included in the epilepsy group (Kløve & Doehring 1962, Meier & French 1965, Matthews & Kløve 1968, Mignone et al 1970, Glass & Matson 1973) totalling 450 patients, reported that the depression scores were raised in people with epilepsy.

Dodrill & Batzell (1986) in a similar type of investigation reported on 17 studies which evaluated interictal behavioural features of patients with epilepsy using standardised objective measures including the MMPI, the CCEI, the PSE, the Eysenck Personality Inventory, the General Hospital Questionnaire, the Bear-Fedio Personal Inventory, the Fear Inventory and the Washington Psychosocial Seizure Inventory, comparing the index group with individuals with cerebral disorders other than epilepsy, those with chronic medical non-neurological problems, and normal volunteers. In addition, they performed an analysis on the majority of MMPI studies included in the Whitman et al (1984) study, plus several additional ones. There was only *partial* agreement between the two studies in that Dodrill & Batzell (1986) concluded that people with epilepsy demonstrated more emotional and psychiatric problems than normal persons, and more difficulties than other patient groups having non-neurological disorders, but having approximately the same incidence of these problems as persons with other neurological disorders. Secondly, they suggested that increased emotional and psychiatric problems were not found among patients with temporal lobe epilepsy when compared to patients with other types of epilepsy, although they acknowledged that there were some behavioural characteristics which appeared in a small proportion of these patients. The authors moreover suggested that the number of seizure types was far more relevant to emotional/psychiatric problems in epilepsy than was the particular seizure type. The patients with TLE often have more than one seizure type and therefore as a consequence appear to be more maladjusted. They also speculated as to the origin of emotional and psychiatric difficulties in people with epilepsy, and suggested that, according to MMPI analyses, patients with generalised tonic clonic seizures had no worse adjustment than patients with partial seizures. This argues against an environmental hypothesis (which would attribute adjustment problems in people with epilepsy to the responses of society). The most likely factor in the aetiology would therefore be biological. Finally they noted, in addition, a tendency for impairment on neuropsychological tests to be associated with emotional and psychiatric problems in people with epilepsy.

de Angelis & Vizioli (1983) using the CCEI and the Zung Depression Inventory, compared the depression scores of two groups of patients with epilepsy (primary generalised and temporal lobe epilepsy) with a cohort of patients with syncopal attacks and another group with chronic non-neurological diseases, although the precise diagnoses were not specified. Their results showed that the groups with epilepsy scored no higher than the control groups.

Several investigations based on clinical judgement have also reported depression to be a common symptom or illness in adult patients with epilepsy (Dominian et al 1963, Currie et al 1971, Dalby 1971, Taylor 1972, Betts 1974, Serafetinides 1975, Gunn 1977, Toone & Driver 1980), while others described that children with epilepsy were particularly prone to depression (Mellor et al 1974, Pazzangia & Frank-Pazzangia 1976).

Hancock & Bevilacqua (1971) reported four female patients with localised temporal lobe dysrythmias (3 = left; 1 = bilateral) who had attendant feelings of anxiety, depressive mood, suicidal ideation and/or attempts, emotional lability, one patient's father having committed suicide. They had all, in addition, presented with, on occasions, dizziness, amnesia, tinnitus, vertigo and/or headaches. Neurological examinations were unremarkable, but all patients had abnormal EEGs localised to the temporal lobes.

Schofield & Duane (1986) studied the psychiatric morbidity amongst neurological referrals to a liaison service and found that the most common conditions were epilepsy, parkinsonism and cervical spondylosis. Amongst the 30 patients with epilepsy, some were found to have no formal clinical psychiatric diagnosis: of those who did qualify for a diagnosis 13 (43%) were found to have a depressive illness.

Finally, the complexity and difficulties found in the relationship between depression and epilepsy can be further illustrated by four case reports and an investigation. Thus, Bacon & Benedek (1982) reported a 26 year old male patient who developed a mild depressive illness (requiring psychotherapy) and 'spells' at the age of 24 years, and after 2 years, experiencing typical grand mal seizures. His personality was noted to change in that he developed unusual affective states, decreased attentiveness and alternating lethargic and excitable periods. Following a latent period after a major seizure, he developed a psychotic illness during which he displayed rapidly fluctuating bizarre emotions with a basically euphoric affect accompanied by anxiety, automatisms, and a grandiose delusional system embracing religious and mystical ideas: an epileptic focus was identified in the right temporal lobe.

Maurice-Williams & Sinar (1984) documented the case of a 62 year old woman who presented with focal epilepsy (left fronto-temporal) and an agitated depression. She had had a previous history of depression which necessitated treatment with ECT. Because of the severity and intractability of the depression and repeated suicidal attempts, a leucotomy was performed which led to a dramatic improvement in her depression, although her epilepsy remained unchanged. Twenty-three years later her seizures became worse and, on reinvestigation, a large left frontal meningioma was discovered and removed. One year after removal of the tumour she was reported as being well, with no seizures and no depression.

A 24 year old male patient who reported a life long history of temper outbursts and a changing pattern of mood changes, consistent with bipolar disorder was described by Pellegrini et al (1984). There was no clinical evidence of epilepsy and an EEG showed bilateral paroxysmal bursts of 5–6 HZ spikes and slow wave activity. Family history revealed epilepsy (n = 2), abnormal EEGs (n = 4) and affective disturbance (n = 4) in the seven members of the nuclear family besides the patient. A diagnosis of complex partial seizures was made, and all symptoms responded to anticonvulsant (phenytoin) medication.

Rubin et al (1985) reported a 38 year old woman with a depressive syndrome, meeting DSM. III criteria for melancholia with mood congruent somatic delusions, involving alterations of body parts (e.g. that her eyes became sockets when she slept) who had no prior history of psychiatric illness nor seizure disorder. She was unresponsive to the antidepressant buproprion combined with lithium carbonate, but following the occurrence of two grand mal seizures, probably precipitated by her medication, she experienced rapid improvement of both depression and psychotic symptoms.

Finally, Silberman et al (1985) addressed the converse phenomenon; namely the occurrence of transient sensory, cognitive and affective changes resembling those described by people with epilepsy, in patients with affective illness. Forty-four patients with a history of affective illness (34 = bipolar; 10 = unipolar major depressive disorder) who were euthymic or only mildly symptomatic, and who had no history of seizure disorder and no seizure activity on the EEG were investigated as the index group. The second group consisted of 37 patients with a diagnosis of complex partial seizures, while a third control group comprised 30 hypertensive patients with no history of psychiatric nor neurological disorder. Results showed that transient visual, auditory and olfactory hallucinations, epigastric symptoms, illusions of significance, derealisation, jumbled thoughts and amnesia, were significantly more common in the two patient groups and more so in people with epilepsy. In addition, for both patient groups, symptoms were more frequent during episodes of illness such as seizures in the case of epilepsy.

From the review it is clear therefore that further controlled studies should be undertaken to determine more exactly the prevalence of depression in people with epilepsy compared to other chronic diseases. However, regardless of the source of referral, namely psychiatric, neurological or general practice, the majority of findings are remarkably consistent in highlighting the fact that *depressive symptomatology* is common in patients with epilepsy.

Several investigations have explored specific aspects of the depression encountered in people with epilepsy. Two studies based on clinial judgement have addressed the question of the type of depression found in people with epilepsy. Thus, Mulder & Daly (1952) described 'reactive' depression in 16 of 62 patients, while Betts (1974) reported more 'endogenous' depression in 22 of 72 patients with epilepsy in a psychiatric hospital. Others have noticed possible links between the depression and epilepsy, in that several authors have noted a decrease in seizure frequency prior to the onset of the depressive illness (Dongier 1959–60, Flor-Henry 1969, Betts 1974, Standage & Fenton 1975). Flor-Henry (1969) suggested that when patients had a combination of temporal lobe epilepsy and psychosis, a dominant-side pathology was more likely to be related to a schizophreniform presentation, while a non-dominant abnormality to a manic depressive psychosis. While the former suggestion has been reaffirmed by several authors, the association of affective illness and the non-dominant hemisphere has been noted by only a few authors (for review see Trimble & Robertson 1987).

Two studies have examined fear, both ictal and inter-ictal, and its relationship to psychopathology. Thus, Hermann et al (1982) investigated 11 patients with temoporal lobe epilepsy and ictal fear, and 28 controls (14 with TLE without ictal fear, and 14 with primary generalised epilepsy) using the MMPI, and results indicated that patients who experience ictal fear have a higher risk of psychopathology, scoring higher on five subscales including depression.

Mittan (1984) constructed a 23-item scale derived from the Sepulveda Epilepsy battery and the Washington Psychosocial Seizure Inventory to assess 321 patients' fears about their epilepsy and, in this cohort, also measured psychopathology using standardised rating scales. The 'high fear' group (n = 98) scored significantly higher on the Depression Adjective Checklist, all six subscales of the Hostility and Direction of Hostility Questionnaire (HDHQ) and the MMPI than the 'low fear' group. In contrast, the 'low fear' group (n = 116) scored within normal limits when compared with test norms. Mittan (1984) suggested therefore that the level of patients' fears may be a strong predictor of the presence of psychopathology.

Nielsen & Kristensen (1981) assessed 42 patients with temporal lobe epilepsy (L = 23; R = 19), using the Bear-Fedio Inventory, and left sided foci patients' scored significantly higher than right sided subjects on the traits 'depression' and 'emotionality' combined.

Perini & Mendius (1983) specifically addressed the laterality question, evaluating 11 left sided and 13 right sided patients with uncontrolled complex partial seizures, comparing them with 19 matched controls, using the Emotions Profile Index and the Bear-Fedio Inventory. Laterality of the epileptogenic lesion was based on the side of seizure onset during closed-circuit EEG telemetry monitoring. Left patients scored higher than controls on depression from the Emotions Profile Index, and higher than both right patients and controls on the aggression, depression and guilt measures of the Bear-Fedio Inventory.

In a second study, Perini & Mendius (1984) evaluated 20 patients with complex partial seizures (9 with left and 8 with right temporal lobe foci) and 19 matched control subjects using the BDI, the Columbia Mania-Depression Scale, and the State-Trait Anxiety Inventory, again testing specifically the laterality hypothesis. Lateralisation of the epileptic focus was determined by sophisticated means, including standard wake-sleep EEG's with nasopharyngeal electrodes, closed circuit television-EEG telementry recordings, on all except three patients, stereotaxic depth EEG, positron computed tomography and thiopental activation. All epileptic patients as a group scored significantly higher on the BDI, on the depression items of the Columbia M-D Scales and on the State-Trait Anxiety Inventory than controls, the manic scores not being significantly different. Left patients scored significantly higher than controls on all scales but mania, and higher than right patients on depression, as measured on the BDI, as well as on trait anxiety. Left sided patients scored non-significantly higher than right patients on the Columbia Depression Scales. Right sided patients did not differ significantly from controls on any measure. When a score of 10 was used as a cut off indicative of depression as measured by the BDI, significantly more left patients (56%) were depressed compared to right patients (0%) and controls (11%).

Camfield et al (1984) studied 27 children with lateralised temporal lobe epilepsy (14 = right; 13 = left), with the parents completing the Personality Inventory for Children (PIC), two of the 13 scales being depression and anxiety. No significant left-right differences were found on the PIC scores.

The personality characteristics of epileptic patients were examined by Brandt et al (1985) who also addressed the laterality hypothesis and the question as to whether people with TLE had specific behavioural and ideational characteristics. They administered the Bear-Fedio Inventory to 47 patients with complex partial seizures with temporal lobe foci (L = 28; R = 19), 10 patients with primary generalised epilepsy and 14 normal controls without histories of neurological disorder, the latter being recruited by postal advertisement. Subjects were chosen without regard to psychiatric history, although those clinically psychotic at the time of the study were excluded. All of the patients were receiving therapeutic doses of anticonvulsants and none had toxic blood levels. Analyses showed that the groups differed significantly on seven traits including humourlessness, sadness and obsessionalism. Left temporal lobe epileptics and generalised seizure patients were most different from controls, while the right temporal lobe epileptics had only slightly elevated profiles, not differing from controls on any of the 18 traits. With the exception of the trait of humourlessness, the left and right temporal lobe epileptics did not differ from each other and so did not support the laterality hypothesis of sadness/mood being associated with the right temporal lobe. They suggested that the disruption of left-hemisphere functioning, whether due to a left temporal; focus or to the propagation of centrencephalic discharges through left temporal/limbic structures, is a key issue with regards to the interictal personality syndrome.

Roy (1979) assessed a consecutive series of 42 patients admitted to hospital (23 = neurology or neurosurgery; 19 = psychiatric) for investigation and treatment of their epilepsy using the HDRS, dividing them into two groups: 23 with affective symptoms (HDRS score 9 or above) and 19 with a HDRS score below 9. The two groups were compared in respect of the epileptic and neurotic history, as well as with regard to data from several mood and personality questionnaires. Results showed no difference in the mean ages of the groups nor the age of onset nor duration of epilepsy. No difference was found between affective symptoms and type of epilepsy. Significantly, more in the group with affective symptoms (N = 17) had a past history of neurotic disorder than those without (N = 1), while the group with affective symptoms scored significantly higher on the following rating scales: the HDRS, the Wakefield Self-Assessment Depression Inventory, the Salkind Morbid Anxiety Inventory, the total hostility score from the HDHQ, the neuroticism score of the Eysenck Personality Inventory and the 30 item Goldberg General Health Questionnaire.

In a survey of psychiatric in—and out-patients with epilepsy, Palia & Harper (1986) assessed 53 who had an IQ of over 70 using the HDRS, the BDI and the Newcastle Diagnostic Index. Results showed that 17 patients were judged as clinically depressed, with a mean HDRS score of 21 and a mean BDI score of 32. Most (N = 12) were classified as non-endogenous on the Newcastle Scale. Eighty-eight of the group were female and the mean age was 42.5 years. The depressed patients (the index group) were compared to those who were not depressed. Those who were depressed had experienced significantly more life events during the 3 months preceding the assessment. The index group had a significantly greater past history of depressive illness, deliberate drug overdosage and self harm. Other rating scales were employed to identify specific areas of psychopathology. Thus, on the CCEI, the depressed epileptics scored significantly higher than their counterparts on the subscales of anxiety, phobias, obsessionalism, somatic and depression, with the mean scores well above those found in the normal population. On the Bear-Fedio inventory the depressed epileptics scored significantly higher on sadness, obsessionalism, dependence and altered sexual interest, while non-depressed epileptics scored higher on 'paranoid' traits. Electroencephalographic studies were employed to assess possible neurophysiological factors contributing towards the depression, addressing specifically the laterality hypothesis. Of those with focal abnormalities (n = 4) 36% (n = 4) had left, 18% (n = 2) right and 45% (n = 5) bilateral fronto-temporal foci. The type of epilepsy amongst the depressed group was generalised in six and partial in 11 patients. Serum folate levels were lower in the epileptics with psychiatric disorders than a group without psychiatric disorders, but there was no significant difference between the depressed and non-depressed group.

Two studies have addressed the question of the phenomenology of depressive illness in people with epilepsy, using currently accepted entry diagnostic criteria and standardised rating scales, in addition to exploring possible relationships between the two conditions.

Mendez et al (1986) compared 20 depressed epileptics (mean HDRS 21.7) with 20 depressed patients without epilepsy (mean HDRS 24.7), all of whom satisfied DSM. III criteria for major depression. Both groups were inpatients in a psychiatric hospital and were comparable with respect to personal and socio-economic factors, the control subjects having no complicating medical or neurological illnesses. Personal and family histories were documented, while behaviour and mood were evaluated using a locally devised questionnaire, the HDRS and the Brief Psychiatric Rating Scale. Quantitative scores of depression were obtained from information gained using all three methods of assessment. Special investigations included serum anticonvulsant levels and an EEG. Results showed that the control patients without epilepsy (47.5 years as compared to 40.3 years) were significantly older, but analysis of variance revealed no statistically significant age effects. Male patients predominated in both groups (index = 15; control = 19), the majority of patients were right handed (index = 18; control = 17) and equal numbers of patients (n = 15) in both groups had made previous suicidal attempts. Significant differences between the two groups were that more control patients (n = 11) than index patients (n = 3) had a family history of depression, while more index patients (n = 14) than control patients (n = 6) had psychotic features, such as persecutory auditory hallucinations, delusions and paranoid ideation. These acute agitated *peri-ictal* psychoses were associated with an increase in seizure frequency, usually as a result of non-compliance with medication or alcohol abuse. Among the 20 patients with a combined diagnosis of depression and epilepsy, 16 had complex partial seizures, 15 proceeding to secondary generalisation. No associations were found between depression and seizure freqency or the duration of depression and serum anticonvulsant dosages or levels. Neither did the aetiology of the epilepsy nor the presence of an aura bear any relationship to the depression. Focal changes on the EEG were evident in 15 patients, of which 10 were on the left, 9 being in the temporal area: 1 patient had a right temporal focus while 4 had bilateral temporal foci. The phenomenology of the depression in both groups was characterised by anhedonia, a disturbance of sleep and appetite, fatigue, hyposexuality, psychomotor retardation, and crying. Patients with epilepsy, however, exhibited significantly more psychotic behaviour, paranoia, irritability, humourlessness, an abnormal affect described as 'less depressed than detached or distant', with a greater past history of chronic dysthymia and significantly less self pity, brooding, guilt, somatisation, anxiety and hopelessness than did control subjects.

Robertson et al (1987) screened 80 consecutive adult patients referred to a neuropsychiatric department with a clinical diagnosis of both epilepsy and depression, and 66 who fulfilled epilepsy criteria, the Research Diagnostic Criteria for major depressive disorder, and who scored over 12 on the HDRS were included in the investigation. Patients were interviewed, seizure frequency documented and hand preference assessed by means of the Annett hand preference questionnaire. The epilepsy diagnoses and the EEG assessments of patients and 66 age and sex-matched control subjects with epilepsy, but no history of psychiatric illness, were made by two independent physicians blind to all other details of the patients. Other special investigations included CT Scans. Sixty-six patients qualified for entry into the study, of whom 46 were female, 59 right handed, with a mean age of 38 years (18–67). Sixteen patients (25%) had a family history of psychopathology, with depression being the most common diagnosis (23 relatives); 43 patients (65%) had a past history of depression while 13 were psychotic, as defined by mood congruent hallucinations and/or delusions, a recognised sub-category of the RDC. Only two patients gave a history of bipolar disorder. Half of the patients were receiving two anticonvulsant agents, 27 being on monotherapy, with carbamazepine and phenytoin being the most prescribed drugs. Twenty-five patients had complex partial secondary generalised seizures, 20 had partial complex seizures, 9 had secondary generalised seizures, while 8 had primary generalised seizures and 1 was unclassified due to insufficient information. In both the index and control groups, the majority of the EEG assessments showed temporal lobe abnormalities (index = 26; control = 16), followed by diffuse generalised abnormalities (index = 18; control = 21). Statistical analysis revealed no significant differences between patient and control groups: among those with temporal lobe abnormalities, there was a bias to the left, which was most marked in the patient group. The severity of the depression was moderate, with the mean BDI score being 24.85, the mean LPD score being 12.73, the 17 item HDRS mean being 19.62 and the 21 item HDRS mean being 21.88. The number of patients who were rated as endogenous on the Newcastle Scale was 28 (42.4%) and on the LPD, 25 (37.09%): 12 patients were rated as endogenous on both rating scales. Attendant features of the depression were high state anxiety (measured on the Spielberger Scale), high neuroticism (measured on the Eysenck Personality Inventory) and high hostility (measured on the HDHQ), especially the intropunitive scores of self-criticism and guilt. The duration of epilepsy correlated significantly with the severity of the depression, and an association was found between complex partial seizures and a past history of depression. No other significant relationships emerged between depression and epilepsy variables. Thus, the type, severity and features of depression were not influenced by the age of onset of epilepsy, the type of epilepsy, the site of a focal lesion, the seizure frequency nor the red blood cell nor serum folic acid. An exception was the effect of anticonvulsant medication and mood, in that several significant relationships emerged. Patients receiving phenobarbitone were more depressed than those not receiving the drug, while patients on carbamazepine were less depressed and had lower trait anxiety. There were significant negative correlations between trait anxiety scores and both carbamazepine dose and level.

The quest for biological markers, and measurable abnormalities in today's field of psychiatry to identify types of illness is borne out by the vast literature on the subject (Loosen & Prange 1982, Braddock 1986). One of the popular 'diagnaostic tests' for the *presence* of depressive illness is the Dexamethasone Suppression Test (DST), although it has frequently been claimed to be a laboratory marker for specifically endogenous depression (Braddock 1986).

Little is known about the use of biological markers to identify depression in patients with epilepsy. Robertson et al (1986) evaluated the use of the DST in patients with depression and epilepsy, and three groups were studied. The first consisted of 15 patients with epilepsy who also fulfilled RDC for major depressive disorder, and all of whom scored over 12 on the HDRS, and whose mean BDI score was 24.5 (13–39) and mean LPD score 12.7 (6–17). The second (control group A) comprised 14 patients with epilepsy who were not depressed as defined by the Levine Pilowsky Questionnaire (mean BDI 6.8; mean LPD 4.4) but who were receiving anticonvulsants which induced hepatic enzyme systems. The third group (control group B) consisted of 10 non-depressed epileptic patients as defined by the Levine Pilowsky Questionnaire (mean BDI score 10.0; mean Levine Pilowsky score 5.8) on monotherapy with sodium valproate, an anticonvulsant reported as not having caused hepatic enzyme induction. A standard DST was performed (Carroll 1982) and suppression was defined as a post-dexamethasone cortisol value of 49 ng/ml or less. Results showed that all the depressed epileptic patients and all non-depressed epileptic patients (control Group A) who were receiving anticonvulsants which induce hepatic enzymes, failed to suppress cortisol after dexamethasone administration. Three of the non-depressed epileptic patients on sodium valproate monotherapy suppressed cortisol, while 7 failed to do so (Fisher Exact Probability Test; $p = 0.013$). All three groups had high post DST cortisol levels as follows: depressed epileptics 144 ng/ml; non-depressed control group A, 173 ng/ml and sodium valproate patients, control group B, 92 ng/ml. Thus, it can be seen that patients on sodium valproate monotherapy had lower post-DST cortisol levels than either of the other two groups, which reached significance even when the 3 patients in the group who fully suppressed cortisol were excluded from the analysis. No link between non-suppressability after the DST and seizure type was found. It was therefore concluded that the DST does not seem likely to be of value in the assessment of depressive illness in patients with epilepsy on anticonvulsants (Robertson et al 1986). This non-suppression is unlikely to be due only to anticonvulsants, as not only did seven patients on sodium valproate fail to suppress, but others (Gallagher et al 1984) have suggested that ACTH and cortisol secretion are abnormal in patients with temporal lobe epilepsy. Since the DST appears unhelpful as a biological marker for depression in people with epilepsy, further attempts to examine neuroendocrine alterations in this population could be undertaken: for example, following up the expanding literature on abnormalities of TSH (thyroid stimulating hormone) release in depression after provocative tests (Loosen & Prange 1982).

## Suicide and parasuicide

The importance of suicide when discussing depression cannot be overstressed. According to figures from the Registrar-General, the crude suicide rate for men in England and Wales is approximately 9.7 per 100 000 and for women 6.2 per 100 000 (averages for 1974–8) (Kreitman 1983). Patients with affective illness are particularly at risk, as those treated by psychiatrists for manic-depressive psychosis and reactive depression have approximately 30 times the risk of death by suicide compared to the general population. In people with epilepsy, suicide and attempted suicide are also over-represented. Thus there is a general consensus that the risk of suicide in people with epilepsy is four to five times greater than that of the general population (Barraclough 1981, Matthews & Barabas 1981, Wannamaker 1983) while those with TLE have an increased risk of approximately 25 times that expected (Barraclough 1981). Two investigations have reported a 5–7% increase in self poisoning (parasuicide) in people with epilepsy, finding that repeated attempts were common, with barbiturates being implicated in particular (Mackay 1979, Hawton et al 1980).

**Management**

Depressive phenomena are common in people with epilepsy and the treatment should initially be directed towards the identification of the problem and its possible cause. Thus, if a patient is undergoing a depressive reaction on acquiring the label of epilepsy, the support and help of a social worker, especially one who has knowledge of and experience in epilepsy, can help the person 'work through' his or her grief (Betts 1981). As several studies have indicated that a high seizure frequency interferes with psychosocial functioning, which may masquerade as depression, behavioural methods of decreasing seizure frequency ought to be considered. Thus, as Temkin & Davis (1984) have shown high stress levels and stressful events are associated with more frequent seizures, attempts should be aimed at decreasing seizures and stress. Indeed, using biofeedback techniques, operant conditioning may be beneficial for reducing seizure frequency (Lubar et al 1981), while there has also been a suggestion (Sunder 1983) that a standardised treatment programme of progressive relaxation is beneficial in psychosocial functioning in people with epilepsy.

Only one investigation of psychotherapeutic techniques in treating the depressive phenomena seen in association with epilepsy has been published. Thus, Davis et al (1984) undertook a controlled randomised study using cognitive and behavioural treatment methods to treat depressed affect in 13 adult people with epilepsy (treatment group n = 8: control group n = 5). Treatment consisted of 6 weekly 2-hour 'classes' led by professional social workers. The subjects were assessed pre- and post-treatment using standardised rating scales such as the Depression Adjective Checklist (DACL), the Hudson Generalised Contentment Scale (GCS), the BDI and the Community Adjustment Questionnaire (CAQ) which consists of 10 subscales including anxiety, depression and anger. Assessment was followed by didactic, skill-building excercises and homework projects directed towards increasing subjects' skills in using specific cognitive-behavioural techniques for the treatment of depression which included increasing pleasant events; increasing physical exercise; increasing assertivensss; identifying self-talk including faulty belief systems; thought stopping; and increasing positive cognitions such as coping and self-reinforcing statements. Results showed significant decreases in dysphoria/depression on the DACL and the GCS, significant reductions in anger and anxiety/stress, and increases in social activities rated on the CAQ among subjects in the treatment group when compared to the control group. Similar trends were noted on the BDI and the depression scale of the CAQ. The authors (Davis et al 1984) acknowledge the small sample sizes, that the groups were not homogeneous with regard to epilepsy variables such as duration, type and frequency of attacks, and the fact that all scales used were self-report. Nonetheless, the results are positive and encouraging, despite the reservations mentioned. When considering the use of behavioural techniques in people with epilepsy it is important to take into account variables which may affect the patient. For example, Gay (1984) studied the effects of anti-epileptic drugs on operant responding/reinforcement in mentally retarded epileptic persons and reported that patients on phenobarbitone performed worse than those receiving phenytoin or valproate.

Psychotherapy is important in the treatment of people with depression, especially when one considers the psychosocial models of depression when applied to people with epilepsy, and the literature on stigma and epilepsy. One may opt for supportive therapy alone or, as recent evidence has shown, a combination of formal psychotherapy (such as cognitive, interpersonal, or behavioural approaches) and antidepressants is more effective than either treatment alone for the ambulatory nonbipolar depressive (Weissman 1981). The use of antidepressants in people with epilepsy, must however, be carried out with care (vide infra).

As many reports indicate, depressive symptoms are associated with low folate levels. Folic acid supplements are indicated if the patient's folic acid levels are abnormally low, as replacement therapy in patients with epilepsy is associated with a particular effect on drive, mood and sociability (Reynolds 1967). Another method of tackling the depression may be the use of S-Adenosylmethionine (SAM) which has been shown to have antidepressant properties (Reynolds et al 1984). This is particularly important in view of the fact that the metabolism and functions of folic acid are intimately related to SAM and methylation (Reynolds et al 1984).

Assessment and rationalisation of the patients' anticonvulsant regimen is also important. Shorvon & Reynolds (1977) emphasise the lack of evidence that two or more anticonvulsant drugs are more effective than one in treating seizures, while about 7.3% of all patients receiving multiple anticonvulsants have some form of toxicity, be it mild or severe, acute or chronic (Hooshmand 1974).

In addition, a review of early studies (1940–1975) suggests that anticonvulsants have adverse effects on the mental state of epileptic patients, with some showing evidence of overt psychiatric illness (Trimble & Reynolds 1976). More recently, improvement in the mental state of patients with a reduction of polypharmacy using standarised methods of assessment has been reported (Thompson & Trimble 1982). Subsequent studies have confirmed this finding. Thus, Giordani et al (1983) reported significant improvement in scores in 25 patients with refractory seizures when anticonvulsant drugs were reduced in number, including measures associated with problem-solving and psychomotor speed (Digit Symbol, Block Design): in addition, a significant improvement in Digit Symbol and Finger tapping (indication of motor speed) were found when barbiturates specifically were discontinued.

In another study (Albright & Bruni 1985), withdrawal of phenobarbitone or primidone in an attempt to convert patients on anticonvulsant polytherapy to monotherapy, resulted in patients being more alert and with improved concentration and overall functioning.

Taking all evidence into account, it seems fair to say that a reduction of anticonvulsants, with particular reference to phenobarbitone with its sedative and depressing side effects, is therefore important. If a patient has been seizure free for 2 or 3 years, there may be arguments for discontinuing anticonvulsant medication, and this is well covered by Chadwick & Reynolds (1985).

If monotherapy is possible and all other factors, such as type of epilepsy, are taken into account, carbamazepine would seem the most appropriate drug. This would be in keeping with the literature of its efficacy as an antidepressant in depressed people without epilepsy (Folks et al 1982, Neumann et al 1984, Roy-Byrne et al 1985, Sethi & Tiwari 1984), as having a prophylactic effect in manic-depressive illness

(Ballenger & Post 1980, Okuma et al 1981, Placidi et al 1984) and having a psychotropic effect in people with epilepsy (Dalby 1971, Dodrill & Troupin 1977, Marjerrison et al 1968, Rodin & Schmaltz 1984, Andrews et al 1986, Robertson et al 1987).

Although seizure control is good in most patients with epilepsy, a chronic intractable disorder develops in about 25% (Reynolds et al 1983). If a patient has refractory epilepsy and depressive symptoms, and is already on one anticonvulsant, adjunctive therapy with clobazam may be appropriate, as positive psychotropic effects of the drug have been documented when used as adjunctive therapy. Robertson (1986b) noted in a literature review, that many studies reported an improvement in demeanour and a feeling of general 'well being' in patients receiving clobazam. Others reported psychomotor arousal, with increased alertness, attention, ability to think faster, decreased anxiety, a reduction in 'nervousness' and improved sleep pattern. To complement these clinical impressions several investigations using standardised procedures have reported less anxiety and tension, increased alertness or minimal or no cognitive impairment compared to other anticonvulsants or to 1,4-benzodiazepines.

What is the role of antidepressants in the treatment of the person who has depression and epilepsy? There are three main issues which need to be considered: the effects of the antidepressants on the seizure threshold, antidepressant — anticonvulsant interactions, and efficacy of the antidepressant in the setting of depression and epilepsy.

It is well known that virtually all non-monoamine oxidase inhibitor antidepressants lower the seizure threshold (Trimble 1978), but to varying degrees. Table 10.3 shows the common antidepressants and some of their properties. Included are the number of cases of convulsions reported to the Committee on Safety of Medicines (CSM) until February 1984 (Edwards 1985). Of note is that nomifensine and zimelidine have been withdrawn due to side effects other than seizures, and tofenacin due to lack of commercial viability. In more recent studies on experimental animals, imipramine, and chlorimipramine and maprotiline were shown to be equally epileptogenic; nomfensine was, in contrast, found not to affect the seizure threshold (Trimble et al 1977). Jobe et al (1984) in rat models, noted that imipramine and desipramine were anticonvulsant at lower doses and proconvulsant at higher doses — the protective effects being greater for imipramine.

Luchins et al (1984) studied the epileptogenic potential of various antidepressants in vitro, examining their effect on spike activity in guinea pig hippocampal sites. Of drugs in use today, imipramine, amitriptyline, nortriptyline, maprotiline and desipramine increased spike activity in a descending order of effect. Doxepin increased spike activity at lower, but reduced it at higher concentrations. Protriptyline and trimipramine reduced spike activity with rising concentrations, while viloxazine had also decreased neuronal excitability with increasing doses. Mianserin produced no significant effect on spike activity.

Studies on patient populations also give some idea as to the relative effect of antidepressants on the seizure threshold. There are difficulties however because of differences in side effect reporting, patient populations and study designs. Crome & Newman (1977) investigated 547 cases of poisoning with antidepressants and documented the frequency of seizures which showed maprotiline to be implicated the most (20–25% of 41 and 48 cases), followed by nortriptyline and imipramine, fits being found in both of these in over 20% of cases. Seizures were found in only 8% of amitriptyline overdoses, while antidepressants not leading to seizures were trimipramine, chlorimipramine, doxepin and mianserin. Trazodone has been noted in two published case reports from the USA (Bowdan 1983, Lefkowitz et al 1985), and 45 reports to the manufacturers in the USA (Hohly & Martin 1986) to cause seizures. Maprotiline has been implicated in at least 98 cases of seizures in the USA (Dessain et al 1986), but it was noted that two-thirds of the patients received dosages in excess of 200 mg daily, outside the dosage guidelines (see Table 10.3). Wall et al (1985, 1986) reported two patients who developed affective symptomatology such as panic attacks, anxiety, episodes of depression and suicidal ideation following right temporal lobe surgery, and which were successfully treated with imipramine. No mention of seizures was made.

It has been suggested following a literature review concerning seizures and viloxazine, that viloxazine is probably less epileptogenic than conventional tricyclics (Edwards et al 1984), while a new suggested antidepressant, lovoxamine, caused no epileptiform activity in patients treated with the agent (Cilasun et al 1986). Fluvoxamine, a highly selective serotonin reuptake inhibitor, was introduced into the United Kingdom in January 1987. It has been used as an antidepressant in Europe in 7 countries for some time, including Switzerland for 4 years, totalling over half a million prescriptions. One patient took an overdose of 96 tablets with resulting sedation, but no seizures. Twelve patients in total (internationally) have had seizures when receiving fluvoxamine: most had epilepsy and the fits were not attributed to the drug (Personal communication — 1987 — Duphar Laboratories, Southampton, England). Moreover, results on experimental animals indicate that fluvoxamine has no convulsant properties, being similar to nomifensine and no different from controls in that respect (Krijzer et al 1984). On the other hand, Chlorimipramine (Setiey & Courjon 1978) and imipramine (Fromm et al 1978) have been shown to be efficacious in treating generalised absence seizures.

Two studies have examined the effect of antidepressants in people with depression and epilepsy, addressing not only effects on the seizure threshold, but also the efficacy of the antidepressants. Following a report that doxepin prevented seizures induced by pentylenetetrazol or electroshock in mice (Pinder et al 1977), it became the most widely prescribed antidepressant to be prescribed in an epilepsy clinic, prompting Ojemann et al (1983) to conduct a retrospective study on the effect of doxepin on seizures and mood in 47 depressed epileptics who had been given the antidepressant over the preceding 3 years. Depression was diagnosed according to the DSM. III criteria, and had been present for at least 1 year in all patients. Confirmed seizure disorder and frequency, and an adequate follow up time (mean 6.8 months) were available for 19 patients of whom 13 were female and 6 male, with a mean age of 35 years (range 16–58) and a mean duration of epilepsy 17 years (range 3–46). Thirteen patients had complex partial seizures with secondary generalisation. As the investigation was retrospective, the anticonvulsant dosage over the study period was not always constant in each patient. Doxepin was given for a mean of 7.5 months), (range 2–22) at a mean dosage of 161 mg daily (range 10–500). However, results showed that depression improved in all 17 patients (excellent $n = 10$; good $n = 22$; mild $n = 5$). In addition, when compared to the control period, seizure frequency decreased in 15 patients, was unchanged in 2 and increased in 2 (statistically significant at the 1% level, sign test). Moreover, the degree of improvement was greater than 50% in more than one half of the patients and in 10, occurred without associated

**Table 10.3** Common antidepressants. (Robertson 1983, Edwards 1985). Grouping of drugs from Spencer (1977), Silverstone & Turner (1978)

| Group | Subgroup | Generic name | Proprietary names | Year introduced to UK | % Prescriptions of market share (1979) | Usual daily dose (mg) | Onset of action | Sedative stimulant | Number of patients with convulsions (CSM 1984) | Average no. cases of convulsions notified per year |
|---|---|---|---|---|---|---|---|---|---|---|
| 1. Monoamine reuptake inhibitors (MARI) | (i) Bicyclic | Viloxazine | Vivalan | 1974 | • • • | 100–300 | 5–10 days | Sedative < Amitrip | 5 | 0.6 |
| | | Zimelidine | Zelmid | 1982 | • • • | 50–300 | 2 weeks | Non-sedative | 22 | 11.0 |
| | (ii) Tricyclics | Amitriptyline | Domical<br>Elavil<br>Endep<br>Lentizol<br>Tryptanol<br>Tryptizol<br>Saroten | 1961 | 34.2 | 75–200 | 10–30 days | Sedative | 27 | 1.2 |
| | | Butriptyline | Evadyne | 1975 | • • • | 50–150 | 7–14 days | Sedative | 1 | 0.1 |
| | | Clomipramine (Chlorimipramine) | Anafranil | 1970 | 5.5 | 50–150 | i.v. 5 days | Sedative | 24 | 2.2 |
| | | Desipramine | Norpramine<br>Pertofran | 1962 | • • • | 75–200 | 2–7 days | Mildly sedative | 3 | 0.2 |
| | | Dothiepin | Prothiaden | 1969 | 13.3 | 75–150 | 7–10 days | Sedative ≡ to Amitrip | 17 | 1.1 |
| | | Doxepin | Adapin<br>Sinequan | 1969 | 3.9 | 75–150 | few days to 2 weeks | Sedative ≡ to Amitrip | 5 | 0.4 |
| | | Imipramine | Berkomine<br>Imavate<br>Janimine<br>Praminil<br>Presamine<br>Tofranil | 1959 | 13.5 | 75–200 | up to 4 weeks | Sedative < Amitrip | 15 | 0.8 |
| | | Lofepramine | Deprimil<br>Gamanil | 1983 | • • • | 140–210 | 2–5 days | Non-sedative | 2 | 2.0 |
| | | Nortriptyline | Allegron<br>Aventyl<br>Pamelor | 1963 | 2.2 | 75–200 | 3–5 days | Sedative < Amitrip | 8 | 0.4 |
| | | Protriptyline | Concordin<br>Triptil<br>Vivactil | 1967 | 0.5 | 15–60 | Within 1 week | Mild stimulant | 1 | 0.1 |
| | | Trimipramine | Surmontil | 1966 | 7.1 | 50–100 | 7–10 days | Sedative > Amitrip | 4 | 0.3 |
| | (iii) Tricyclic related | Dibenzepin | Noveril | 1970 | • • • | 240–480 | 10–14 days | Sedative | | |
| | | Iprindole | Prondol | 1968 | 0.3 | 45–90 | 1–2 weeks | Sedative < Amitrip | 1 | 0.1 |
| | | Opipramol | Insidon | 1971 | • • • | 100–300 | 10 days | Sedative | | |

| | | | | | | | | | | |
|---|---|---|---|---|---|---|---|---|---|---|
| | (iv) Tetracyclics | Maprotiline | Ludiomil | 1975 | 3.6 | 50–150 | 1–2 weeks | Sedative < Amitrip | 122 | 13.6 |
| | | Mianserin | Bolvidon<br>Lantanon<br>Norval<br>Tolvin | 1976 | 5.8 | 20–60 | 1–2 weeks | Sedative | 62 | 7.8 |
| 2. Monoamine oxidase inhibitors (MAOI) | (i) Hydrazines<br>a. With acute stimulant effects | Iproniazid<br>Isocarboxazid<br>Phenelzine | Marsilid<br>Marplan<br>Nardil | 1957<br>1960<br>1959 | ● ● ●<br>0.3<br>1.3 | 50–75<br>20–40<br>30–60 | 2–3 weeks<br>1–4 weeks | Stimulant<br>Stimulant<br>Stimulant | 0<br>0<br>4 | 0.0<br>0.0<br>0.2 |
| | b. Without acute stimulant effects<br>(ii) Non-Hydrazines | Nialamide<br>Tranylcypro-mine | Niamid<br>Parnate | 1959<br>1960 | 0.3 | 50–150<br>10–30 | 14 days–3 weeks<br>7 days–3 weeks | Non-stimulant<br>Stimulant | 2 | 0.0 |
| | a. With acute stimulant effects<br>b. Without acute stimulant effects | Pargyline | Eutonyl | | | 25–50 | | Non-stimulant | | |
| 3. Naturally occurring agents | (i) Amino acid precursors of transmitters | L Tryptophan | Optimax<br>Pacitron | 1971 | 1.3 | 3000–6000 | 3–4 weeks | Sedative | 2 | 0.2 |
| | (ii) Lithium salts | | Camcolit<br>Liskonum<br>Priadel | 1964 | 2.2 | 250–2000 | Acute 3–7 days mania<br>1–2 weeks (depression)<br>Prophylaxis up to 12 months | Non-sedative | 5 | 0.3 |
| 4. Amphetamine related sympatho-mimetic agents | (i) Releasers of non-granular amine stores | (+)-Amphetamine (dexamphetamine) | Dexedrine | | | 5–60 | Uncertain | Stimulant | | |
| | (ii) Releasers of granular and non-granular amine stores | Methylphenidate | Ritalin | 1955 | | 20–30 | 15–45 min | Stimulant | | |
| 5. Miscel-laneous | | Flupenthixol | Fluanxol | 1973 | ● ● ● | 2–3<br>1–2 | 3 days | Non-sedative | | |
| | | Nomifensine | Alival<br>Merital | 1977 | 2.6 | 50–150 | 7–10 days | Mild stimulant | 5 | 0.7 |
| | | Tofenacin | Elamol | 1971 | ● ● ● | 240 | 4–7 days | Unapplic-able | 0 | 0.0 |
| | | Trazodone | Desyrel<br>Molipaxin | 1980 | | 50–600 | 10–30 days (11) | Sedative | 8 | 2.0 |
| | | Fluvoxamine | Faverin<br>Floxyfrau<br>Dumyrox | 1987 | ● ● ● | 100–300 | 10 days | Non-sedative | See text | 0.0 |

Key: > more than; < less than; ≡ similar to; CSM, Committee on Safety of Medicine. Shares marked ● ● ● total less than 1.4% between them.

changes in type or dose of anticonvulsant drugs. The decrease in fit frequency was apparent for both complex partial and generalised tonic clonic seizures. Ojemann et al (1983) suggested that the reduction in seizure frequency may have been due to a direct anticonvulsant affect of doxepin, an indirect effect due to improved mood, due to drug interactions or hepatic enzyme induction with resultant potentiation of anticonvulsants or a combination of factors. They noted that the antidepressant effect may be directly due to the chemical intervention by doxepin or due to the added effects of counselling and informal psychotherapy from which the patients in the study benefited.

Robertson & Trimble (1985) conducted a randomised double-blind placebo controlled antidepressant trial in 42 patients satisfying RDC criteria for major depressive disorder, scoring over 15 on the HDRS and satisfying accepted criteria for epilepsy (Pond et al 1960, Hopkins & Scambler, 1977). Pre-treatment and throughout the trial, patients were assessed using the HDRS, the BDI and the Spielberger State Anxiety Inventory. The dose of the active drug was 25 mg tid., which was doubled in non-responders on the active drug after 6 weeks. At that point, a further 6 week follow up was carried out. Serum antidepressant and anticonvulsant levels were assessed throughout, and seizure frequency documented. Results indicated that using all three rating scales, there was a significant decrease in scores over the 6 weeks (HDRS, $p < 0.001$; BDI, $P < 0.0001$; Spielberger State Scale, $p < 0.001$), but no significant differences between either of the drugs or placebo emerged. There were no significant differences in the serum amitriptyline or nomifensine levels between weeks 2,4 and 6 of the double-blind trial, nor were there significant differences between any of the serum anticonvulsant levels of the patients on any of the treatment agents between weeks 2–6. Moreover, no significant associations between anticonvulsants and antidepressant levels were found. Seizure frequencies of patients showed large variation, but there were no statistical differences in fit frequency between placebo, amitriptyline and nomifensine groups. At 12 weeks nomifensine was superior to amitriptyline, but as this was based on small numbers it may well have been due to chance. Secondly, it may have been on differential drug effect. A third possibility is that, in spite of randomisation, significantly fewer patients in the amitriptyline group (only one) were classified as endogenously depressed on the Newcastle Scale, and the literature indicates that endogenous depression is more likely to respond to biological treatments (Meyer-Gross et al 1974, Bielski & Friedel 1976).

Anticonvulsants and antidepressants can affect each other's levels, as hepatic enzyme induction by anticonvulsants may result in a reduction in serum antidepressant levels (Richens et al 1983). Thus phenytoin, phenobarbitone, primidone and carbamazepine, which are powerful inducers of hepatic enzymes, can result in an enhanced clearance of agents which are metabolised by the system (Perucca & Richens 1977). For example, Richens et al (1983) performed a simple dose study of mianserin in healthy volunteers and patients with epilepsy who were taking one or more enzyme-inducing anticonvulsants. Results showed that mianserin levels were lower and the plasma half-life shorter in the patients. Conversely, anticonvulsant levels can be affected by antidepressants. Phenytoin levels may be increased by imipramine, nortriptyline and viloxazine (Perucca & Richens 1977), while carbamazepine toxicity has been caused by viloxazine (Pisani et al 1984, 1986).

What conclusions can be drawn from the data, given the inherent problems? The antidepressants most likely to be implicated with seizures are maprotiline, mianserin, trazodone and chlorimipramine, while the drugs which are less likely to be associated are doxepin, fluvoxamine, viloxazine, protriptyline, butriptyline and the MAOI's: no seizures have ever been reported in associated with iproniazid, isocarboxazid, and tranylcypromine. Viloxazine should probably be avoided, however, because of its potential to cause anticonvulsant toxicity. Thus, at present doxepin, fluvoxamine protriptyline, nortriptyline and the MAOI's appear to be safest. In addition, it may be wise to prescribe a non-sedating or less sedative antidepressant (see Table 10.3), as most anticonvulsants which the patient will be taking have sedative side effects. Having said this, many clinicians prefer to use antidepressants they know well, and commence with small doses (see Table 10.3), increasing the dose gradually.

The role of ECT in the depressed epileptic remains an enigma to those unacquainted with the problem. Betts (1981) makes the point that epileptic depression can be rather resistant to conventional antidepressant treatment and may need ECT to clear it. Clinically, this is particularly important to consider when suicide is a real danger, or in cases of severe paranoid agitation in which the patient's seizure frequency appears to have diminished prior to the onset of the depression. Paradoxically, some of these patients appear to have a particularly high seizure threshold during the administration of ECT (RTC Pratt, personal communication) and they do not readily produce a seizure in response to the electric shock. This may be partly explained by the fact that there is increasing evidence that ECT has significant anticonvulsant properties, and results in decreased neural metabolic activity. It has been suggested that these effects are due to enhanced gamma-aminobutyric acid (GABA) transmission (Sackeim et al 1983).

## DISCUSSION AND CONCLUSION

The conclusion from the review is that depressive symptomatology occurs frequently in people with epilepsy. Several studies using standardised rating scales have found the depression scores to range from moderate to severe and to compare favourably with studies on depressed patients without epilepsy (Beck et al 1961, Mowbray 1972, Metcalfe & Goldman 1965, Levine 1975, Bailey & Coppen 1976, Bech et al 1979, Pilowsky 1979). Thus, although only two studies specifically addressed depressive illness in the context of epilepsy and employed entry criteria, many of the patients included in the review would probably have qualified for a depressive illness. There was some consensus of opinion on several issues. A number of variables have been postulated with regard to the pathogenesis of depression and several predisposing or provoking factors include genetic endowment, patients' fears, social stigmatisation, adverse life events and a past history of depressive illness. The phenomenology of the depression does not seem intimately linked with epilepsy variables with some exceptions. Thus, anticonvulsants can affect the mental state, and the longer the duration of epilepsy the more severe the depression. The majority of studies demonstrated involvement of the left hemisphere, with some emphasis on the temporal lobe/complex partial seizure patients. Whether this is specific as suggested by Mendez et al (1986), or because the left hemisphere and frontotemporal areas seem particularly vulnerable as far as psychopathology is concerned, as evidenced by studies on head injury (Lishman 1968, Robinson & Szetcha 1981), stroke patients (Robinson et al 1984), patients with epilepsy (Bingley 1958, Taylor 1972, Stores 1978, Pritchard et al 1980), or because when focal abnormalities are found, foci on the left side appear to be more common (Scott 1985), is as yet uncertain.

An attractive model which could be considered is that proposed by Akiskal & McKinney (1975), who view depressive illness as a 'psychobiological final common pathway' and the culmination of various processes which converge on those areas of the diencephalon that modulate arousal, mood, motivation and psychomotor function. They take the view that the specific form that the depressive illness will take in a given individual depends on the interaction of several factors which has relevance to this review and topic: (1) genetic vulnerability (as suggested by some studies); (2) developmental events (and their disruption by epileptic seizures); (3) psychosocial events (such as stigma and other issues discussed); physiological stressors (again, for example, a seizure), which impinge on diencephalic function, and (5) personality traits. In many studies trait anxiety, obsessionality, neuroticism and hostility were much higher when compared with other populations and only some but not all of these, could have been accounted for by depressive illness (Robertson 1983), as in most studies the reporting of their symptomatology was not measured in the context of illness.

The treatment of the depression should therefore be tailored to the individual, and in all cases supportive psychotherapy is imperative. Thereafter rationalisation of anticonvulsant therapy and institution of monotherapy, possibly with carbamazepine, could be instituted. Depending on the severity of the illness, on provoking factors, and the expertise of the clinician, formal psychotherapy, such as cognitive or behavioural approaches, the prescription of appropriate antidepressants or even ECT may be appropriate.

*Acknowledgements*
I would like to express my gratitude to Mrs Penny Nicholson for her invaluable help in preparing the manuscript.

## REFERENCES

Abramson L Y, Seligman M E P, Teasdale J D 1978 Learned helplessness in humans: critique and reformulation. Journal of Abnormal Psychology 87: 49–74

Akiskal H S, McKinney W T Jr 1975 Overview of recent research in depression. Archives of General Psychiatry 32: 285–305

Albright P, Bruni J 1985 Reduction of polypharmacy in epileptic patients. Archives of Neurology 42: 797–799

Allen M G, Cohen S, Pollin W, Greenspan S I 1974 Affective illness in veteran twins: a diagnostic review. American Journal of Psychiatry 131: 1234–1239

American Psychiatric Association 1980 DSM. III — Diagnostic and statistical manual of psychiatric disorders, 3rd edn. American Psychiatric Association, Washington D.C.

Andreason N C 1982 Concepts and classification of depression. In: Paykel E S (ed) Handbook of affective disorders. Churchill Livingstone, Edinburgh

Andrews D G, Bullen J D, Tomlinson L, Elwes R D C, Reynolds E H 1986 A comparative study of the cognitive effects of Phenytoin and Carbamazepine in new referrals with epilepsy. Epilepsia 27: 128–134

Angelis G de, Vizioli R 1983 Epilepsy and depression. In: Parsonage M, Grant R H E, Craig A, Ward A A J Jr (eds). Advances in epileptology: XIVth Epilepsy International Symposium. Raven Press, New York, p 203–206

Bacon P D, Benedek E P 1982 Epileptic psychosis and insanity: case study and review. Bulletin of the AAPL 10: 3: 203–210

Bagley C 1972 Social prejudice and the adjustment of people with epilepsy. Epilepsia 13: 33–45

Bailey J, Coppen A 1976 A comparison between the Hamilton Rating Scale and the Beck Inventory in the measurement of depression. British Journal of Psychiatry 128: 486–489

Ballenger J C, Post R M 1980 Carbamazepine (Tegretol) in manic-depressive illnesss: a new treatment. American Journal of Psychiatry 137: 782–790

Barham G F 1907 Notes on the management and treatment of the epileptic insane, with special reference to the NaCl-free (or hypo-chlorisation) diet. Journal of Mental Science 53: 361–367

Barraclough B 1981 Suicide and epilepsy. In: Reynolds E H, Trimble M R (eds) Epilepsy and psychiatry. Churchill Livingstone, Edinburgh, p 72–76

Baugh L D H 1908 Observations on insane epileptics treated under hospital principles. Journal of Mental Science 54: 518–528

Bear D M, Fedio P 1977 Quantitative analysis of interictal behavior in temporal lobe epilepsy. Archives of Neurology 34: 454–467

Bech P, Bolwig T G, Kramp P, Rafaelsen O J 1979 The Bech Rafaelson mania scale and the Hamilton Depression Scale. Acta Psychiatrica Scandinavica 59: 420–430

Beck A T, Ward C H, Mendelson N, Mock J, Erbaugh J 1961 An inventory for measuring depression. Archives of General Psychiatry 4: 561–571

Beran R G, Read T 1981 Patient perspectives of epilepsy. Clinical and Experimental Neurology 17: 56–69

Bertelsen A, Harvald B, Hauge N 1977 A Danish twin study of manic depressive disorders. British Journal of Psychiatry 130: 330–351

Betts T A 1974 A follow-up study of a cohort of patients with epilepsy admitted to psychiatric care in an English city. In: Harris P, Mawdsley C (eds) Epilepsy: Proceedings of the Hans Berger Centenary Symposium. Churchill Livingstone, Edinburgh, p 326–338

Betts T A 1981 Depression, anxiety and epilepsy. In: Reynolds E H, Trimble M R (eds) Epilepsy and psychiatry. Churchill Livingstone, Edinburgh, p 60–71

Betts T A 1982 Psychiatry and epilepsy: part one. In: Laidlaw J, Richens A eds A textbook of epilepsy 2nd edn. Churchill Livingstone, Edinburgh, p 227–270

Bielski R J, Friedel R O 1976 Prediction of tricyclic antidepressant response. A critical review. Archives of General Psychiatry, 33: 1479–1489

Bingley T 1958 Mental symptoms in temporal lobe epilepsy and temporal lobe gliomas. Acta Psychiatrica et Neurologica Scandinavica, 33: (Suppl. 120), 1–151

Blanchet P, Frommer G P 1986 Mood change preceding epileptic seizures. Journal of Nervous and Mental Disease 174: 471–476

Bowdan N D 1983 Seizure possibly caused by Trazodone HCL. American Journal of Psychiatry 140: 642

Bowman K M, Rose M 1951 A criticism of the terms 'psychosis, 'psychoneurosis' and 'neurosis'. American Journal of Psychiatry 108: 161–166

Braddock L 1986 The dexamethasone suppression test. Fact and artefact. British Journal of Psychiatry 148: 363–374

Brandt J, Seidman L J, Kohl D 1985 Personality characteristics of epileptic patients: A controlled study of generalized and temporal lobe cases. Journal of Clinical and Experimental Neuropsychology 7: 25–38

Britten N, Wadsworth M E J, Fenwick P B C 1984 Stigma in patients with early epilepsy: a national longitudinal study. Journal of Epidemiology and Community Health 38: 291–295

Broughton R J, Guberman A, Roberts 1984 Comparison of the psychosocial effects of epilepsy and narcolepsy/cataplexy: A controlled study. Epilepsia 25: 423–433

Brown G W, Craig T K J, Harris T O 1985 Depression: distress or disease? Some epidemiological considerations. British Journal of Psychiatry 147: 612–622

Brown S W, McGowan M E L, Reynolds E H 1986 The influence of seizure type and medication on psychiatric symptoms in epileptic patients. British Journal of Psychiatry 148: 300–304

Bruens J H 1971 Psychosis in epilepsy. Psychiatria, Neurologia Neurochirurgia 74: 175–192

Callaghan N, Mitchel R, Cotter P 1969 The relationship of serum folic acid and vitamin B12 levels to psychosis in epilepsy. Irish journal of Medical Science 28: 497–505

Camfield P R, Gates R, Ronen G, Camfield C, Ferguson A, MacDonald G W 1984 Comparison of cognitive ability, personality profile, and school success in epileptic children with pure right versus left temporal lobe EEG foci. Annals of Neurology 15: 122–126

Carney M W P, Sheffield B S 1972 Depression and the Newcastle Scales: their relationship to Hamilton's Scale. British Journal of Psychiatry 121: 35–40

Carney M W P, Roth N, Garside R S 1965 The diagnosis of depressive syndromes and the prediction of ECT responses. British Journal of Psychiatry 111: 659–674

Carroll B J 1982 The dexamethasone suppression test for melancholia. British Journal of Psychiatry 140: 292–304

Chadwick D, Reynolds E H 1985 When do epileptic patients need treatment? Starting and stopping medication. British Medical Journal 290: 1885–1888

Cilasun J, Edwards J G, Sedgwick E M 1986 Electroencephalographic changes during treatment with clovoxamine fumarate. Neuropharmacology 25: 665–667

Clayton P J, Halikas J A, Maurice W L 1972 The depression of widowhood. British Journal of Psychiatry 120: 71–78

Coppen A J 1972 Indoleamines and affective disorders. Journal of Psychiatric Research 9: 163–171

Crome P, Newman B 1977 Poisoning with maprotiline and mianserin. British Medical Journal ii: 260

Crome P, Newman B 1979 The problem of tricyclic antidepressant poisoning. Postgraduate Medical Journal 55: 528–532

Crunelli V, Cervo L, Samanin R 1981 Evidence for a preferential role of central noradrenergic neurons in electrically induced convulsions and activity of various aniconvulsants in the rat. In: Morselli P L, Lloyd K G, Loscher W (eds) Neurotransmitters, seizures and epilepsy. Raven Press, New York, p 195–202

Cummings J L, Mendez M F 1984 Secondary mania with focal cerebrovascular lesions. American Journal of Psychiatry 141: 1084–1087

Currie S, Heathfield K W G, Henson R A, Scott D F 1971 Clinical course and prognosis of temporal lobe epilepsy; a survey of 666 patients. Brain 94: 173–190

Dalby M A 1971 Antiepileptic and psychotropic effect of carbamazepine, (Tegretol) in the treatment of psychomotor epilepsy. Epilepsia 12: 325–333

Danesi M A 1984 Patient perspectives on epilepsy in a developing country. Epilepsia 25: 184–190

Danesi M A, Odusote K A, Roberts O O, Adu E O 1981 Social problems of adolescent and adult epileptics in a developing country, as seen in Lagos, Nigeria. Epilepsia 689–696

Dansky L V, Andermann E, Andermann F 1980 Marriage and fertility in epileptic patients. Epilepsia 21: 261–271

Davis G R, Armstrong H E, Donovan D M, Temkin N R 1984 Cognitive-behavioral treatment of depressed affect among epileptics: Preliminary findings. Journal of Clinical Psychology 4: 930–935

Dessain E C, Schatzberg A F, Woods B T, Cole J O 1986 Maprotiline treatment in depression. Archives of General Psychiatry 43: 86–90

Dikmen S, Hermann B P, Wilensky A J, Rainwater G 1983 Validity of the Minnesota Multiphasic Personality Inventory (MMPI) to psychopathology in patients with epilepsy. Journal of Nervous and Mental Disease 171: 114–122

Dodrill C B, Breyer D N, Diamond M B, Dubinsky B L, Geary B B 1984a Psychosocial problems among adults with epilepsy. Epilepsia 25: 168–175

Dodrill C B, Beier R, Kasparick M, Tacke I, Tacke U, Tan S Y 1984b Psychosocial problems in adults with epilepsy: Comparison of findings from four countries. Epilepsia 25: 176–183

Dodrill C B, Batzel L W 19896 Interictal behavioral features of patients with epilepsy. Epilepsia 27: (Suppl. 2): S64–S76

Dodrill C B, Troupin A S 1977 Psychotropic effects of carbamazepine in epilepsy: a double-blind comparison with phenytoin. Neurology 27: 1023–1028

Dominian J, Serafetinides E A, Dewhurst M 1963 A follow-up study of late onset epilepsy: II: psychiatric and social findings. British Medical Journal 1: 431–435

Dongier S 1959/1960 Statistical study of clinical and electroencephalographic manifestations of 536 psychotic episodes occurring in 516 epileptics between clinical seizures. Epilepsia 1: 117–142

Edeh J, Toone B K. (1985) Antiepileptic therapy, folate deficiency and psychiatric morbidity: a general practice survey. Epilepsia 26; 434–440.

Edwards J G 1985 Antidepressants and seizures: Epidemiological and clinical aspects. In: Trimble M R (ed) The psychopharmacology of epilepsy. Wiley, Chichester, p 119–139

Edwards J G, Glen-Bott M 1984 Does viloxazine have epileptogenic properties? Journal of Neurology, Neurosurgery and Psychiatry 47: 960–964

Feighner J P, Robins E, Guze S B, Woodruff R A, Winokur G, Mundz R 1972 Diagnostic criteria for use in psychiatric research. Archives of General Psychiatry 26: 57–63

Fenton G W 1986 Minor psychiatric morbidity in people with epilepsy: evidence for a gender difference. Presented at the Annual Meeting of the Royal College of Psychiatrists, 8–10th July, 1986, Southampton, United Kingdom

Ficol M, Ramani V, Herron C 1984 Episodic fear in epilepsy. Epilepsia 25: 669–670

Flor-Henry P 1969 Psychosis and temporal lobe epilepsy: a controlled investigation. Epilepsia 10: 363–395

Folks D G, King L D, Dowdy S B, Petrie W N, Jack R A, Koomen J C, Swenson B R, Edwards P 1982 Carbamazepine treatment of selected affectively disordered inpatients. American Journal of Psychiatry, 139: 115–117

Frank J D 1961 Persuasion and healing. Hopkins Press, Baltimore
Fromm G H, Wuessel H B, Glass J D, Alvin J D, Van Horn G 1978 Imipramine in absence and myoclonic — astatic seizures. Neurology 28: 953–957
Gallagher B B, Murvin A, Flanigin H F, King D W, Luney D 1984 Pituitary and adrenal function in epileptic patients. Epilepsia 25(6): 683–689
Gay P E 1984 Effects of antioepileptic drugs and seizure type on operant responding in mentally retarded persons. Epilepsia 25: 377–386
Gerner R H, Hare T A 1981 CSF GABA in normal subjects and patients with depression, schizophrenia, mania and anorexia nervosa. American Journal of Psychiatry 138: 1098–1101
Giordani B, Sackellares J C, Miller S, Berent S, Sutula T, Seidenberg M, Boll T J, O'Leary D, Dreifuss F E 1983 Improvement in neuropsychological performance in patients with refractory seizures after intensive diagnostic and therapeutic intervention. Neurology 33: 489–493
Glass D H, Mattson R H 1973 Psychopathology and emotional precipitation of seizures in temporal lobe and nontemporal lobe epileptics. Proceedings of the 81st Annual Convention of the American Psychological Association 8: 425–426
Goodwin F K, Post R M, Dunner D L, Gordon E K 1973 Cerebrospinal fluid amine metabolism in affective illness: the probenecid technique. American Journal of Psychiatry 130: 73–79
Gough K R, Read A E, McCarthy C F, Waters A H 1963 Megaloblastic anaemia due to nutritional deficiency of folic acid. Quarterly Journal of Medicine 32: 243–256
Graham B, Freemon F R 1982 Continuous psychomotor seizures presenting as longstanding mental illness. Southern Medical Journal 75: 505–506
Greenberg D B, Hochberg F H, Murray G B 1984 The theme of death in complex partial seizures. American Journal of Psychiatry 141: 12 1587–1589
Gudmundson G 1966 Epilepsy in Iceland. A clinical and epidemiological investigation. Acta Neurologica Scandinavica 43 (Suppl. 25): 1–124
Guerrant J, Anderson W W, Fischer A, Weinstein M R, Jaros R M, Deskins A 1962 Personality in Epilepsy, Charles C Thomas: Springfield Illinois
Gunn J 1977 Epileptics in prison. Academic Press, London
Gupta A K, Jeavons P M, Hughes R C, Covanis A 1983 Aura in temporal lobe epilepsy: clinical and electroencephalographic correlation. Journal of Neurology, Neurosurgery and Psychiatry 46: 1079–1083
Guze S, Robins E 1970 Suicide and primary affective disorder. British Journal of Psychiatry 117: 437–438
Hamilton M 1982 Symptoms and assessment of depression. In: Paykel E S (ed) Handbook of affective disorders. Churchill Livingstone, Edinburgh, p 3–11
Hancock J C, Bevilacqua A R 1971 Temporal lobe dysrhythmia and impulsive or suicidal behavior: preliminary report. Southern Medical Journal 64: 1189–1193
Hauck G 1968 The attitude towards epilepsy of the general population of Germany and the USA Nervenarzt 39: 181–183
Hawton K, Fagg J, Marsack P 1980 Association between epilepsy and attempted suicide. Journal of Neurology, Neurosurgery and Psychiatry 43: 168–170
Henriksen G F 1973 Status epilepticus partialis with fear as clinical expression: report of a case and ictal EEG findings. Epilepsia 14: 39–46
Hermann B P 1979 Psychopathology in epilepsy and learned helplessness. Medical Hypotheses 5: 723–729
Hermann B P, Chabria S 1980 Interictal psychopathology in patients with ictal fear: examples of sensory-limbic hyperconnection? Archives of Neurology 37: 6678–668
Hermann B P, Dikmen S, Schwartz M S, Karnes W E 1982 Interictal psychopathology in patients with ictal fear: A quantitative investigation. Neurology 32: 7–11
Hohly E K, Martin R L 1986 Increased seizure duration during ECT with Trazodone administration. American Journal of Psychiatry 143: 1326
Hooshmand H 1974 The toxic effects of anticonvulsants: General principles. Pediatrics 53: 551–556
Hopkins A, Scambler G 1977 How doctors deal with epilepsy. Lancet i: 183–186
Jaffe R 1963 Ictal behaviour disturbance as the only manifestation of seizure disorder. Journal of Nervous and Mental Disease 134: 470–476
Jensen O N, Olesen O V 1969 Folic acid and anticonvulsant drugs. Archives of Neurology 21: 208–214
Jobe P C, Woods T W, Dailey J W 1984 Pro-convulsant and anticonvulsant affects of tricyclic antidepressants in genetically epilepsy-prone rats. In: Porter R J, Mattson J, Richard H, Ward A A Jr, Dam M (eds) Advances in epileptology: 15th Epilepsy International Symposium, Raven Press, New York p 187–191
Jones R 1912 The relation of epilepsy to insanity and its treatment. Practitioner 89: 772–792
Kendell R E 1976 The classification of depressions: a review of contemporary confusion. British Journal of Psychiatry 129: 15–28
Kendell R E, Gourlay J 1970 The clinical distinction between psychotic and neurotic depressions. British Journal of Psychiatry 117: 257–266

Kiloh L G, Garside R F 1963 The independence of neurotic depression and endogenous depression. British Journal of Psychiatry 109: 451–463
Kiloh L G, Andrews G, Nielson N, Bianchi G N 1972 The relationship of the syndromes called endogenous and neurotic depression. British Journal of Psychiatry 121: 183–196
Kløve H, Doehring D G 1962 MMPI in epileptic groups with differential etiology. Journal of Clinical Psychology 18: 149–153
Kogeorgos J, Fonagy P, Scott D F 1962 Psychiatric symptom patterns of chronic epileptics attending a neurological clinic: a controlled investigation. British Journal of Psychiatry 140: 236–243
Kraeplin E 1921 Manic depressive insanity and paranoia. Translated by Barclay R M, Robertson G. M. Livingstone: Edinburgh
Kreitman N 1983 Suicide and parasuicide. In: Kendell R E, Zealley A K (eds) Companion to psychiatric studies, 3rd ed Churchill Livingstone, Edinburgh p 396–411
Krijzer F, Snelder N, Bradford D 1984 Comparison of the (pro) convulsive properties of fluvoxamine and clovoxamine with eight other antidepressants in the animal module. Neuropsychobiology, 12: 249–254
Leestma J E, Kalelkar M B, Teas S S, Jay G W, Hughes J R 1984 Sudden unexpected death associated with seizures: Analysis of 66 cases. Epilepsia 25: 84–88
Lefkowitz D, Kilgo G, Lee S 1985 Seizures and Trazodone therapy. Archives of General Psychiatry 42: 523
Lehmann H E 1959 Psychiatric concepts of depression: nomenclature and classification. Canadian Psychiatric Association Journal 4: Special Suppl S1–S112
Leonhard K 1959 Aufteilung der endogenes psychosen. Cited in Kendell 1976
Levine S 1975 A controlled comparison of maprotiline (Ludiomil) with imipramine avoiding observer bias. Journal of International Medical Research 3: suppl 2: 75–78
Lewis A J 1934 Melancholia: a historical review. Journal of Mental Science 80: 1–42
Lim J, Yagnik P, Schraeder P, Wheeler S 1986 Ictal catatonia as a manifestation of nonconvulsive status epilepticus. Journal of Neurology, Neurosurgery and Psychiatry 49: 833–836
Lishman W A 1968 Brain damage in relation to psychiatric disability after head injury. British Journal of Psychiatry 114: 373–410
Loosen P T, Prange A J Jr 1982 Serum thyrotropin response to thyrotropin-releasing hormone in psychiatric patients: a review. American Journal of Psychiatry 139: 405–416
Lubar J F, Shabsin H S, Natelson S E 1981 EEG operant conditioning in intractable epileptics. Archives of Neurology 38: 700–704
Luchins D J, Oliver A P, Wyatt R J 1984 Seizures with antidepressants: An in vitro technique to assess relative risk. Epilepsia 25(1): 25–32
Mackay A 1979 Self-poisoning — a complication of epilepsy. British Journal of Psychiatry 134: 277–282
Maier S F, Seligman M E P 1976 Learned helplessness: theory and evidence. Journal of Experimental Psychology: General 105: 3
Mannheimer E, Pakesch F, Reimer E E, Vetter H 1952 Die Hamatologischen Komplikationen der Epilepsiebehandlung mit Hydantoinkorpern. Medizinische Klinik 47: 1397–1401
Margalit M, Heiman T 1983 Anxiety and self-dissatisfaction in epileptic children. Journal of Social Psychiatry 29: 220–224
Marjerrison G, Jedlicki S N, Keogh R P, Hrychuk W, Poulakakis G N 1968 Carbamazepine: behavioural, anticonvulsant and EEG effects in chronically hospitalised epileptics. Diseases of the Nervous System 29: 133–136
Matthews C H G, Kløve H 1968 MMPI performances in major motor, psychomotor and mixed seizure classifications of known and unknown etiology. Epilepsia 9: 43–53
Matthews W S, Barabas G 1981 Suicide and epilepsy: a review of the literature. Psychosomatics 22: 515–524
Maurice-Williams R S, Sinar E J 1984 Depression caused by an intracranial meningioma relieved by leucotomy prior to diagnosis of the tumour. Journal of Neurology, Neurosurgery and Psychiatry 47: 884–887
Maynert E W, Marczynsk T J, Browning R A 1975 The role of the neurotransmitters in the epilepsies. Advances in Neurology 13: 79–147
Meier M J, French L A 1965 Some personality correlates of unilateral and bilateral EEG abnormalities in psychomotor epilepsy. Journal of Clinical Psychology 1: 3–9
Meldrum B S 1975 Epilepsy and gamma-aminobutyric acid-mediated inhibition. In: Pfeiffer C C, Smythies J R (eds) International Review of Neurobiology. Academic Press, New York, p 1–36
Mellor D H, Lowit I, Hall D J 1974 Are epileptic children behaviourly different from other children. In: Harris P, Mawdsley C (eds) Epilepsy: Proceedings of the Hans Berger Centenary Symposium. Churchill Livingstone, Edinburgh, p 313–316

Mendels J, Cochrane C 1986 The nosology of depression: the endogenous — reactive concept. American Journal of Psychiatry 124: May suppl 1–11
Mendez M F, Cummings J L, Benson D F 1986 Depression in epilepsy. Archives of Neurology 43: 766–770
Metcalfe M, Goldman E 1965 Validation of an inventory for measuring depression. British Journal of Psychiatry 111: 240–242
Meyer J E, Meyer R 1987 Self portrayal by a depressed poet: a contribution to the clinical biography of William Cowper. American Journal of Psychiatry 144: 127–132
Meyer-Gross, Slater E, Roth N 1974 In: Slater E, Roth M (eds) Clinical psychiatry. Bailliere, Tindall and Cassell, London
Mignone R J, Donnelly E F, Sadowsky D 1970 Psychological and neurological comparisons of psychomotor and non-psychomotor epileptic patients. Epilepsia 11: 345–359
Mittan R J 1984 Patient's fears about seizures may predict presence and absence of psychopathology. Epilepsia 25: 648
Modlin H C 1960 A study of the MMPI in clinical practice. In: Welsh G S, Dahlstrom W G (eds) Basic Readings on the MMPI in Psychology and Medicine. University of Minnesota Press, Minneapolis, p 388–402
Mowbray R M 1972 Rating scales for depression. In: Davies B, Carroll B J, Mowbray R M (eds) Depressive illness. Some research studies, Thomas, Springfield, Illinois, p 278–308
Mulder D W, Daly D 1952 Psychiatric symptoms associated with lesions of the temporal lobe. Journal of the American Medical Association 150: 173–176
Neumann J, Seidel K, Wunderlich H P 1984 Comparative studies of the effect of carbamazepine 1 and trimipramine 2 in depression. In: Emrich H N, Okuma T, Muller A A (eds) Anticonvulsants in affective disorders. Elsevier Science, Excerpta Medica, Amsterdam
Nielsen H, Kristensen O 1981 Personality correlates of sphenoidal EEG-foci in temporal lobe epilepsy. Acta Neurologica Scandinavica 64: 289–300
Ojemann L M, Friel P N, Trejo W J, Dudley D L 1983 Effect of doxepin on seizure frequency in depressed epileptic patients. Neurology 33: 646–648
Okuma T, Inanaga K, Otsuki S et al 1981 A preliminary double-blind study of the efficacy of carbamazepine in prophyllaxis of manic depressive illness. Psychopharmacology 73: 95–96
Palia S S, Harper M A 1986 Mood disorders in epilepsy: a survey of psychiatric patients. Presented at the Annual meeting of the Royal College of Psychiatrists, The University of Southampton, 8–10 July, 1986 United Kingdom
Pazzangia P, Frank-Pazzangia L 1976 Record in grade school of pupils with epilepsy: An epidemiological study. Epilepsia 17: 361–366
Pellegrini A, Lippmann S B, Crump G, Manshadi M 1984 Psychiatric aspects of complex partial seizures: case report. Journal of Clincal Psychiatry 45: 6, 269–271
Perini G, Mendius R 1984 Depression and anxiety in complex partial seizures. Journal of Nervous and Mental Disease 172: 287–290
Perini G, Suny M D, Mendius R 1983 Interictal emotions and behavioral profiles in left and right temporal lobe epileptics. Psychosomatic Medicine 45: 1, 83
Perris C 1966 A study of bipolar (manic depressive) and unipolar recurrent depressive psychoses. Acta Psychiatrica Scandinavica Suppl 194
Perucca E, Richens A 1977 Interaction between phenytoin and imipramine. British Journal of Clinical Pharmacology 4: 485–486
Pilowsky I 1979 Further validation of a questionnaire method for classifying depression illness. Journal of Affective Disorders 1: 179–185
Pinder R M, Brogden R N, Speight T M, Avery G S 1977 Doxepin up-to-date: a review of its pharmacologaical properties and therapeutic efficacy with particular reference to depression. Drugs 13: 161–218
Pisani F, Narbone M C, Fazio et al 1984 Effect of Viloxazine on serum carbamazepine levels in epileptic patients. Epilepsia 25: 482–485
Pisani F, Fazio A, Oteri G et al 1986 Carbamazepine-viloxazine interaction in patients with epilepsy Journal of Neurology, Neurosurgery and Psychiatry 49: 1142–1145
Placidi G F, Lenzi A, Rampello E, Andreani M F, Cassano G B, Grossi E 1984 Long-term double-blind prospective study on carbamazepine versus lithium in bipolar and schizo-affective disorders: preliminary results. In: Emrich H N, Okuma T, Muller A A (eds) Anticonvulsants in affective disorders. Elsevier, Excerpta Medica, Amsterdam, p 188–197
Pond D A, Bidwell B H, Stein L 1960 A survey of epilepsy in 14 general practices: demographic and medical data. Journal of Neurology, Neurosurgery and Psychiatry 63: 217–236
Pritchard P B, Lombroso C T, McIntyre M 1980 Psychological complications of temporal lobe epilepsy. Neurology 30: 227–232

Reynolds E H 1967 Effects of folic acid on the mental state and fit frequency of drug-treated epileptic patients. Lancet i: 1086–1088
Reynolds E H 1975 Chronic antiepileptic toxicity: a review. Epilepsia 16: 319–352
Reynolds E H 1983 Why does epilepsy become intractable? Prevention of chronic epilepsy. Lancet: 952–954
Reynolds E H, Elwes R D C, Shorvon S D 1983 Why does epilepsy become intractable? — Prevention of chronic epilepsy. Lancet, Oct. 22: 952–954
Reynolds E H 1985 Folic acid and neuropsychiatry. Presented at the Symposium on Folates at the 1st Congress of the Mediterranean Society of Therapy, Florence. Farmagi and Terapia 163–168
Reynolds E H, Milner G, Matthews D M, Chanarin I 1966 Anticonvulsant therapy, megaloblastic haemopoiesis and folic acid metabolism. Quarterly Journal of Medicine 35: 521–537
Reynolds E H, Preece J M, Bailey J, Coppen A 1970 Folate deficiency in depressive illness. British Journal of Psychiatry 117: 287–292
Reynolds E H, Carney M W P, Toone B K 1984 Methylation and mood. Lancet ii: 196–197
Reynolds J R 1861 Epilepsy: its symptoms, treatment and relation to the chronic convulsive diseases. Churchill, London
Richens A, Nawishy S, Trimble M 1983 Antidepressant drugs, convulsions and epilepsy. British Journal of Clinical Pharmacology 15: 295–298
Robertson M M 1983 Depression in patients with epilepsy. M D Thesis, University of Cape Town, South Africa
Robertson M M 1986a Ictal and interictal depression in patients with epilepsy: In: Trimble M R, Bolwig T G (eds) Aspects of epilepsy and psychiatry. Wiley p 213–234
Robertson M M 1986b Current status of the 1,4 and 1,5 benzodiazepines in the treatment of epilepsy: the place of clobazam. Epilepsia 27: Suppl 1 S27–S41
Robertson M M, Trimble M R 1985 The treatment of depression in patients with epilepsy. A double-blind trial. Journal of Affective Disorders 9: 127–136
Robertson M M, Coppen A, Trimble M R 1986 The dexamethasone suppression test in medicated epileptic patients. Biological Psychiatry 21: 225–228
Robertson M M, Trimble M R, Townsend H R A 1987 The phenomenology of depression in epilepsy. Epilepsia 28: 364–372
Robins E, Munoz R A, Martin S, Gentry K A 1972 Primary and secondary affective disorders. In: Zubin J, Freyhan F A (eds) Disorders of mood. Hopkins Press, Baltimore, p 33–45
Robinson R G, Szetela B 1981 Mood change following left hemispheric brain injury. Annals of Neurology 9, 5: 447–453
Robinson R G, Kubos K L, Starr L B, Rao K, Price T R 1984 Mood disorders in stroke patients. Brain 107: 81–93
Rodin E, Schmaltz S 1983 Folate levels in epileptic patients. In: Parsonage M, Grant R H E, Craig A G, Ward A A (eds) Advances in epileptology: XIVth Epilepsy International Symposium. Raven Press, New York, p 143–153
Rodin E, Schmaltz S 1984 The Bear-Fedio personality inventory and temporal lobe epilepsy. Neurology 34: 591–596
Rodin E A, Katz M, Lennox K 1976 Differences between patients with temporal lobe seizures and those with other forms of epileptic attacks. Epilepsia 17: 313–320
Roy A 1979 Some determinants of affective symptoms in epileptics. Canadian Journal of Psychiatry 24: 554–556
Roy-Byrne P, Uhde T W, Post R M, Joffe R T 1984 Relationship of response to sleep deprivation and carbamazepine in depressed patients. Acta Psychiatrica Scandinavica 69: 379–382
Rubin A L, Charney D S, Price L H, Heninger G R 1985 Rapid improvement of delusional depression following drug-induced seizures: Case report. Journal of Clinical Psychiatry 46: 146–147
Rutter M, Graham P, Yule W 1970 A neuropsychiatric study in childhood. Clinics in Developmental Medicine Nos 35/36
Ryan R, Kemper K, Emlen A C 1980 The stigma of epilepsy as a self-concept. Epilepsia 21: 433–444
Sackeim H A, Decina P, Prohovnik I, Malitz S, Resor S R 1983 Anticonvulsant and antidepressant properties of electroconvulsive therapy: A proposed mechanism of action. Biological Psychiatry 18: 1301–1310
Schildkraut J J 1965 The catecholamine hypothesis of affective disorders: a review of supporting evidence. American Journal of Psychiatry 122: 509–522
Schofield A, Duane A 1986 0rganic pathology and psychiatric morbidity in neurological referrals to a consultation/liaison service. Presented at the Royal College of Psychiatrists Annual Meeting, 8–10th July 1986 Southampton, United Kingdom
Schutte W 1968 Epilepsy from the patients point of view. Nervenarzt 39: 296–301
Scott D F 1985 Left and right cerebral hemisphere differences in the occurrence of epilepsy. British Journal of Medical Psychology 58: 189–192
Seligman M E P 1975 Helplessness. Freeman, San Fransisco

Serafetinides E A 1975 Psychosocial aspects of neurosurgical management of epilepsy. In: Purpura D P, Penry U K (eds) Advances in neurology, vol 8. Raven Press, New York, p 323
Sethi B B, Tiwari S C 1984 Carbamazepine in affective disorders. In: Emrich H M, Okuma T, Muller A A (eds) Anticonvulsants in affective disorders. Elsevier Publishers, Excerpta Medica, Holland
Setiey A, Courjon J 1978 Clomipramine et petit mal. Lyon Medical 239: 751–754
Shorvon S D, Reynolds E H 1977 Unnecessary polypharmacy for epilepsy. British Medical Journal i: 1635–1637
Silberman E K, Post R M, Nurnberger J, Theodore W, Boulenger J P 1985 Transient sensory, cognitive and affective phenomena in affective-illness. British Journal of Psychiatry 146: 81–89
Slater E, Cowie V 1971 The genetics of mental disorders. Oxford University Press: London
Snaith R P 1987 The concepts of mild depression. British Journal of Psychiatry 150: 387–393
Snaith R P, Mehta S, Raby A H 1970 Serum folate and vitamin B12 in epileptics with and without mental illness. British Journal of Psychiatry 116: 179–183
Snyder M 1983 Effect of relaxation on psychosocial functioning in persons with epilepsy. Journal of Neurosurgical Nursing 15, 4: 250–255
Spitzer R L, Endicott J, Woodruff R A, Andreasen N 1977 Classification of mood disorders. In: Usdin G (ed) Depression clinical, biological and psychological perspectives. Brunner-Mazel, New York, p 73–103
Spitzer R L, Endicott J, Robins E 1978 Research diagnostic criteria. Rationale and reliability. Archives of General Psychiatry 35: 773–782
Standage K F, Fenton G W 1975 Psychiatric symptom profiles of patients with epilepsy: a controlled investigation. Psychological Medicine 5: 152–160
Stevens J R 1975 Interictal clinical manifestations of complex partial seizures. In: Penry J K, Daly D D (eds) Advances in neurology. Raven Press, New York
Stores G 1978 School children with epilepsy at risk for learning and behavioural problems. Developmental Medicine and Child Neurology 20: 502–508
Tasini M 1986 Complex partial seizures in a patient receiving Trazodone. Journal of Clinical Psychiatry 47: 6, 318–319
Taylor D C 1971 Ontongenesis of chronic epileptic psychoses: a reanalysis. Psychological Medicine 1: 247–253
Taylor D C 1972 Mental state and temporal lobe epilepsy: a correlative account of 100 patients treated surgically. Epilepsia 13: 727–765
Temkin N R, Davis G R 1984 Stress as a risk factor for seizures among adults with epilepsy. Epilepsia 25: 450–456
Temkin O 1971 The falling sickness (2nd edn revised). John Hopkins Press, Baltimore
Thompson P J, Trimble M R 1982 Anticonvulsant drugs and cognitive functions. Epilepsia 23: 531–544
Toone B K, Driver N V 1980 Psychosis and epilepsy. Research and Clinical Forums 2: 121–127
Trimble M 1978 Non-monoamine oxidase inhibitor antidepressants and epilepsy: a review. Epilepsia 19: 241–250
Trimble M R, Perez M M 1982a Quantification of psychopathology in adult patients with epilepsy. In: Kulig B M, Meinardi H, Stores G (eds) Epilepsy and behaviour '79 and Proceedings of WOPSASSEPY I 1980 Swets and Zeitlinger, Lisse, p 118–126
Trimble M R, Perez M M 1982b The phenomenology of the chronic psychoses of epilepsy. Advances in Biological Psychiatry, 8: 98–105
Trimble M R, Reynolds E H 1976 Anticonvulsant drugs and mental symptoms: a review. Psychological Medicine 6: 169–178
Trimble M R, Robertson M M 1987 Laterality and psychopathology: recent findings in epilepsy. In: Flor-Henry P, Gruzelier J (eds) Cerebral dynamics, laterality and psychopathology vol 3. Elsevier, North Holland, p 359–369
Trimble M, Anlezark G, Meldrum B 1977 Seizure activity in photosensitive baboons following antidepressant drugs and the role of serotoninergic mechanisms. Psychopharmacology 51: 159–164
Trimble M R, Corbett J A, Donaldson D 1980 Folic acid and mental symptoms in children with epilepsy. Journal of Neurology Neurosurgery and Psychiatry 43: 1030–1034
Tucker W M, Forster F M 1950 Petit mal epilepsy occurring in status. Archives of Neurological Psychiatry 64: 823–827
Wada J A, Balzamo E, Meldrum B S, Naquet R 1972 Behavioural and electrographic effects of L-5-hydroxytrytophan and D,L-parachlorophenylalanine on an epileptic Senegalese baboon (Papio papio). Electroencephalography and Clinical Neurophysiology 33: 520–526
Wall M, Tuchman M, Mielke D 1985 Panic attacks and temporal lobe seizures associated with a right temporal lobe arteriovenous malformation: case report. Journal of Clinical Psychiatry 46: 143–145

Wall M, Mielke D, Luther J S 1986 Panic attacks and psychomotor seizures following right temporal lobectomy. Journal of Clinical Psychiatry 47: 4, 219
Wannamaker B B 1983 Unexplained mortality in epilepsy. A perspective on death of persons with epilepsy. Presented at the 15th Epilepsy International Symposium, Washington D C, September 1983
Weil A A 1955 Depressive reactions associated with temporal lobe-uncinate seizures. Journal of Nervous and Mental Disease 121: 505–510
Weil A A 1959 Ictal emotions occurring in temporal lobe dysfunction. Archives of Neurology 1: 87–97
Weissman M N 1981 Antidepressants and psychotherapy in depression. Advances in Biological Psychiatry 7: 230–239
Wells C E 1975 Transient ictal psychosis. Archives of General Psychiatry, 32: 1201–1203
White E W 1900 Epilepsy associated with insanity. Journal of Mental Science 46: 73–79
Whitman S, Hermann B P, Gordon A C 1984 Psychopathology in epilepsy: how great is the risk. Biological Psychiatry 19, 2: 213–236
Williams F 1956 The structure of emotions reflected in epileptic experiences. Brain 79: 29–67
Wing J K, Mann S A, Leff, J P, Nixon J M 1978 The concept of a 'case' in psychiatric population surveys. Psychological Medicine 8: 203–217
Zigmund A S, Snaith R P 1983 The hospital anxiety and depression scale. Acta Psychiatrica Scandinavica 67: 361–370

# 11. Epilepsy and the law

*P. Fenwick*

Ignorance, superstition and misunderstanding have ensured that epilepsy, throughout its history, has inspired fear and derision in those witnessing an attack and that epileptics have suffered discrimination, both socially and legally. Temkin (1945) quotes the Babylonian code of Hammurabi, in approximately 2000 B.C., as protecting the interests of slave buyers against the possibility of a slave developing epilepsy within a month of purchase. The vendor was required to give a money-back guarantee in the case of a slave developing bennu (epilepsy) within a month of purchase.

## DISCRIMINATION AGAINST PEOPLE WITH EPILEPSY

Gunn (1981) has given a historical background to the legal discrimination against people with epilepsy. He records that Sweden, in 1757, was probably the first country in modern times to legislate against marriage for those with epilepsy. Indeed, many US states still have laws making such marriages illegal, void or voidable on their statute books, though they are not enforced. In many states, sterilisation of epileptics, either voluntarily or by court order, has also been practised. Some countries, for example Australia, still refuse immigration visas to people with epilepsy.

However, a Gallup poll survey between 1969 and 1979 has shown a noticeable change in attitudes towards epilepsy reflecting a growing public understanding of and knowledge about epilepsy. In 1969, only 57% of people thought people with epilepsy 'should be employed like other people,' as compared to 78% in 1979. In 1969, 68%, and in 1979 80%, would not object to having their 'children associate with people who had fits.' It is to be hoped that this trend will continue at an even faster pace.

## EPILEPSY AND THE CRIMINAL LAW

The basis of English law is the doctrine of *mens rea* — 'Actus non facit reum nisi mens sit rea' — the deed does not make a man guilty unless his mind is guilty. For to convict a man for an offence that he does not know he is committing and is unable to prevent, goes against the spirit of English justice and brings the law into contempt.

Everyone who has reached the age of discretion is, unless the contrary is proved, presumed by law to be sane and to be accountable for his actions. Unless the offence is a statutory one which carries an absolute liability (e.g. driving with a raised blood alcohol level), the doctrine of *mens rea*, or the presence of a guilty mind, can only be negated by three major considerations. Firstly, that the mind is not guilty because it is innocent: secondly, because the mind is diseased, and thirdly, because at the time of the act there was an absence of mind.

The defence of innocence is seldom used: it is applied sometimes to mental subnormality, but is of little relevance to epilepsy. Disease of the mind legally rests on the McNaghten Rule which arose as a consequence of the case of Daniel McNaghten who was tried in 1843. Following this case it was established that for a defence on the grounds of insanity to be successful it must be clearly proved that *at the time of committing the act the party accused was labouring under such a defect of reason, from disease of the mind, as not to know the nature and quality of the act he was doing, or, if he did know it, that he did not know he was doing what was wrong.*

This defence can be used by patients with epilepsy only if at the time they commit an offence, they have an associated mental illness. It might thus be used in epileptic patients who have for example, either a postictal or an inter-ictal paranoid psychosis and who at the time they commit their crime are suffering from an insane delusion. In these circumstances, epilepsy is very little different from any other functional psychotic illness and the rules applying to epileptics are no different from those applying to the mentally ill population as a whole.

**The defence of automatism**

However, when we consider the third category of defence — that no mind was present at the time of the act — the law relating to epilepsy is distinct. For during an epileptic seizure the mind is absent and so any action carried out is automatic. An act carried out in the absence of mind is known legally as an automatic act, and the defence of automatism may be established.

It is important to understand, so that there is no subsequent confusion, that the legal definition of automatism, and the medical definition of automatism, are quite different. This is largely because the law has to deal with the protection of the public as well as the rights of the individual, whereas medicine's primary concern is with brain mechanisms, their disorder and cure. Thus although both the law and medicine use the same word they mean different things.

**Definitions of epileptic automatism**

An epileptic automatism is defined medically as:

> 'A state of clouding of consciousness which occurs during or immediately after a seizure, during which the individual retains control of posture and muscle tone, but performs simple or complex movements without being aware of what is happening. The impairment of awareness varies. A variety of initial phenomena before the interruption of consciousness and the onset of automatic behaviour may occur.'
>
> Fenton (1972)

By that definition, automatisms are really very common. They can be sub-divided into two groups: ictal automatisms, which occur during a fit, and post-ictal automatisms, occurring after a fit.

The accepted legal definition of automatisms is that given by Viscount Kilmuir L.C. in the House of Lords Appeal in the case of Bratty v. Attorney General for Northern Ireland, and is as follows:

> 'The state of person who, though capable of action, is not conscious of what he is doing . . . it means unconscious, involuntary action and it is a defence because the mind does not go with what is being done.'

Viscount Kilmuir continued:

> 'This is very like the words of the learned President of the Court of Appeal of New Zealand (Gresson P.) in Reg. v. Cottle where he said: 'With respect, I would myself prefer to explain automatism simply as action without any knowledge of acting, or action with no consciousness of doing what was being done.'
>
> Bratty (1961)

Although this definition is apparently very close to the medical definition, the law, unlike medicine, defines two types of automatisms: sane (*automatism simpliciter*), for example, sleepwalking, and insane (*automatism due to disease of the mind*), for example, resulting from arteriosclerosis. Either kind of automatism can be put forward as a defence and if accepted by the Court will enable the defendent to plead not guilty. However, the consequences of a successful defence are quite different in the two cases. In the case of a non-insane automatism, the defendent will walk free from the court. But in the case of an insane automatism the defendent must be compulsorily committed to a mental hospital, possibly for an indefinite period, at the discretion of the Home Secretary.

**Sane and insane automatism**

The distinction between insane and non-insane automatism is arbitrary and makes little medical sense. A brief look at several legal cases which have tried to categorise epileptic automatisms, shows the extent of the confusion.

*Epilepsy is automatism simpliciter: Regina v. Charlson*

In the case of Reg. v. Charlson (1955), epilepsy was defined as a non-insane automatism. At the trial of Charlson, the following facts were admitted.

> 'The accused, who was a shopkeeper, lived in a house, the backroom windows of which overlooked a river 2 feet deep. The accused called his 10 year old son Peter into the back room, telling him that there was a rat to be seen standing on a stone in the river. When the boy came to the window, the accused picked up a wooden mallet from the floor, and struck the boy twice on the head, breaking the skin of the scalp and causing blood to flow . . . The accused thereupon picked the boy up and threw him out of the window.' (p 317)

In his summing up, Mr Justice Barry said:

> 'If he struck his son with the mallet, knowing what he was doing, and by those blows caused the injuries, then he is guilty . . . If he did not know what he was doing, if his actions were purely automatic, and his mind had no control over the movement of his limbs, if he was *in the same position as a person in an epileptic fit*, then no responsibility rests upon him at all, and the proper verdict is, not guilty.' (p 325)

There was thus no doubt at that time that epilepsy was a sane automatism requiring an acquittal.

*Automatism due to disease of the brain is insane automatism: Reg. v. Kemp*

In the case of Reg. v. Kemp (1956), held before Mr Justice Devlin, it was held that an automatic act could be a disease of the mind. Kemp was accused of causing grievous bodily harm to his wife.

> 'During one night he made an entirely motiveless and irrational attack upon his wife, striking her with a hammer with such violence as to cause a grievous wound.
>
> The accused suffered from a physical disease, namely arteriosclerosis, or hardening of the arteries ... It is a well recognised consequence of arteriosclerosis that it may lead to a congestion of blood in the brain due to a sudden rise of blood pressure. As a result of such a congestion, the accused suffered a temporary lapse of consciousness, so that he was not conscious when he picked up the hammer or that he was striking his wife with it. In that mental condition he was not responsible for his actions.' (p 400)

In his further discussion of the case Mr Justice Devlin continued:

> 'The broad submission that was made to me on behalf of the accused was that this is a physical disease and not a mental disease; arteriosclerosis is a physical condition primarily and not a mental condition. But that argument does not go so far as to suggest that for the purpose of the law diseases that affect the mind can be divided into those that are physical in origin and those that are mental in origin. There is such a distinction medically . . . (p 406). The distinction between the two categories is quite irrelevant for the purposes of the law, which is not concerned with the origin of the disease, or the cause of it, but simply with the mental condition which has brought about the act. It does not matter for the purpose of the law, whether the defect of reason is due to degeneration of the brain or to some other form of mental derangement. That may be a matter of importance medically, but it is of no importance to the law, which merely has to consider the state of mind in which the accused is, not how he got there . . . (p 407). Hardening of the arteries is a disease which is shown on the evidence to be capable of affecting the mind in such a way as to cause a defect, *temporarily* or permanently, of its reasoning, understanding and so on, and so is in my judgement a disease of the mind which comes within the meaning of the Rules.' (p 408)

*Epileptic automatism is disease of the mind: Bratty v. Att. General*

Thus a malfunction of the brain leading to an automatic act was seen to be a disease of the mind even if it was temporary. So it was not surprising that when epilepsy was put forward as *automatism simpliciter* in the case of Bratty v. The Attorney General of Northern Ireland (1961) this was disallowed. Bratty was charged with killing a girl whom he had taken for a ride in his car. He maintained that a 'blackness' came over him at the time of the killing, and that he did not know what he was doing. The medical evidence suggested that he might be suffering from psychomotor epilepsy, although a close reading of the medical history could not possibly support this. The defence asked the jury to acquit the accused on a plea of automatism, or to find him guilty of manslaughter, or to find him not guilty by reason of insanity.

The trial judge discounted the plea of automatism for lack of evidence, and Bratty was convicted of murder.

The case on appeal reached the House of Lords, on the question of whether or not the trial judge was correct in dismissing the plea of automatism. It is of interest that it was in this case that the medical profession themselves suggested that epilepsy was a disease of the mind.

Lord Denning, in his opinion said:

> 'This brings me to the root of the question in the present case: was a proper foundation laid here for the defence of automatism, apart from the plea of insanity? There was the evidence of George Bratty himself, that he could not remember anything because "this blackness was over me". He said, "I did not realise exactly what I was doing," and added afterwards, "I didn't know what I was doing. I didn't realise anything." He said he had four or five times previously had "feelings of blackness", and frequent headaches. There was evidence, too, of his odd behaviour at times, his mental backwardness and his religious leanings. Added to this there was the medical evidence. Dr Sax, who was called on his behalf, said there was a possibility that he was suffering from psychomotor epilepsy. It was, he said, practically the only possibility that occurred to him. Dr Walker, his general practitioner, said you could not leave the possibility out of account. Dr Robinson, a specialist, who gave evidence on behalf of the Crown, said he thought it was extremely unlikely that it was an epileptic attack, but one could not rule it out. *All the doctors agreed that psychomotor epilepsy, if it exists, is a defect of reason due to disease of the mind*: (my italics) and the judge accepted this view. No other cause was canvassed.
>
> 'In those circumstances, I am clearly of the opinion that, if the act of George Bratty was an involuntary act, as the defence suggested, the evidence attributed it solely to a disease of the mind and the only defence open was the defence of insanity. There was no evidence of automatism apart from insanity.' (Bratty, p 105)

Lord Denning discussed Mr Justice Barry's statement that epilepsy was automatism simpliciter and not a disease of the mind (insane automatism). He said:

> 'that in Charlson's case, Barry J. seems to have assumed that other diseases such as epilepsy or cerebral tumour are not diseases of the mind, even when they are such as to manifest themselves in violence. I do not agree with this. It seems to me that any mental disorder which has manifested itself in violence and is prone to recur, is a disease of the mind. At any rate, it is the sort of disease for which a person should be detained in hospital rather than being given an unqualified acquittal.' (Bratty, p 102–103)

The implications of this case are clearly that, from both the medical and legal points of view, an epileptic seizure should be considered a disease of the mind, and crimes committed during an epileptic seizure could not use the defence of automatism simpliciter.

*Appeal — epileptic automatism as disease of the mind: Reg. v. Sullivan*
From the medical point of view, the case of Bratty v. the Attorney General for Northern Ireland was unsatisfactory as a foundation case on which to base the concept that a violent act occurring during an epileptic seizure was an insane automatism. A detailed reading of the accounts of the offence produces very little medical evidence that the act was, in fact, committed during an epileptic seizure. Indeed, the defence recognised this by running simultaneously the defence of automatism, insanity or manslaughter. It was also unsatisfactory from the legal point of view, as additional legal points were being tested besides that of automatism. It was thus in the case of Regina v. Sullivan (1983) that the argument about whether an epileptic automatism was a sane or an insane automatism was first put to the test.

Sullivan, a man of previous good character, was an epileptic who suffered partial complex seizures with occasional secondary generalisation from the age of eight. He had had two severe head injuries which have resulted in widespread brain damage and some degree of personality change. His major attacks ceased in 1979, and only the partial complex seizures remained. These seizures spread rapidly and bilaterally into both amygdala and hippocampal structures, so that Sullivan had no memory for the seizure or events immediately after the seizure.

During a partial complex seizure Sullivan attacked and seriously injured an elderly neighbour. The seizure and the attack were witnessed, and both prosecution and defence accepted that there was no medical doubt that the assault took place during an epileptic automatism. Sullivan wished to establish the defence of the sane automatism (automatism simpliciter), and pleaded not guilty. The trial judge, His Honour Judge Lymbery, ruled that this plea was not available to the defence, and that if Mr Sullivan carried out the act during an epileptic fit, then he must plead not guilty because of automatism due to disease of the mind. If Mr Sullivan had pleaded 'insane automatism' and his plea had succeeded, as it undoubtedly would, it would have meant that the court would have had to send him to hospital, possibly a special hospital. Mr Sullivan's defence lawyers were not willing to risk this possibility, and so Mr Sullivan was persuaded to plead guilty to an act which he could not remember committing and over which he had no control. Because of the difficulty Mr Sullivan was placed in by not being allowed the plea of non-insane automatism, the case went forward to the Court of Appeal and finally to the House of Lords. In both cases the Appeal was rejected, thus confirming that in legal terms epilepsy is a disease of the mind and that a criminal act perpetrated during an epileptic seizure is an insane automatism. (Fenwick & Fenwick 1985, p 7).

Commenting on the verdict of the House of Lords, Mr Lionel Swift who presented the Appeal, said:

> 'From the point of view of the administration of the law and justice to epileptics and others, the reasoning of the House of Lords is, with respect, impeccable ... It matters not whether the impairment (of mind) is organic, as in epilepsy, or functional. It matters not whether the impairment is permanent or transient, or capable of control by drugs. Provided that (impairment) is his condition at the material times, he comes within the definition of being temporarily insane. At the time he committed the act, Sullivan was completely unaware of what he was doing, therefore, he was insane at the time.' (p. 10)

*Present definition of sane and insane automatism: Reg. v. Quick*

The definition of automatism simpliciter was re-defined in the case of Reg. v. Quick (1973). Quick, a nurse at a mental hospital, was charged with assaulting a patient while hypoglycaemic due to the effects of insulin. Quick was a diabetic, and on the morning of the assault he had taken his insulin as prescribed, drunk a quantity of spirits, but had eaten little food. He had no recollection of the assault. The trial judge, quite logically in view of Lord Denning's judgment in the Bratty case, felt that the defence of automatism simpliciter was not available to Quick but that he must plead automatism due to a disease of the mind. This was, however, reversed in the Court of Appeal. The Court of Appeal judges quoted Lord Denning's discussion in the case of Bratty, quoted above, and they go on to say:

> 'If that opinion is right, and there are no restricting qualifications which ought to be applied to it, Quick was setting up a defence of insanity. He may have been, at the material time, in a condition of mental disorder manifesting itself in violence. Such manifestations had occurred before and might recur. The difficulty arises as soon as the question is asked, whether he should be detained in a mental hospital. No mental hospital would admit a diabetic merely because he had a low blood sugar reaction; and common sense is affronted by the prospect of a diabetic being sent to such a hospital, when in most cases the disordered mental condition can be rectified quickly by pushing a lump of sugar or a teaspoonful of glucose, into the patient's mouth.' (p. 31)

Thus, the Appeal Court countered Lord Denning's argument that a disordered mind leading to an automatic act which was prone to recur must be a disease of the mind.

The Appeal Court also dealt with Justice Devlin's comments in the case of Kemp, (Reg. v. Kemp, p 407), which had stressed the importance of the accused's state of mind at the time of the act, and not the underlying physiological mechanisms.

> 'Applied without qualification of any kind, Devlin J's statement of the law would have some surprising consequences. Take the not uncommon case of the rugby player who gets a kick on the head early in the game and plays on to the end in a state of automatism. If, while he was in that state, he assaulted the referee, it is difficult to envisage any court adjudging that he was not guilty by reason of insanity. Another type of case that could occur is that of the dental patient who kicks out while coming round from an anaesthetic. The law could be in a defective state if a patient accused of assaulting a dental nurse by kicking her while regaining consciousness could only excuse himself by raising the defence of insanity.' (Reg. v. Quick, 1973 p 31)

They concluded . . .

> 'In this case Quick's alleged mental condition, if it ever existed, was not caused by his diabetes but by his use of the insulin prescribed by his doctor. Such malfunctioning of his mind as there was, was caused by an external factor and not by a bodily disorder in the nature of a disease which disturbed the working of his mind.'

Thus the defence of automatism simpliciter should have been allowed to Quick.

This case defines the present standing of the difference between sane and insane automatism. Automatism simpliciter occurs when the mind is disordered by an *external factor* such as an injection of insulin, a blow on the head, or the injection of an anaesthetic. An insane automatism occurs when the mind is disordered due to an *intrinsic factor* which leads to a situation that is prone to recur and may result in violence. Any organic condition of the brain or the body resulting in a disorder of the mind, even if temporary, is therefore legally an insane automatism. This clearly leads to differences which appear to be nonsensical. For example, a violent act committed while the mind is disordered due to an excess of insulin is automatism simpliciter if the insulin is injected, while it is an insane automatism if the insulin comes from an insulinoma of the pancreas. It is my opinion that the distinction between sane and insane automatism is meaningless, and probably best abandoned altogether. The drawing of an arbitrary line always leads to confusion.

## EPILEPSY AND CRIMINALITY

Not infrequently, forensic psychiatrists are called upon to decide whether or not a crime has been committed during an epileptic seizure, and whether or not the defence of automatism is one that can be substantiated by the medical facts of the case. Usually the offence is fairly trivial, for example shoplifting during either a post-ictal confusional state or during the automatism of a partial complex seizure. Occasionally, however, defendents may claim the defence of epileptic automatism when there is little evidence to support this. The psychiatrist should satisfy himself on the following six points before going to court to substantiate the diagnosis of epileptic automatism.

1. The patient should be a known epileptic. It is clearly unlikely that a crime will be committed during a first seizure. Thus, unless there is overwhelming evidence, the diagnosis of epilepsy should be rejected if the act is said to have occurred during a first seizure. The case of epilepsy is strengthened if there is evidence that the patient is either subject to ictal or post-ictal automatisms, and that the behaviour described during the crime is consistent with behaviour that has been previously described during such an automatism.

2. The act should be out of character for the individual and inappropriate for the circumstances. Clearly, if the defendent is habitually aggressive and commits a violent and aggressive crime, it is much more difficult to substantiate the diagnosis of epileptic automatism than if the act occurred in a patient who was mild mannered and tolerant. It is also important that the act should be inappropriate in the circumstances in which it occurred. A violent act of automatism during a fight, although it may occur, is less likely to persuade the court than one which occurs during a Sunday stroll.

3. There must be no evidence of premeditation or concealment. An epileptic automatism must arise de novo from ongoing behaviour. If there is any suggestion that there was a preplanning for the act, then it is not possible to substantiate a diagnosis of automatism. Concealment is also unlikely after an automatism. On regaining consciousness a patient emerges from a state of confusion or amnesia and thus he is unlikely to register the full meaning of the events which have occurred. His natural

response to such a situation is immediately to seek help, and not to conceal the evidence of any crime.

4. If a witness is available, they should report a disorder of consciousness at the time of the act. Unfortunately, witnesses are not always available, but when they are, detailed questioning about the defendent's behaviour to establish a disorder of consciousness is essential. Features to seek are those of automatism; staring eyes, glassy look, stereotyped movements, confusion, and evidence that the person was out of touch with his surroundings.

5. Because the act occurs during an automatism or a post-ictal confusional state, a disorder of memory is the rule. It is unlikely that an epileptic automatism can occur in the setting of clear consciousness. Thus, memory for the act should be impaired. It is essential that there is no loss of memory antedating the event. During a seizure, loss of memory starts with the onset of the seizure and not before it. Thus any loss of memory which antedates the episode is a point against it being an epileptic automatism.

6. The diagnosis of automatism is a clinical diagnosis. Although weight will clearly be given to abnormal investigations, such as a focal lesion on the CT scan or evidence of focal neuropsychological deficit or of generalized or focal EEG epileptiform discharges, none of these make the diagnosis of epilepsy. Epilepsy is a clinical diagnosis and any physician who enters court unable to substantiate the diagnosis on clinical grounds alone is likely to find himself in trouble.

## EPILEPSY AND DRIVING

Attacks of unconsciousness are potentially dangerous for anyone who is in charge of a machine. This is particularly so when the machine is a motor vehicle on the public roads. Driving is one of the most important skills of modern life. In the UK there are 24 million licence holders — nearly half the adult population, and for many of these driving is an essential part of their employment, and on it their livelihood depends. Estimates suggest that about 130 000 epileptics are potential drivers, so the problem is one of considerable size. Not only are attacks of unconsciousness due to epilepsy a possibility while driving, but so are drowsiness and sleep, which may be induced by anticonvulsant medication. In an analysis of 1605 road accidents involving collapse at the wheel, approximately 38% were thought to be due to epilepsy. (Godwin-Austen & Espir 1983). The rate of accidents amongst licenced drivers with epilepsy is 1.3–2.0 times greater than their age-matched controls without epilepsy (Hormia 1961, Millingen 1976).

Unfortunately, there is also evidence that many patients with epilepsy have deliberately concealed their epilepsy from the licensing authorities. Many medical practitioners have only a sketchy knowledge of the driving regulations, as was shown by a questionnaire survey by Harvey and Hopkins reported in 1983. For a review see Godwin-Austen & Espir (1983), p 9–15. The law relating to driving licences was recently amended with effect from the 21st April 1982 and defines the conditions under which an epileptic patient may and may not drive.

1. Any fit after the age of 5 prevents the holding during the person's lifetime of a heavy goods vehicle (HGV) licence, or a public service vehicle licence. Heavy goods

vehicles are responsible for 70% more deaths than lighter vehicles, and thus it is logical that restrictions in this area should be more severe (Godwin-Austen & Espir 1983). Fits after the age of 5 are also an absolute bar to becoming a commercial airline pilot.

2. Any person who has an epileptic seizure may not drive until they have had 2 seizure-free years, either with or without anticonvulsant medication.

3. If a person's seizures only occur during sleep, then they can drive providing they have had no daytime seizures within the last 3 years, either with or without anticonvulsant medication.

The Royal Automobile Club of Great Britain will only issue racing and rallying licences to patients with epilepsy if they have been seizure free and off drugs for 5 years.

The Civil Aviation Authority will only issue commercial pilot's licences under the same conditions as for commercial lorry drivers.

4. Should a patient who holds a driving licence have his medication changed or withdrawn, then he should inform the Driving Licensing Authority. This is the generally accepted view although it is little publicised, and it is also generally accepted that a period of 6–12 months off driving should follow such a change (British Medical Journal 1976).

5. There is a statutory requirement, as part of the privilege of holding a driving licence, that the driving licencing authorities must be informed should the patient have any medical condition which might impair their capacity to drive. This is particularly so with regards to epilepsy. In the UK, but not in other places in the world such as America, there is no statutory requirement for the doctor to report that a patient who is having seizures still holds a driving licence. Whether or not the doctor informs the authorities will depend on good medical practice and is usually a question of personal medical ethics. However, a doctor should draw any epileptic patients' attention to the law and advise them not to drive (Godwin-Austen & Espir 1983, p 1–2).

The diagnosis of epilepsy is not trivial, especially if the patient is a driver whose livelihood depends on a vehicle licence. It is therefore essential that time should be set aside during the interview in which the diagnosis of epilepsy is made known to any patient, and in subsequent follow-up sessions, to counsel and support them about difficulties arising through the loss of their licence. It is a sad fact that many patients with epilepsy do still drive, and the consequences of having an accident are severe, as the patient is uninsured and will be personally liable for any damage claims arising (Godwin-Austen & Espir 1983).

## CONCLUSION

Patients with epilepsy have been discriminated against throughout the centuries, and this is certainly true as regards the law. For an epileptic fit to be called a disease of the mind heightens the stigma. It is unreasonable that patients with epilepsy should have to carry the additional burden that whenever they have a fit they are, in law, insane, even though this will not be formally recognised unless they offend during a fit. The law on automatism as it now stands is illogical, leads to much hardship and suffering, and so clearly needs revision.

## REFERENCES

Bratty 1961 In: 46 Cr. App. R. 1, 7, 8; (1963) A.C. at p 401
Bratty v. Attorney General for Northern Ireland. Northern Ireland Law Reports 1961. p 78–110
British Medical Journal 1976 Leader i: 1235–1236
Fenton G 1972 Epilepsy and automatism. British Journal of Hospital Medicine. January
Fenwick P, Fenwick E (eds) 1985 Epilepsy and the law — a medical symposium on the current law International Congress and Symposium Series Number 81. Royal Society of Medicine, London
Godwin-Austen R B, Espir M L E (eds) 1983 Driving and epilepsy — and other causes of impaired consciousness. Royal Society of Medicine International Congress and Symposium Series. No. 60 The Royal Society of Medicine, London
Gunn J 1981 Medico-legal aspects of epilepsy. In: Reynolds E H, Trimble M R (eds) Epilepsy and psychiatry ch 13. Churchill Livingstone, Edinburgh
Hormia A 1961 Acta Scandanavica Suppl. 150: 210–212
Millingen K S 1976 Proceedings of the Australian Association of Neurologists 13: 67–72
Regina v. Charlson 1955 March 29th 1 Weekly Law Reports pp. 317–325
Regina v. Kemp 1957 The Law Reports. 1Q.B. Queen's Bench Division. p 399–408
Regina v. Quick 1973 3 Weekly Law Reports. p 26–36

# 12. Epilepsy and the law: a commentary from the United States perspective

*R. P. Schmidt B. J. Wilder*

As Dr Fenwick notes, epileptic persons have been subject to personal and institutionalized discrimination throughout the history of the disorder. Fortunately, public attitudes are changing, and the fear provoked by a seizure or by associating with an epileptic patient has lessened. Much of the legislation limiting full civil rights of the person with seizures has been repealed. Thus, in the United States the last law limiting the right of epileptic persons to marry was repealed in 1982. Three states have retained legislation permitting involuntary sterilization; in two of these it is limited to those who are committed for institutionalized care. An epileptic person with controlled seizures can be licensed to drive in each of the 50 states and other jurisdictions.

In the past 20 years there has been extensive legislation affecting the rights of the handicapped to fair consideration for education, employment, access to public accommodations, vocational rehabilitation, and other benefits of affirmative action programs. The Epilepsy Foundation of America, Inc., has published a comprehensive review of the legal rights of persons with epilepsy (1985) with sections describing federal and state laws applicable to the rights and opportunities for patients with seizures. Although it is not feasible to review the full nature of this legislation, several of its most important positions will be outlined.

The Developmental Disabilities and Bill of Rights Act of 1975, amended in 1978, provides funds to the states for special programs. States must comply with federal standards. The Act specifically targets services for those with severe disability with onset before age 21 and likely to continue indefinitely with substantial functional limitation in three or more defined areas of life activity and with needs for extended or life-long care. Although specific disorders are not named, the severely handicapped epileptic child may be eligible for special services provided by state programs.

The Education of the Handicapped Act of 1975, as amended, is designed to assure the rights of handicapped children to meaningful public education. Epileptic children whose condition adversely affects educational performance may be eligible for services, including special education at no cost to parents. Administration of 'related services', such as medication, may be required. Further, it is mandated that handicapped children receive services in the least restricted environment including the possibility of portions of their education in regular classrooms with non-handicapped children.

The Rehabilitation Act of 1973, amended in 1978, provides important and far-reaching rights to handicapped individuals, including those with epilepsy. Additional state legislation expands upon federal legislation and may affect those who are not protected by federal law. Federal law requires affirmative action in hiring individuals who are qualified and prohibits categorical discrimination against those whose handicap does not constitute a bona fide impediment to work. It also provides processes of complaint and appeal, and sanctions may be applied to the employer. Reasonable accommodation may be required for the handicapped individual who is able to perform the essential functions of the job. An important portion addresses pre-employment inquiries which may limit the employer's ability to deny employment categorically to persons with epilepsy. The employer may require medical examination as a condition of employment only if all employees are required to undergo such examination and if the results of the examination are not used for discrimination.

There is an extensive body of case law and administrative procedures which further define the full effect of this legislation and its various sections. Although qualified epileptic individuals continue to be affected by discriminatory practices, there has been substantial improvement in employment opportunity and redress.

## DRIVING LICENSE

It is now possible for persons with epilepsy to obtain a driving license in each state and all political jurisdictions of the United States. Federal law prohibits epileptics from operating trucks engaged in interstate commerce. In general, laws and regulations appear to be more liberal in the United States than in the United Kingdom. Epileptic drivers do have an increased accident rate as reflected in two United States studies (Crancer & McMurray 1968, Waller 1965). In general, the accident rate is roughly equal to that among patients with diabetes mellitus or less than twice that of drivers not handicapped. Many accidents involving the driver having a seizure involve unlicensed drivers or those who have concealed epilepsy on application.

Most states require a fixed period, usually 1 year, of freedom from seizures for licensure. Usually, a medical statement of safety and treatment is necessary, and evaluation by a specialist may be required. Many states have medical advisory boards, members of which may assist in initial evaluation and in appeals by those who have been denied licensure. Nine states require physicians to report epileptic patients to licensing authorities or other state agencies. This is opposed by medical groups and voluntary health organizations, partly on the basis of confidentiality of the physician-patient relationship. It is incumbent upon the physician to warn patients with epilepsy not to drive if seizures are uncontrolled. Protection against lawsuit is specifically provided in other states should it be necessary for the physician to inform authorities of an unsafe driver. Further, failure to warn or to notify may be cause for legal action irrespective of statute. There may be prohibitions against driving if medication is being changed or discontinued.

Applications for licensure are not uniform, but all require some statement of health and conditions which affect ability to drive.

There may be provision for limited or restricted licensure, such as those which would confine driving privilege to daylight hours, only to and from work, or to less traveled roads. Restriction may be further tailored to those patients whose seizures occur only during sleep or who may have sufficient warning to avoid being at the wheel at the time of a seizure. Most states restrict licensing for commercial driving such as trucks or buses.

Spudis et al (1986) have proposed a system of classification for use in judging limitations of drivers with epilepsy. Their recommendations include a variable time interval from last attack to return to driving, based upon predicted likelihood of recurrence accord to their classification scheme. This may be as short as 4 months for isolated seizures associated with transient disease. In general, it appears that many states are moving from a requirement of a fixed period of freedom from seizures prior to driving, to more individualized evaluations permitting shorter periods before licensure in exceptional instances. Such individualization will place an increased responsibility upon physicians. Improved and comprehensive epidemiological studies are needed to evaluate relative risks as more drivers are licensed through liberalized regulation and as drug management improves.

## THE EPILEPSY DEFENSE

The relationship between epilepsy and violent behavior remains disputed. The prevalence of epilepsy is increased several fold in prison populations (Gunn & Fenton 1971, Whitman et al 1984) but with little or no relationship between epilepsy and the type of crime leading to conviction. Further, prevalence of epilepsy among prisoners appears to be little different than in the socio-economic groups represented by the prison population. The act, violent or otherwise, leading to criminal trial is only rarely related directly to a seizure. Epilepsy is more common among those with organic brain disease which may lead to limited capacity and contribute to aggressive or anti-social behavior. Problems arise when abnormalities of behavior are related solely to epilepsy. The specificity of behavioral and psychological abnormalities associated with seizure types or brain regions of origin is controversial as are the personality characterizations reported in patients with temporal lobe epilepsy (Dodrill & Batzel 1986). The extensive literature on the relationship between epilepsy and violence and its apparent confusing nature may facilitate the occurrence of conflicting medical testimony before the law.

Violence or aggressive acts have been documented occasionally during epileptic automatisms or in post-ictal states. In the most careful observations of seizures associated with violence, ictal or postictal, directed violence is unusual (Delgado-Escueta et al 1981). Aggression or violence is most often non-directed or resistive in type. Complex, premeditated, or coordinated crime or violence is not compatible with what is medically known about epileptic automatisms.

Fenwick has presented an interesting and comprehensive review of the epilepsy defense in the United Kingdom. We share the confusion over the differences between medical and legal terminology and in the circular reasoning which may equate seizures with 'insanity' although the patient is 'sane'.

Treiman (1986) has recently reviewed medical and legal issues of epilepsy and violence from a United States perspective. He notes an apparent increased use of the 'epilepsy defense' against accusation of crime of murder or homicide, citing 19 newspaper reports between 1980–1984.

Treiman has further tabulated 75 crimes from appellate court literature in which epilepsy was used as a defense stating that it was successful only in one. In once instance, the accused shot and killed the alleged assassin of President Kennedy in full view of millions of people observing the event on television. One of us had the opportunity of reviewing the medical records and EEG on this individual before trial, and it was his impression that the diagnosis of epilepsy was unlikely, although competent and respected neurologists testified on both sides of the issue. Another widely publicized case is cited by Treiman as an instance in which a 15 year old youth was shot and killed by a police officer with little evidence of provocation. He was acquitted by the jury on the basis of insanity with a claimed psychomoter seizure at the time of the shooting (with supportive medical testimony) despite a normal EEG and lack of a seizure history. Since he was found 'insane' by the court, he was committed to custody and very shortly thereafter found 'sane' by examining psychiatrists and subsequently released by court order. The same district attorney who prosecuted the case in court against the epileptic 'insanity' defense again fought against his release because he was found 'sane'.

The McNaghten rule continues to be the guiding principle in United States Courts for pleas of not guilty by reason of insanity. As cited by Treiman (1986), several modifications have occurred. The United States Court of Appeals of the District of Columbia Circuit, held 'that an accused is not guilty if his unlawful act was a product of mental disease or mental deficit' (the Durham test). In 1966, the Model Penal Code of the American Law Institute was accepted by the court: 'an accused is not responsible for criminal conduct if at the time of such conduct as a result of mental disease or defect he lacks substantial capacity either to appreciate the criminality (wrongfulness) of his conduct or to conform his conduct to the requirements of law' (Freeman rule). Another decision, analogous to the *automatism simpliciter*, a California court accepted the 'unconscious defense' based on the conept that individuals cannot be held legally liable for their actions if the actions were committed at the time of unconsciousness. Treiman further states, '—to the extent that a violent criminal act has occurred as a result of an epileptic seizure and clearly at a time when a patient has had an alteration of consciousness as a result of a seizure, then that individual should not be found guilty of a criminal act.'

Fenwick documents the infrequency of criminal acts which can be established to occur during epileptic seizures. Further, the defense of an epileptic person who becomes psychotic whether associated with epilepsy or not differs little from the defense of psychotic individuals without epilepsy and need not be related to the seizure itself and differs, as such, from the 'epilepsy defense' in which the accused is personally responsible for his actions between attacks.

Fenwick has provided a set of criteria which may guide the examining physician called upon to examine or provide testimony with respect to allegations of crime occurring during an epileptic automatism (ictal or post-ictal). These are eminently reasonable and highly recommended.

Delgado-Escueta et al (1981), repeated by Treiman (1986), recommends criteria as follows: (1) The diagnosis of epilepsy should be established by at least one neurologist with special competence in epilepsy. (2) The presence of epileptic automatisms should be documented by the case history and closed circuit TV-EEG. (3) The presence of aggression during epileptic automatisms should be verified by video-recorded seizure in which ictal epileptiform patterns are also recorded on the EEG. (4) The aggressive or violent act should be characteristic of the patient's habitual seizure as elicited in the history. (5) A clinical judgment should be made by the neurologist attesting to the possibility that the act was part of a seizure.

## REFERENCES

Crancer A Jr, McMurray T 1968 Accident and violation rates of Washington's medically restricted drivers. Journal of the American Medical Association 205: 272–276.

Delgado-Escueta A V, Mattson R H, King L et al 1981 The nature of aggression during epileptic seizures. New England Journal of Medicine 305: 711–716

Dodrill C B, Batzel L W 1986 Interictal behavioral features of patients with epilepsy. Epilepsia (suppl 2): S64–S76

Epilepsy Foundation of America 1985 The legal rights of persons with epilepsy. Landover, Md

Gunn J, Fenton G 1971 Epilepsy, automatism, and crime. Lancet 1: 1173–1176

Spudis E V, Penry J K, Gibson P 1986 Driving impairment caused by episodic brain dysfunction: restrictions for epilepsy and syncope. Archives of Neurology 43: 558–564

Treiman D M 1986 Epilepsy and violence: medical and legal issues. Epilepsia 27 (suppl 2): S77–S104

Waller J A 1965 Chronic medical conditions and traffic safety: review of the California experience. New England Journal of Medicine 273: 1413–1420

Whitman S, Coleman T E, Patmon C et al 1984 Epilepsy in prison: elevated prevalence and no relationship to violence. Neurology 34: 775–782

# Index


absence seizures
childhood, 73
clinical trials for, 168
juvenile, 73–4
S-adenosylmethionine therapy, 225
adults
drug withdrawal in, 80–1
seizure recurrence in, EEGs predicting, 72, 80–1
after discharges(s) (AD), generation of, kindling and, 24, 27, 28, 29
after discharge threshold, 24, 25
age, amino acid levels in CSF/plasma related to, 52–3
aggregates, transmission between, 2–3, 4
AIDS, toxoplasmosis in, 150, 153
ambulatory EEG (cassette) monitoring, 83–4, 84
amino acid
abnormalities in epilepsy, 45–57
in animals, 46–7
in humans, 47–57
levels, in CSF/plasma, 50–7
metabolism, in brain, 50–2
γ-aminobutyric acid, *see* GABA
2-amino-7-phosphono-heptanoic acid (2-APH) actions, 7, 8
amitriptyline therapy, assessment, 230
amoebic encephalitis, primary, 152
amygdala (-induced) kindled seizures, 24, 25, 29
antiepileptic drug effects on, 36
staging, 22, 26
anomalies, syndromes of, antiepileptic drugs associated with, 96–100
antidepressant drugs, 225–31
effects on convulsions, 226, 228–9, 230, 231
therapy, 225, 225–31
antiepileptic/anticonvulsant drugs, 36, 77–82, 93–103, 110–13, 114–17, 161–78
antidepressant drug interactions with, 230
concentrations and dosage, 110–13, 171
effects
on amino acid levels in plasma/CSF, 53, 54–5, 56
on EEG, 77–80
on hepatic enzymes, 223, 230
on kindling/kindled seizures, 36
on mental states of epileptics, 225, 231
history of development, 161–5
new, 161–78
clinical testing, *see* clinical trials
development strategies, 165–7
need for, 161
antiepileptic/anticonvulsant drugs (*contd.*)
prospective, 175–8
structures, 164
teratogenicity/dysmorphogenicity, 93–103, 112, 114–17
mechanisms, 100–2
therapy/management using, 110–13, 161–78, 225–6
multiple (drugs), 116
in pregnancy, *see* pregnancy, antiepileptic drugs in
withdrawal
advisability, 82
EEG before and after, predictive value, 81–2
Antiepileptic Drug Development Program, 165, 166
arene oxide formation, 100–1
arrest of seizures, 32–3
aspartate
CSF levels, epilepsy related to, 57
drugs diminishing the actions of, 167
automatism, 242–9
defence of, 242, 243–8
epileptic, 242–3, 244–7
definitions, 242–3
diagnosis by psychiatrists, 248–9
sane and insane, 243–8
automatism simpliciter, 243, 244, 245, 247, 248
autoradiography of brain sections, measurements using, 5–6

baboon, photically seizure-susceptible, 10, 11
amino acid changes in, 46
baby care by epileptic mothers, 117–18
background activity in EEGs, antiepileptic drug effects on, 78, 79, 80
barbiturates
teratogenicity, 116, *see also specific drugs*
therapy, 161–2, 163
withdrawal, 225
basal ganglia
focal stimulation in, effects, 13
in neonatal seizures, 9
Bear-Fidio Inventory, 207
epilepsy-related depression studies using, 214, 216, 219, 220
Beck Depression Inventory (BDI), 207
epilepsy-related depression studies using, 219, 220, 222, 223, 224, 230
behavioural manifestations, *see also* depression
of corpus callosotomy, 200

behavioural manifestations (*contd.*)
  of seizures/convulsions/epilepsy, 22, 24, 25, 26, 35–7
    legal defence attributed to, 242–8, 255–6
benzodiazepine receptors, changes with kindling, 30–1
benzodiazepine syndromes, 99
benzonidazol therapy, 143
biological markers of depression, 222–3
bleeding, *see* haemorrhage
blinding in clinical trials, 172–3
blood
  features and tests
    in cysticercosis, 134
    in malaria, 146–7
  flow, regional, autoradiographic measurement, 5–6
blood/brain barrier, damaged, 52
blood/brain exchange of amino acids, 50–1
blood/CSF exchange of amino acids, 51
brain
  amino acid changes in
    in human epileptic tissue, 47–50
    in seizure-prone animals, 46–7
  amino acid metabolism, 50–2
  disease of the, automatism due to, 244
  function, long-term changes, with kindling, 33
  space/volume, extracellular, 51–2
brain/blood barrier and exchange, *see entries under* blood/brain
brain/CSF exchange of amino acids, 51
brain stem, generalised epilepsy initiated within, 12
brain stem seizures in man, 14–15
breast feeding by epileptic mothers, 117
Brief Psychiatric Rating, 221
bromide salts therapy, 161

CA3 region, interictal events in, 2, 3
callosotomy, *see* corpus callosotomy
carbamazapine
  effects of
    antidepressant, 222, 225–6
    on EEG, 79
    on kindling/kindled seizures, 36
    teratogenic, 116
  therapy, 225–6
    in clinical trials, 170–1
    concentration (of drug) during, 111
    in malaria, 149
cardiac defects/rate, *see entries under* heart
case reports in epilepsy-related depression, 217–18
catecholaminergic involvement in kindled seizures, 30
central-midtemporal spikes, benign childhood epilepsy with, EEG findings in, 74
central nervous system
  kindled seizure susceptibility, 26
  parasitosis of the, *see* parasitosis
  recurrent seizure susceptibility, 24–5
centrencephalic theory, 12
cerebrospinal fluid
  amino acid changes in, in seizure-susceptible animals, 46–7
  amino acid levels in, 50–4, 55–7
    epilepsy related to, 55–7
    factors affecting, 52–4
  in cysticercosis, 132–3, 134–5
  in schistosomiasis, 125
cerebrospinal fluid/blood exchange of amino acids, 51
cerebrospinal fluid/brain exchange of amino acids, 51
cessation of seizures, 32–3
Chagas' disease, *see* trypanosomiasis
childbearing years, treatment of epileptic women during, 118–19
childhood absence epilepsy, EEG findings, 73
childhood epilepsy, benign, with central-midtemporal spikes, EEG findings, 74
children
  corpus callosotomy in, 201
  drug withdrawal in, 81
  malaria in, 145
  recurrence of seizures in, predicting, 71–2, 81
chloroquine-resistant *Palasmodium falciparum*, 147, 148
chloroquine therapy in malaria, 148
  side-effects, 149
choline acetyl transferase, 30
cholinergic system, kindling and the, 27, 30
classification
  of depressive illnesses, 206–7
  of seizure types, *see* types of seizure
cleft lip and palate malformations, antiepileptic drug-associated, 95–6
clinical course of parasitosis of the CNS, 125–53 *passim*
clinical drug trials, 167–75
  bias control, 171–5
    introducing, 173–4
  concommitant medication in, 170–1
  dose, 171
  exclusion criteria, 169–70
  patients in, 167–9
Clinical Interview Schedule (CIS), 215
clobazam therapy, 226
clonazepam effects on EEG, 79–80
clonic convulsions, 4–5, *see also* tonic-clonic seizures
clonic motor activity, 4
colliculus, inferior, sound-induced seizures and the, 11–12
Columbia Mania-Depression Scales, 219
commisurotomy, 181–202, *see also* corpus callosotomy
  central, 183–4, 190, 191, 192, 193, 194
  complete, 183, 184, 189, 191, 193
  frontal, 183, 184
  literature review on, 189–94
Community Adjustment Questionnaire, 224
complex partial seizures, *see* partial seizures

computerised tomography in cysticercosis, 128–37 *passim*
concommitant medications in clinical trials, 170–1
congenital malformations, antiepileptic drug-associated, 93–6, 114–17
congenital toxoplasmosis, 150
corpus callosotomy, 181–202
  comparison with other procedures, 188–201
  development, 181–4
  expectations, 184–5
  judging outcome, 185
  mechanisms of actions, 195
  operative complications, 186–7
  operative technique, 183–4
  partial vs. total, 201
corpus callosum, kindling, 24, 25
cortically-induced kindled seizures, antiepileptic drug effects, 36
cortico-reticular theory, 13–14
cortisol value, dexamethasone-related, 223
criminal law, epilepsy and, 241–8
criminality, epilepsy and, 248
Crown Crisp Experiential Index (CCEI), 207
  epilepsy-related depression studies using, 214, 215, 216, 220
cyst(s)
  in cysticercosis, 128, 135, 136
  in hydatid disease, 126, 127
cysticercosis, 128–38
  classification, 132
  diagnosis, 134–5
  epidemiology and microbiology, 128
  management, 127, 135–7, 153
  pathophysiology and clinical course, 128–32
  prognosis, 137–8

defence (legal), relating to epilepsy, 242, 243–8, 255–6
delivery, labour and, 117
depression, 205–32
  aetiology and pathogenesis, 208–11, 231–2
  biological markers, 223
  biological theories of, 210–11
  bipolar vs. unipolar, 207
  classification, 206–7
  endogenous vs. non-endogenous, 207
  in epilepsy, 208–32
    management, 224–31, 232
    types of, 211, 211–22
  history, 205
  meaning of, 205
  measurement, 207–8
  primary vs. secondary, 206–7
  psychosocial models of, 208–10
  type A (psychotic) vs. type B (neurotic), 207
Depression Adjective Checklist, 219, 224
depth electrodes, 85
Development Disabilities and Bill of Rights Act (1975 and 1978), 253
Dexamethasone Suppression Test, 222–3
diagnosis
  of epilepsy, 63–86
diagnosis (*contd.*)
    driving and the, 250
    EEG in, 63–86
    in women of childbearing ages, 118
  of epileptic automatism, 248–9
  of parasitosis of the CNS, 125–53
diazepam effects on kindling/kindled seizures, 36
diet, amino acid levels in CSF/plasma related to, 53
discharge patterns, EEG, short-term variability, 77
discrimination against epileptic persons, 241
dogs, seizure-susceptible, amino acid changes in, 46–7
dose
  in clinical trials, 171
  concentration related to, 111–13 *passim*
double-blind clinical trials, 173
doxepin therapy, 227–30
driving, epilepsy and, 249–50, 254–5
Drug Amendments Act (1982), 165
drug management
  antiepileptic, *see* antiepileptic drugs
  of depresion, 225–31, *see also* antidepressant drugs
  of parasitosis of the CNS, 126–53 *passim*
dysmorphogenic drugs, *see* teratogenic drugs

echinococcosis, *see* hydatid disease
Education of the Handicapped Act (1975), 253
electrical kindling
  in animals, 23
  in humans, 34
electroconvulsive therapy of depressed epileptics, 231
electrodes for EEGs
  additional, 67–8
  in presurgical evaluation, 85
electroencephalogram, 63–86
  abnormalities in non-epileptics, 69–70
  of depressives, 212, 213, 217, 219
  in diagnosis and management of epilepsy, 63–86
  drug-induced changes, 77–80
  in generalised epilepsy, 12–13
  in long-term follow-up, 75–7
  long-term monitoring, 82–5
  normal, in epileptics, 70–1
  post commissurectomy/corpus callosotomy, 184, 185–6, 187, 189–94, 195
  recording, duration, 63–4
  recurrent seizure risk predicted by, 71–2, 81–2
  sensitivity and specificity, 68–71
  in specific epileptic syndromes, 73–4
  standard, obtaining maximum yield with, 63–8
electroencephalogram monitoring, long-term, 82–5
electroencephalogram/video monitoring, 82–3, 84
Emotions Profile Index, 219
encephalitic cysticercosis, 128–9, 135
encephalitis, primary amoebic, 152
enkephalins, kindling and the involvement of, 31
*Entamoeba histolytica* infection of the CNS, 152
enzymes, hepatic, anticonvulsants inducing, 223, 230

Epilepsy Branch of the NINCDS, drug trials conducted by, 165, 166
Epilepsy Foundation of America, Inc., review of legal rights of persons with epilepsy published by, 253
epileptiform patterns and activity, 70, 71
  definition, 69
  during drug withdrawal, 81
  in long-term follow-up, 76
  maximising yield of, 63–8
  in non-epileptics, 69–70
epileptogenesis, 1–15
  kindling in, *see* kindling
  secondary, 34–5
epoxide(s), teratogencity, 100, 102
epoxide hydrolase, defects, drug teratogenicity related to, 100, 101
erythrocytes in malaria, 146
estrogen levels in pregnancy, 110
ethosuximide, 163
  effects
    on EEG, 80
    on kindling/kindled seizures, 36
  structure, 164
excitatory transmitter levels
  in control tissue, 49
  in epileptic tissue, 48
  in plasma, 54
Eysenck Personality Inventory, 216, 221

facial malformations and anomalies, antiepileptic drugs associated with, 95–100
fear, 218–19
  ictal, 218
Fear Inventory, 216
febrile seizures, seizure recurrence with, EEGs predicting, 72
felbamate, 175
fetal (drug-associated) malformations/anomalies/syndromes, 93–6, 114–17
fetus, effect of seizures on, 113–14
flunarizine, 175
fluvoxamine therapy, 227
focal (motor) seizures, 4–6
  more intense, after corpus callosotomy, 197
  secondary generalisation, 9–10
  spread, 4–6, 9–10
    intracortical, 4
    subortical, 4–5
  transition from generalised seizures to, 34
foci
  epileptic
    amino acid changes in, 47–8
    bilaterally independent, corpus callosotomy with, 199
  kindling, 26–9
folic acid
  levels, depression related to, 210–11, 215, 225
  supplementation, antiepileptic drug-associated congenital malformations and the effects of, 116–17
follow-up, long-term, EEG role in, 75–7
frequency of seizures
  clinical drug tests and, 168
  post-corpus callosotomy, 185
  in pregnancy, 109–10

GABA (γ-aminobutyric acid)
  abnormalities
    in humans, 48, 49–50
    in seizure susceptible animals, 46, 47
  involvement of
    in kindling, 27–8
    in seizures, 32
  levels in brain/CSF/plasma, 52, 53, 54
  neuronal inhibition mediated by, drug development involving use of, 166
GABA agonist activity, 4, 7, 8
  sound-induced seizures and, 11
GABA antagonist activity, 4, 8, 9
  sound-induced seizures and, 11, 11–12
GABA-ergic system
  drug development involving use of, 166
  involvement of (in epilepsy), 45, 50
    in seizure arrest, 32
    in seizure initiation and spread, 4, 7, 27–8, 30–1
GABA receptor density in epileptic patients, 50
GABA-T (transaminase)
  activity in epileptics, 49
  inhibitors, effects on GABA levels, 53
Gabapentin, 176
General Hospital Questionnaire, epilepsy-related depression studies using, 214, 216
Generalised Contentment Scale, 224
generalised seizures and epilepsy, 12–14, 34, 73–4
  corpus callosotomy for, 197–8, 198
  EEG findings in, 73–4, 197, 198
  primary, 197–8
  secondary, 9–10, 29–31
  transition to focal seizures, 34
genetic influences on antiepileptic drug-associated congenital malformations, 100, 101, 117
gerbils, seizure-susceptible, amino acid changes in, 47
globus pallidus, 7–8, 13
glucose, metabolic rate for, autoradiographic measurement, 5–6
glutamate
  drugs diminishing the actions of, 167
  levels, epilepsy related to
    in CSF, 56–7
    in plasma, 55
glutamate decarboxylase activity
  in epileptic humans, 49–50
  in seizure-susceptible gerbils, 47
glycine levels in epileptic tissue, 48–9

haemorrhage/bleeding
  intracranial/intracerebral, 113
  neonatal, 117
half-controlled trials, 173
Hamilton Depression Rating Scale (HDRS), 207

Hamilton Depression Rating Scale (HDRS) (*contd.*)
  epilepsy-related depression studies using, 220, 221, 222, 223, 230
heart
  defects, congenital, antiepileptic drug-associated, 96
  rate, fetal, 113
hemiplegia, infantile, corpus callosotomy with, 199
hepatic enzymes, anticonvulsants inducing, 223, 230
hippocampus, kindling, 28
hormonal changes in pregnancy, 110
Hospital Anxiety Depression Scale, 208
Hostility and Direction of Hostility Questionnaire (HDHQ), 219, 220
hydantoin(s), development, 163
hydantoin syndrome, fetal, 97, 98–9, 116
hydatid disease (hydatidosis; echinococcosis), 126–8
  diagnosis, 127
  epidemiology and microbiology, 126
  management and prognosis, 127, 153
  pathophysiology and clinical course, 126
hyperventilation response, 64
hypoglycaemia in malaria, 144, 149
hypsarrhythmia during long-term follow-up, 76

ictal(peri-) depression, 211–13
ictal discharges, 2–3
ictal fear, 218
imaging techniques, 1, *see also specific techniques*
  in cysticercosis, 135
infancy, benign myoclonic epilepsy in, EEG findings with, 73
infant care by epileptic mothers, 117–18
infantile hemiplegia, corpus callosotomy with, 199
inhibitory transmitters, 45
  levels
    in 'control' tissue, 49
    in epileptic tissue, 48, 48–9
    in plasma, 54
initiation of seizure activity, 1–15, *see also* epileptogenesis
  pharmacology, 3–4
intelligence quotient, corpus callosotomy and, 199
intensive EEG/video monitoring, 82–3, 84
interictal depression, 213–23
interictal discharges, 2–3
intracranial/intracerebral haemorrhage in fetus, 113

Jacksonian seizures, *see* focal motor seizures
juvenile absence epilepsy, EEG findings, 73–4
juvenile myoclonic epilepsy, EEG findings, 74

Kefaurer-Harris Amendment, 165
kidney failure in malaria, 144
kindled seizures
  antiepileptic drug effects on, 36
  behavioural manifestations, 24, 25, 26
kindling, 6–7, 21–37
  clinical implications, 33–7
kindling (*contd.*)
  in developing animals, 25–6
  focus, 26–9
  induction, 23
    agents used in, 23
  long-term/permanent effects, 33
  mechanisms, 26–33
  site specificity, 23–4
  species specificity, 22–3
kindling-like processes/mechanisms in humans, 34–5, 37

labour and delivery, 117
lamotrigine, 176
language, corpus callosotomy effects on, 188, 200
law, epilepsy and the, 241–56
legislation, epilepsy-related, 241, 253–4
Lennox-Gastaut syndrome, EEG findings in, 74
Levine Pilowsky Questionnaire (LPD), 207, 208
  epilepsy-related depression studies using, 222, 223
limbic (psychomotor) seizures/epilepsy, 6–9, 21
  legal defence of, 245
localisation of epilepsy, corpus callosotomy used in the, 201
localisation-related epilepsies and syndromes, EEG findings, 74–5
long-term changes in seizures with corpus callosotomy, 198
long-term EEG monitoring, 82–5
long-term follow-up, EEG role in, 75–7
long-term potentiation, 26–7
lymphocyte cytotoxicity, phenytoin birth defects and, 101

McNaghten rule, 242, 256
magnetic resonance imaging in neurocysticercosis, 135, 136, 137, 138, 139
malaria (*P. falciparum*-type), 143–9
  cerebral, 143–4, 145
  clinical course, 144–5
  diagnosis, 144, 147
  epidemiology and microbiology, 143–4
  management, 147–9, 153
  pathophysiology, 145–7
  prognosis, 147
  seizures and, 144–5
malformations, congenital/fetal, antiepileptic drug-associated, 93–6, 114–17
management
  drug, *see* drug management
  of epilepsy/seizures, 109–19, 161–78, 181–202, 224–32
    during childbearing years, 118–19
    EEG in, 63–86
    during pregnancy, 109–19
    surgical, 181–202
  of epilepsy-related depression, 224–31, 232
  of parasitosis of the CNS, 126–53 *passim*
manic-depressive disease, 205
markers, biological, of depression, 222–3
maximal electroshock seizure (MES), 165, 166

melarprosol therapy, 141
memory, corpus callosotomy effects on, 199
mental problems in epilepsy, 205–32, *see also* behavioural manifestations; depression
mephenytoin, teratogenicity, 93
N-methyl-D-aspartate actions, 8–9, 28
N-methyl-D-aspartate antagonist actions, sound-induced seizures and, 12
N-methyl-D-aspartate receptor, 4, 46
  kindling and the involvement of, 28, 33
mice, seizure-susceptible, 11–12
  amino acid changes in, 47
milacemide, 176
mind, diseases of the mind, epileptic automatism as, 241–6
Minesota Multiphasic Personality Inventory (MMPI), 207
  epilepsy-related depression studies using, 214, 215, 216
MK-801, 176
models, seizure, development, 162
monitoring, EEG, long-term, 82–5
monitoring, neurodiagnostic, 82–5
monoamine oxidase inhibitors (MAOI), 229
monoamine reuptake inhibitors (MARI), 228
mood changes preceding seizures, 213
mothers, epileptic, malformations in offspring of, 94–6
motor function, corpus callosotomy effects on, 188, 200
muscimol actions, 7, 8
myoclonic epilepsy
  benign, in infancy, EEG findings, 73
  juvenile, EEG findings, 74
myoclonus of striatal origin, 6

nafimidone, 176
nasopharyngeal electrodes, 67, 68
neonatal seizures, basal ganglia in, 9
neural tube defects, valproic acid-associated, 102, 103, 116
neurocysticercosis, 128, 129, 130, 131, 132, 133, 134, 139
  classification, 133
  diagnosis, 135
  management, 135–7, 139
neurodiagnostic monitoring, long-term, 82–5
neurological function, post-commisurectomy/corpus callosotomy changes in, 187–8, 189–94, 199–200
neurological involvement in parasitosis of CNS, characteristics, 124
neuronal excitation, drugs diminishing, 167
neuronal inhibition, drugs enhancing, 166–7
neuropathology, epilepsy and, 45–6
neurotransmitter systems
  drug development involving the use of, 166
  involvement of (in epilepsy), 45–57
    depression and the, 210
    kindling and the, 27–8, 30–1, 32–3, 33
Newcastle Diagnostic Index, 220
nifurtimox therapy, 143

nomifensine therapy, assessment, 230

occipital spikes, 65
oestrogen levels in pregnancy, 110
operative procedures for epilepsy, 181–202
opiates, kindling and the involvement of, 28, 31, 33
orofacial cleft malformations and anomalies, antiepileptic drug-associated with, 95–100
Org 6370, 177
oxcarbazepine, 177

parasitosis of the CNS, 123–53
  characteristics of epilepsy in, 124
  characteristics of neurological involvement, 124
  countries/regions with high prevalence, 123
parasuicide, 223–4
paroxysmal activity and seizure recurrence prediction, 72
partial seizures
  clinical trials for, 168–9
  complex, 195–6
    depression related to, 219
    in pregnancy, 114
  corpus callosotomy effects on, 195–6, 198
  kindling and, relationship between, 34–7
pathology (neuro-) and epilepsy, 45–6
pathophysiology
  epilepsy and, 46
  of parasitosis of the CNS, 125–53 *passim*
patients in clinical drug trials, 167–9
penicillin, epileptogenic activity, 13
pentylenetetrazol-induced seizures, 14
  screening of new drugs using, 165, 166
peri-ictal depression, 211–13
permanent effects of kindling, 33
Personality Inventory for Children, 219
petit mal, EEG findings, 73
phencyclidine/sigma receptors, 33
phenobarbital
  concentrations, 112
  effects
    on EEG, 80
    on kindling/kindled seizures, 36
  structure, 164
  therapy, 161
    in pregnancy, 112, 115
phenylsuccinimides, development, 163
phenytoin
  analogues, 163
  concentrations, 111
  effects, 36, 79, 100–1
    on EEG, 79
    on kindling/kindled seizures, 36
    tetratogenic, 98, 100–1, 116
  structure, 164
  therapy, 163
    in pregnancy, 111
photic stimulation during EEG, 64–6
photoconvulsive response in patients, 65
photomyoclonic respone, 65
photosensitive epilepsy, 10–12

pilocarpine, limbic seizures induced by, 7–9
pilot studies in clinical trials, 173–4
piriform cortex, kindling and the involvement of, 28–9
plasma amino acid levels, 50, 52, 52–4, 54–5
  epilepsy and, 54–5
  factors affecting 52–4
*Plasmodium*, 143, 147
  *falciparum* malaria, *see* malaria
potentiation, long-term, 26–7
praziquantal therapy, 136, 136–7, 137
predictive value of EEG relating to seizure recurrence, 71–2, 80–2
pregnancy, 109–19
  antiepileptic drugs in, *see* pregnancy, antiepileptic drugs in
  seizures in, 109–10, 113–14
    frequency, 109–10
    management, 109–19
    outcome of births with, 113–14
pregnancy, antiepileptic drugs in, 110–13
  concentration/dosage, 110–13
  risk management, 103
  teratogenicity of, *see* antiepileptic drugs
prepiriform cortex, 8, 9
  kindling and the involvement of, 29
Present State Examination (PSE), 207
  epilepsy-related depression studies using, 214, 216
presurgical evaluation, EEGs for, 85
primidone concentrations during pregnancy, 112
primidone embryopathy, 99
progabide, 177
progesterone effects on seizure frequency, 110
prognosis with parasitosis of the CNS, 126–53 *passim*
prognostic value of EEG, 71–2, 80–2
propagation of seizures, *see* spread
psychiatrist, epileptic automatism diagnosis by, 248–9
psychological problems in epilepsy, 205–32, *see also* behavioural manifestations; depression
psychomotor epilepsy, *see* limbic seizures/epilepsy
psychosocial models of depression, 208–10
psychotherapy for depression, 224–5
pyrimethamine therapy, 151

quinine therapy in malaria, 148

randomization in clinical trials, 172
rats
  amino acid changes in seizure-susceptible, 47
  kindled seizures in, 22, 25–6
  limbic seizures induced in, 7–9
  sound-induced seizures in, 11–12, 47
recording of EEG, duration of, 63–4
recurrent seizures, *see also* status epilepticus
  CNS resistance capacity to, 24–5
  in developing animals, 25–6
  predictive value of EEG, 71–2, 81–2
red cells in malaria, 146
Rehabilitation Act (1973 and 1978), 253
relapse, *see* recurrent seizures
remission with epilepsy, 80–2
renal failure in malaria, 144
risk of recurrent seizures, predictive value of EEG, 71–2, 81–2
rodents, sound-induced seizures in, 11–12, *see also specific rodents*

Schistosomiasis, 124–6
  diagnosis, 125
  epidemiology and microbiology, 124
  management and prognosis, 125, 153
  pathophysiology and clinical course, 125
secondary generalisation of seizures, 9–10, 29–31
seizures, *see specific types*
sensory induction, seizures with, 10–12
Sepulveda Epilepsy battery, 219–20
serum tests in cysticercosis, 134
severity of seizures, quantification, 22
sex, amino acid levels in CSF/plasma related to, 53
sleep
  deprivation, EEG recording with, 66, 67
  natural, EEG recording in, 66
  sedated, EEG recording in, 66–7
sleeping sickness, *see* trypanosomiasis
social visibility, index of, 209
somatostatin, kindling and the involvement of, 31
sound-induced seizures, 10, 11–12
speech, corpus callosotomy effects on, 200
sphenoidal electrodes, 67–8
spike, 12–14
  central-midtemporal, 74
  interictal, 77, 78, 80
  occipital, 65
  patterns
    antiepileptic drug effects, 78
    during long-term follow-up studies, 76, 77
    during long-term neurodiagnostic monitoring, 83
spike-wave discharge, generalised, 78
  antiepileptic drug effects on, 80
Spileberger State-Trait Anxiety Inventory, 214, 219, 230
spina bifida, valproic acid-related, 102, 103
spread/propagation of seizure activity, 1–15, 29–31
  pharmacology, 3–4
staging, amygdala-induced kindled seizures, 22, 26
Standard Psychiatric Interview, 214–15
Standardised Personal Feelings Scale, 213
State-Trait Anxiety Inventory, 214, 219, 230
status epilepticus, 24, *see also* recurrent seizures
  in cysticercosis, 132
  non-convulsive, 75
  in pregnancy, 109, 112–13
steroid therapy
  in cysticercosis, 136
  in malaria, 149
stimulation
  of kindling, electrical, *see* electrical stimulation
  photic, during EEG, 64–6
stopping (spontaneously) of seizures, 32–3
striatum, myoclonus originating from, 6

stroboscopically-stimulated seizures, 10–11
subclinical rhythmic EEG discharge of adults, 70
subdural electrodes, 85
substantia nigra, 13
  activation during kindled seizures, 6–7
  inhibiting role in seizure development, 32
substantia nigra pars reticulata, limbic seizures and the, 7, 8
substantia nigra pars reticulata neurons/cells in seizure arrests, 32
succinimides, development, 163
suicide, 223–4
sulphadizine therapy, 151
suramin therapy, 141
surgical procedures for epilepsy, 181–202
synaptic system in the brain, 1
syndromes, epileptic, EEG findings in, 73–5
syndromes of anomalies, antiepileptic drugs associated with, 96–100

taurine, plasma levels, epilepsy related to, 55
telemetry, radio/cable, EEG/video monitoring using, 82–3
temporal electrodes, lower anterior, 68
temporal lobe epilepsy (TLE), depression with, 212, 214, 216, 218, 219, 219–20
teratogenicity of antiepileptic drugs, *see* antiepileptic drugs
thalamic nuclei, generalised epilepsy and the involvement of, 13
therapy, *see* management
threshold, seizure, antidepressant drug effects on, 226, 226–7
thrombocytopenia in malaria, 146
tissue, epileptic, human, amino acid changes in, 47–50
tomography, computed, in cysticercosis, 128–37 *passim*
tonic-clonic seizures, 12–14
  clinical trials for, 168
  in cysticercosis, 132
toxoplasmosis, 149–51
  acquired, 150–1
  congenital, 150
  diagnosis, 151
  epidemiology and microbiology, 149–50
  management and prognosis, 151, 153
transfer effects, 30
transmitter systems, *see* neurotransmitter systems
treatment, *see* management
trials, drug, *see* clinical drug trials
tricyclic antidepressants, 228
tridione teratogenicity, 115
trimethadione
  structure, 164
  teratogenicity, 94, 97, 97–8
  therapy, 163
trimethadione syndrome, fetal, 97, 97–8
*Trypanosoma*
  *brucei*, 138, 140
  *cruzi*, 141, 143
  *gambiense*, 138, 140, 141
  *rhodesiense*, 138, 140, 141
trypanosomiasis, 138–43
  African, 138–41
    diagnosis, 140
    epidemiology and microbiology, 138–40
    management and prognosis, 141, 153
    pathophysiology and clinical course, 140
  American (Chagas' disease), 141–3
    diagnosis, 142–3
    epidemiology and microbiology, 141
    management and prognosis, 143, 153
    pathophysiology and clinical course, 141–2
types of seizures
  classification, 167
    in women of childbearing age, 118–19
  clinical trials involving, 167, 167–8, 168–9
  number of, emotional/psychiatric problems related to, 216

United Kingdom, epilepsy and the law in, 241–50
United States
  antiepileptic drugs marketed in, 162
  epilepsy and the law in, 253–6

valproate/valproic acid
  concentrations, during pregnancy, 111–12
  effects, 78–9, 101–2, 223
    on EEG, 78–9
    on kindling/kindled seizures, 36
    on plasma amino acid levels, 53, 55
    teratogenic, 97, 99, 101–2, 116
valproate syndrome, fetal, 97, 99
video/EEG monitoring, 82–3, 84
vigabatrin, *see* γ-vinyl GABA
γ-vinyl GABA (vigabatrin), 177
  effects on GABA levels, 52, 53
violent behaviour, epilepsy-related, legal defence attributed to, 242–8, 255–6

Washington Psychosocial Seizure Inventory (WPSI), 210, 216, 219
West syndrome, EEG findings, 74

Yale series of corpus callosotomies, 185–8
  comparison with results from other centres, 188–201
    areas of controversy, 194–201
    areas of agreement, 188–94

zonisamide, 177
Zung depression Inventory, 207
  epilepsy-related depression studies using, 216